Introduction to Organic Mass Spectrometry

Introduction to Organic Mass Spectrometry

Dr. Anees A. Siddiqui
Dept. of Pharmaceutical Chemistry
Jamia Hamdard University
New Delhi-110062 (India)

CBS

CBS Publishers & Distributors Pvt. Ltd.

New Delhi • Bengaluru • Chennai • Kochi • Kolkata • Mumbai
Hyderabad • Nagpur • Patna • Pune • Vijayawada

ISBN: 978-81-239-1937-9

First Edition: 2011
Reprint: 2019

Published by **Satish Kumar Jain** and produced by **Varun Jain** for
CBS Publishers & Distributors Pvt. Ltd.,
4819/XI Prahlad Street, 24 Ansari Road, Daryaganj, New Delhi - 110002
delhi@cbspd.com, cbspubs@airtelmail.in • www.cbspd.com
Ph.: 23289259, 23266861, 23266867 • Fax: 011-23243014

Corporate Office: 204 FIE, Industrial Area, Patparganj, Delhi - 110 092
Ph: 49344934 • Fax: 011-49344935
E-mail: publishing@cbspd.com • publicity@cbspd.com

Branches:

- ***Bengaluru:*** 2975, 17th Cross, K.R. Road, Bansankari 2nd Stage, Bengaluru - 70 • Ph: +91-80-26771678/79 • Fax: +91-80-26771680 E-mail: cbsbng@gmail.com, bangalore@cbspd.com
- ***Chennai:*** No. 7, Subbaraya Street, Shenoy Nagar, Chennai - 600030 Ph: +91-44-26681266, 26680620 • Fax: +91-44-42032115 E-mail: chennai@cbspd.com
- ***Kochi:*** Ashana House, 39/1904, A.M. Thomas Road, Valanjambalam, Ernakulum, Kochi • Ph: +91-484-4059061-65 Fax: +91-484-4059065 • E-mail: cochin@cbspd.com
- ***Kolkata:*** 6-B, Ground Floor, Rameshwar Shaw Road, Kolkata - 700014 Ph: +91-33-22891126/7/8 • E-mail: kolkata@cbspd.com
- ***Mumbai:*** 83-C, Dr. E. Moses Road, Worli, Mumbai - 400018 Ph: +91-9833017933, 022-24902340/41 • E-mail: mumbai@cbspd.com

Representatives:

- Hyderabad: 0-9885175004
- Patna: 0-9334159340
- Jharkhand: 0-9811541605
- Nagpur: 0-9021734563
- Pune: 0-9623451994
- Uttarakhand: 0-9716462459

Printed at:
J.S. Offset Printers, Delhi (India)

PREFACE

Preface

The first edition of the book entitled **"Introduction to Organic Mass Spectrometry"** is compiled to guide the students of various scientific disciplines with a complete overview of the principles, theories and key applications of modern mass spectrometry. All instrumental aspects of mass spectrometry are clearly and concisely described: sources, analyzers and detectors. Tandem mass spectrometry, GC-MS and LC-MS are explained in more detail in a separate chapter. Emphasis is placed throughout the text on optional utilization conditions. Various fragmentation patterns are described together with analytical information that derives from the mass spectra. Large number of mathematical equations and derivations has been avoided and compilation of book has been undertaken to present the field of mass spectrometry in a logical manner. I hope, this book will be an invaluable resource for all undergraduate and postgraduate students using this technique in departments of chemistry, biochemistry, medicine, pharmacology, agriculture, pharmacy and food science. It is also of interest for researchers looking for an overview of the latest techniques and development. Biological mass spectrometry is also included to illustrate the importance of mass spectrometry in clinical medical research. Appendices included in this book provide vide range of informations at a glance.

The author hopes that this book will assist in teaching the subject of mass spectrometry to the students in different levels.

I express my thanks to those authors of articles from which information are collected for compiling this book. I am thankful to their staff members for their suggestions and Mr. S.K. Jain and Mr. Vinod K. Jain of M/s CBS Publishers & Distributors Pvt. Ltd. for bringing out the first edition of this book.

All constructive criticism and comments of this book from students and teachers are most welcome and shall form the base for future editions.

New Delhi **Dr. Anees Ahmad Siddiqui**

CONTENTS

Contents

Preface v

1. Introduction to Mass Spectrometry **1**

1.1 Introduction 1

1.2 History of Mass Spectrometry 2

1.3 Applications 5

2. Introduction to Mass Spectrometer **7**

2.1 Introduction 7

2.2 General Structure of Mass Spectrometer 8

3. Types of Ions **40**

3.1 Molecular ion 40

3.2 Isotopic ions 41

3.3 Fragment ions 44

3.4 Rearrangement ions 45

3.5 Multiple charged ions 45

3.6 Metastable ions 46

3.7 Negative ions 47

3.8 Ions formed by ion molecule interaction 48

4. Determination of Molecular Formula **49**

5. Fragmentation of Organic Compounds **57**

5.1 Introduction 57

5.2 Stevenson's rule 58

5.3 Ions with Odd or Even numbers of electrons 58

5.4 Factors influencing the fragmentation 59

5.5 Handy Rules of Fragmentation 67

6. Fragmentation Patterns for Organic Functional Groups 71
6.1 Hydrocarbon 71
6.2 Hydroxy compounds 82
6.3 Aldehyde 88
6.4 Ketones 90
6.5 Carboxylic acid 94
6.6 Ester 97
6.7 Lactones 102
6.8 Ethers 103
6.9 Amines 105
6.10 Amide 109
6.11 Nitriles 111
6.12 Nitro compounds 113
6.13 Epoxides 114
6.14 Halogenated compounds 115
6.15 Heterocyclic compounds 118
6.16 Natural Products 121

7. Analytical Mass Spectrometry 143
7.1 Qualitative analysis 143
7.2 Quantitative Analysis 146

8. Tandem Mass Spectrometry 149
8.1 Introduction 149
8.2 Applications of Tandem mass spectrometry 150
8.3 MS-MS instrumentation 151

9. Gas Chromatography-Mass Spectrometry (GC-MS) 158
9.1 Introduction 158
9.2 Gas Chromatography 159
9.3 Mass Spectroscopy 160
9.4 GC–MS 161
9.5 Interface used in GC-MS 162
9.6 Limitations of GC-MS 164
9.7 Applications of GC-MS 165

10. Liquid Chromatography/Mass Spectrometry (LC/MS) 166
10.1 Introduction 166
10.2 Interfaces using Desorption Techniques 167
10.3 Interfaces using Aerosols and Additional Ion Generation 168
10.4 Interfaces using Aerosols Incorporating Ion Generation 170
10.5 Applications of LC/MS 171

11. Biological Mass Spectrometry 174
11.1 Introduction 174
11.2 Applications of MS in biological research 174
11.3 Protein Characterization 176

Questions and Solved Exercise 181

Appendices 197
Appendix 1. Websites on Mass Spectrometry 197
Appendix 2. Isotope Masses and Abundances 199
Appendix 3. Intensities of Molecular Ions for Compounds Containing Combinations of Bromine and Chlorine 203
Appendix 4. Mass-to-Charge Ratios of McLafferty Rearrangement Ions for Common Carbonyl Compounds 203
Appendix 5. Primary Fragmentations Associated with Some Common Functional Groups 204
Appendix 6. Fragments Commonly Lost for Molecular Ions 204
Appendix 7. Masses and Possible Structures of Common Fragment Ions 205
Appendix 8. Amino Acid Residue Masses and Modifying Groups 206
Appenix 9. Monosaccharide Residue Masses 207
Appendix 10. Isotopic Abundances for Various Elemental Compositions 208

Index 289

CHAPTER

1

Introduction to Mass Spectrometry

1.1 INTRODUCTION

Mass spectrometry is a sophisticated analytical technique that is used to determine the mass of a compound, identify unknown compounds, and to elucidate the structure & chemical properties of molecules.

Mass spectrometry is the study of systems converting the molecule into gaseous ions, with or without fragmentation, which are separated and then characterized by their mass to charge ratios (m/e) and relative abundances. With the help of masses of fragment, the mass/original structure of molecule is predicted. To illustrate the function of mass spectrometry (Fig 1.1), imagine a stone being projected from a catapult towards a delicate vase (I). On impact the vase is shattered (II). If

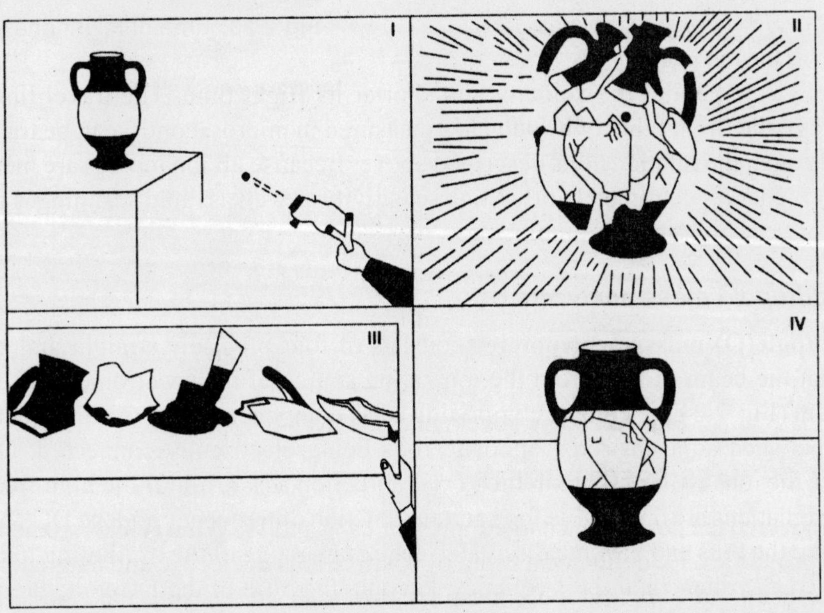

Fig. 1.1. Illustration of the principle of mass spectrometry by electron bombardment.

the pieces are carefully collected (III), the vase can be reconstructed from the fragments (IV). In this example, the vase represents the molecule, the catapult and stone represent the device for making the fragments.

Mass spectrometry is different from most other forms of spectroscopy or spectrometry that are concerned with non-destructive interactions between molecules and electromagnetic radiation. In contrast, mass spectrometry is the study of the effect of ionizing energy on molecules. It depends upon chemical reactions in the gas phase in which sample molecules are consumed during the formation of ionic and neutral species. Although sample is consumed destructively by the mass spectrometer the technique is very sensitive and only trace amounts of material are used in the analysis. A mass spectrometer converts sample molecules into ions in the gas phase, separates them according to their mass to charge ratio (m/e) and sequentially records the individual ion fragment in the form of the mass spectrum. The mass spectrum (Fig 1.2) usually presented as a vertical bar graph in which bar represent an ion (fragment ion) having specific mass to charge ratio and length of bar indicates the relative abundance or relative intensity. The highest peak intensity is counted 100%, and rest of peaks are measured with respect to 100% intensity peak (base peak). For example, in mass spectrum of methyl-t-butyl ketone, the highest peak (base peak) at m/e 57 is taken as 100% intensity peak. The rest of fragment ions peaks e.g. m/e 100, 85, 43, 41, 29 are measured with respect to highest peak, m/e 57.

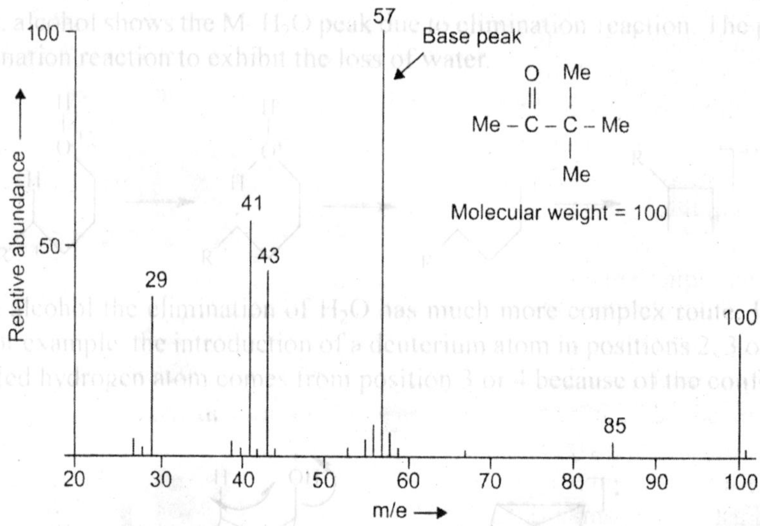

Fig. 1.2. Mass spectrum of Methyl *t*-butyl ketone.

1.2 HISTORY OF MASS SPECTROMETRY

Goldstein discovered the positively charged 'rays' in 1886 and **W. Wien** (1898) studied their electric and magnetic properties. He deflected a beam of positive ions in electric and magnetic fields. In the 1912 **J.J. Thomson** built his 'parabola mass spectrograph' to measure the charge to mass ratio (z/m) for several ionic species. He was able to demonstrate the existence of two isotopes of neon, masses 20 and 22, using a magnetic deflection instrument. In the expression z/m, z is the charge number, i.e. the total charge on an ion divided by the elementary charge (e), and m is the nucleon number, i.e. the sum of the total number of protons and neutrons in an atom, molecule or ion. In modern mass spectrometry, the parameter measured is m/z, rather than z/m.

Thomson student, **Aston** continued the work at Cambridge and built instruments that helped him to establish the presence of isotopes. He was subsequently able to measure the atomic mass of most elements with sufficient accuracy to be able to calculate the 'packing fraction' of their atomic nuclei. The packing fraction is the difference between the accurate atomic mass of the isotope and the nearest whole number divided by the mass number, also known as the mass defect. His work on isotopes also led to his formulation of the **Whole Number Rule** which states that "the mass of the oxygen isotope being defined [as 16], all the other isotopes have masses that are very nearly whole numbers", a rule that was used extensively in the development of nuclear energy.

Aston also obtained accurate measurements of the ratios of the stable isotopes of many of the known elements. At the end of this exciting period of development, Aston was convinced that much of the potential of mass spectrometry had been exploited. It was not until the 1940s that the technique was put to work in elucidating organic structures in the petroleum industry. Ionization was effected by electron 'impact' [now called electron ionization (EI)] for those molecules that could withstand vaporization into the heated and evacuated ion source without decomposition. This limited the practical mass range to less than 1000 daltons (Da)* but yielded useful fragmentations for structure elucidation (see Chapter 2).

By choosing to work with 70 electron volt (eV), many ions were formed with internal energies far in excess of the ionization energy (IE)⁺. These ions decompose rapidly to produce lower mass (fragment) ions and neutral radicals or molecules. During the 1950s, commercial instruments were being built and new applications discovered. One of the earliest of these was the identification of low molecular weight volatile food flavor compounds. Ten years later, the powerful combination of electron ionization mass spectrometry (EIMS) with gas chromatography (GC/MS) led to an explosion of applications where mass spectrometry was used in qualitative and quantitative, chemical and biochemical studies. GC/MS instruments produced enormous amounts of data, which were best handled by computers data acquisition methods. In 1966, **Munson and Field** described chemical ionization (CI) technique. This technique increased the yield of ions representative of the molecular weight of volatile molecules through interactions with reagent gas ions (e.g. CH_5^+ ions from methane) with little excess energy. Other 'soft' ionization techniques such as field desorption (FD) and particle desorption methods based upon ion generation by Cf–252 fast fission products [plasma desorption, (PDMS)] were introduced during the 1970s for nonvolatile compounds. At the same time (and in response to these developments) the instrumental mass range was increased to cope with the larger sample molecule ions now entering the gas phase. This process accelerated in the 1980s with the introduction of Fast Atom Bombardment (FAB) ionization. FAB was the first ionization technique to enable biologists and biochemists routinely to obtain molecular weight information on complex, labile biomolecules, including polypeptides and small proteins.

Ionization from the liquid state, followed by evaporation/desolvation of charged droplets, includes techniques such as ion spray, thermospray (TSP) and electrospray ionization (ESI). These methods

---

* The dalton (Da) is the unit of mass (also known as the mass unit, u) and is 1/12 of the mass of '*C (defined as 12.000000).

⁺ Ionisation energy – minimum energy of excitation of an atom or molecule required to remove an electron in order to produce a positively charged ion.

differed mainly in the manner in which ionisation was initiated. Multiple charged molecular ions could be formed under ESI, facilitating the measurement of high molecular masses, even on conventional instruments (i.e. those with a mass range up to 2000 or 4000 Th). More efficient pumping systems were required to cope with the increased gas volumes generated by vaporising liquids.

Separation techniques such as liquid chromatography and capillary electrophoresis coupled to mass spectrometry (LC/MS and CE/MS respectively) have extended the advantages first associated with the analysis of volatile compounds by GC/MS to compounds of low volatility and high molecular weight. Tandem mass spectrometry (MS/MS) collision-induced dissociation (CID), focal-plane array detectors, ion traps and hybrid instruments are providing a high sensitivity structure elucidation facility for nonvolatile compounds similar to that provided by EIMS of volatiles. Recently, Laser Desorption (LD), and especially Matrix Assisted Laser desorption Ionisation (MALDI), combined with Time-of-Flight (ToF) mass analysis has extended the practical mass range to over 300 000 Da, producing mainly singly–charged molecular ions. Fourier transform mass spectrometry (FTMS), also known as Fourier transform ion cyclotron resonance (FT-CR) mass spectrometry is only slowly entering in the commercial area.

Historical development in Mass spectrometry

19th century

1886: Eugen Goldstein observes canal or positive rays rays.

1898: Wilhelm Wien demonstrates that canal rays can be deflected using strong electric and magnetic fields. He shows that the mass-to-charge ratio of the particles have opposite polarity and is much larger compared to the electron. He also realizes that the particle mass is similar to the one of hydrogen particle.

1898: J. J. Thomson measures the mass-to-charge ratio of electrons.

20th century

1901: Walter Kaufmann uses a mass spectrometer to measure the relativistic mass increase of electrons.

1905: J.J. Thomson begins the study of positive rays.

1906: Thomson is awarded the Nobel Prize in Physics "in recognition of the great merits of his theoretical and experimental investigations on the conduction of electricity by gases"

1913: Thomson is able to separate particles of different mass-to-charge ratios. He separates the ^{20}Ne and the ^{22}Ne isotopes, and he correctly identifies the m/e = 11 signal as a doubly charged ^{22}Ne particle.

1919: Francis Aston constructs the first velocity focusing mass spectrograph with mass resolving power of 130.

1922: Aston is awarded the Nobel Prize in chemistry "for his discovery, by means of his mass spectrograph, of isotopes, in a large number of non–radioactive elements, and for his enunciation of the whole-number rule."

1931: Ernest O. Lawrence invents the cyclotron.

1934: Josef Mattauch and Richard Herzog develop the double-focusing mass spectrograph.

1936: Arthur J. Dempster develops the spark ionization source.
1937: Aston constructs a mass spectrograph with resolving power of 2000.
1939: Lawrence receives the Nobel Prize in Physics for the cyclotron.
1942: Lawrence develops the Calutron for uranium isotope separation.
1946: William Stephens presents the concept of a time-of-flight mass spectrometer.
1956: Fred McLafferty proposes a hydrogen transfer reaction that will come to be known as the McLafferty rearrangement.
1959: Researchers develop a chemical interface for a gas chromatograph to a mass spectrometer.
1966: F.H. Field and M.S.B. Munson develop chemical ionization.
1968: Malcolm Dole develops electrospray ionization.
1969: H.D. Beckey develops field desorption.
1974: Comisarow and Marshall develop Fourier Transform Ion Cyclotron Resonance Mass Spectrometry.
1976: Ronald MacFarlane and co-workers develop plasma desorption mass spectrometry.
1984: John Bennett Fenn and co-workers use electrospray to ionize biomolecules.
1985: Franz Hillenkamp, Michael Karas and co-workers describe and coin the term matrix–assisted laser desorption ionization (MALDI).
1987: Koichi Tanaka uses the "ultra fine metal plus liquid matrix method" to ionize intact proteins.
1989: Wolfgang Paul receives the Nobel Prize in Physics "for the development of the ion trap technique"
1999: Alexander Makarov presents the Orbitrap mass spectrometer.

21st century

2002: John Bennett Fenn and Koichi Tanaka are awarded one–quarter of the Nobel Prize in chemistry each "for the development of soft desorption ionization methods for mass spectrometric analyses of biological macromolecules."

1.3 APPLICATIONS

- **Determine accurate molecular weight** (It is required for *sample confirmation/ purity of a sample/ verifying amino acid substitutions*).
- **Monitoring the reaction** *(monitor enzyme reactions, chemical modification, protein digestion)*
- Online monitoring for fermentations for the biotechnology industry.
- **Determine the Amino acid sequence** (*sequence confirmation,* de novo *characterization of peptides, identification of proteins by database searching with a sequence "tag" from a proteolytic fragment*).
- Determine how drugs are metabolized in the body.
- Detect and identify illegitimate use of drugs in athletes. There is a perfect relationship between **Mass Spectrometry and Olympic Drug Testing.** Anabolic steroids such as testosterone are used to build muscle, analgesics (including narcotics such as morphine) allow injured athletes to continue training, diuretics increase urine production and thus decrease a drug's concen-

tration in the analyzed urine sample, peptide hormones such as human growth hormone stimulate tissue growth, and stimulants (including high levels of caffeine) enhance endurance. Most of the companies use the technique of Liquid chromatography–Mass spectrometry. First a standard anabolic steroid is injected into the machine. The machine recognizes it and develops a curve with peaks. The peaks are then depicted on a timed graph. The data is stored in the computer as a reference. Then an unknown drug is injected into the machine. If it is the same drug as the standard, it appears in the same position at the same time. This immediately tells the technician that the unknown drug has matched a standard drug. The latest devices can even compute the dose of the drug. The amount of drug that can be detected with the latest machines is in nanograms (10^{-9} g).

- Detect and identify the drug of abuse (Forensic analysis)
- Detect the adulteration of honey with corn syrup.
- Detect and identify the toxins/pesticides in case of poisoning
- Determine damage of human or animal genes due to environmental causes
- Determine the age and origins of specimens in geochemistry and archaeology (Radiocarbon dating). Mass spectrometry measures the amount of Carbon 14 (C14) available in living creatures as a measuring stick. All living things maintain a content of carbon 14 in equilibrium with that available in the atmosphere, right up to the moment of death. When an organism dies, the amount of C14 available within it begins to decay at a half life rate of 5730 years; i.e., it takes 5730 years for 1/2 of the C14 available in the organism to decay.
- Detect dioxins in food and humans (The dioxins are produced as a waste product by industrial plants and waste incineration. These may cause hormonal changes, cancer and other severe disorder).
- Locate petroleum deposits by testing rock samples
- To estimate the potentiality of grapes and how it may be transferred into wine is key to grasping enological chemistry. Nowadays, mass spectrometry is a crucial aspect in ensuring the production, the quality, and the safety of grape, wine, and grape derivative products. Mass Spectrometry in Grape and Wine Chemistry examines in depth the relationship between the high structural identification power of mass spectrometry techniques and the chemistry of grapes and wine.
- Test the purity of semi-conductor materials used in making microchips for computers
- Monitor and track air pollutants. Mass spectrometers was used as sensitive chemical warfare detectors to protect troops in war on Iraq.
- The identification and characterization of proteins involved in biological processes
- Find novel proteins in biological samples for use as therapeutic or diagnostic targets
- Detect the presence of amino acid metabolic disorders (PKU, maple syrup urine disease, and homocystinuria) among newborns.

Only a brief introduction to the principles and practice of mass spectrometry is given herein. The reader is directed towards more general books on this subject.

CHAPTER

2

Introduction to Mass Spectrometer

2.1 INTRODUCTION

Mass Spectrometer (MS) is a kind of instrument which uses an analytical technique to measure the mass-to-charge ratio of ions. This analytical technique is known as Mass spectrometry. The mass spectrometer involves the following sequences:

Sequence 1: Ionization

The molecule is ionized by knocking one or more electrons off to give a positive ion. This is true even for things which you would normally expect to form negative ions (chlorine, for example). Mass spectrometers generally work with positive ions.

Note: *It is easy to handle the charged particle in comparison to neutral molecule.*

Sequence 2: Acceleration

The ions are accelerated so that they all have the same kinetic energy.

Sequence 3: Deflection

The ions are then deflected by a magnetic field according to their masses. The lighter they are, the more they are deflected. The amount of deflection also depends on the number of positive charges on the ion - in other words, on how many electrons were knocked off in the first stage. The more the ion is charged, the more it gets deflected.

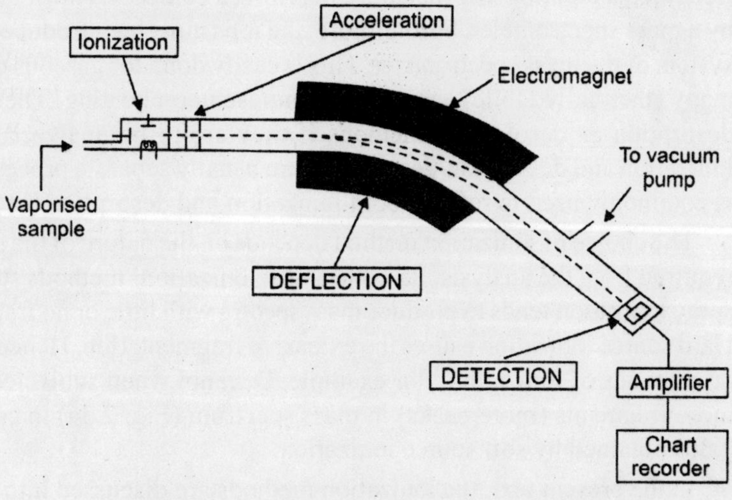

Fig. 2.1. Sequences of mass spectrometry.

Sequence 4: Detection

The beam of ions passing through the machine is detected electrically.

The need for a vacuum

It's important that the ions produced in the ionization chamber have a free run through the machine without hitting air molecules. For this reason, vacuum is needed.

2.2 GENERAL STRUCTURE OF MASS SPECTROMETER

Generally, a typical Mass Spectrometer consists of three parts: an ion source, a mass analyzer and a detector.

The function of the ion source is to produce ions from the sample. The function of the mass analyzer is to separate ions with different mass-to-charge ratios. Then, numbers of different ions are detected by the detector. Finally, the mass spectrum is generated after all the data have been collected. Fig. 2.2 is a schematic diagram of the mass spectrometer.

Apart from the above components, there is a sample inlet system and vacuum system.

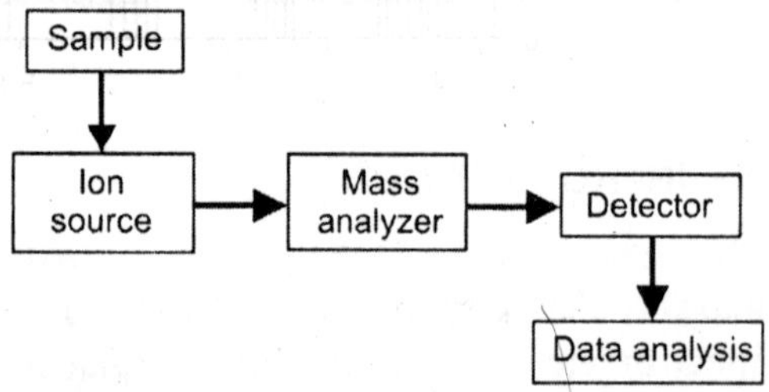

Fig. 2.2. Schematic diagram of mass spectrometer.

2.2.1 Ion Source

A mass spectrometer works by using magnetic and electric field to exert forces on charged particles (ions) for separation in a vacuum. Therefore, a compound must be charged or ionized to be analyzed by a mass spectrometer. Furthermore, the ions must be introduced in the gas phase into the vacuum system of the mass spectrometer. This is easily done for gaseous or heat-volatile samples. However, many (thermally labile) analytes decompose upon heating. These kinds of samples require either desorption or desolvation methods if they are to be analyzed by mass spectrometry. Although ionization and desorption/desolvation are usually separate processes, the term "ionization method" is commonly used to refer to both ionization and desorption (or desolvation) methods.

The choice of ionization method depends on the nature of the sample and the type of information required from the analysis. So-called 'soft ionization' methods such as field desorption and electrospray ionization tends to produce mass spectra with little or no fragment-ion content. Comparatively, Hard source ionization causes the extensive fragmentation. Hence, nature of mass spectrum depends on methods of ionization. For example, Decanol when subjected to hard source ionization shows more fragments (more peaks) in mass spectrum (Fig. 2.3a) in comparison to mass spectrum (Fig. 2.3b) obtained by soft source ionization.

In the present text, the ionization methods are discussed into the gaseous phase and desorption ionization.

2.2.1.1 Gas-Phase Ionization

These methods rely upon ionizing samples in gaseous phase. The samples are usually introduced through a heated batch inlet, or heated direct insertion probe, or a gas chromatograph.

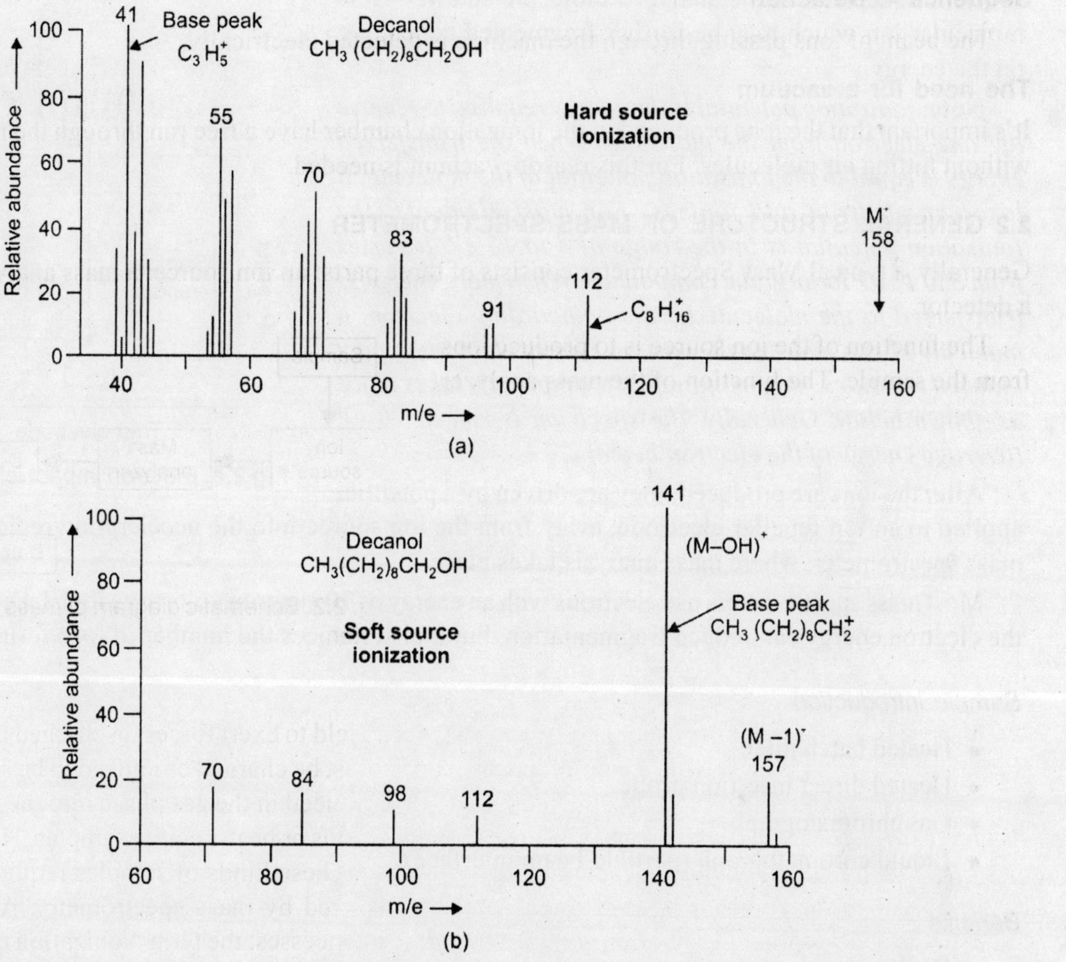

Fig. 2.3. Comparison of mass spectrum (a) hard source ionization, (b) soft source ionization.

2.2.1.1.1. Electron Ionization (EI)

It, also referred to as electron impact ionization, is the oldest and best-characterized of all the ionization methods. The process is a relatively harsh form of ionization producing a wide range of molecular fragments. EI is best suited to relatively non-polar, volatile samples. The electron impact source (Fig. 2.4) consists of a heated tungsten or rhenium filament that produces electrons which are accelerated to another electrode called the ion trap. Sample vapor diffuses into the electron beam and become ionized and fragmented. The size of fragment depends on the electron energy which is controlled by the accelerating potential on the ion trap electrode. Low energy electrons produce molecular ions and larger fragments, whereas high energy electrons produce many smaller fragments and possibly no molecular ions. The following gas phase reaction describes the electron ionization process:

$$M + e^- \longrightarrow M^{+\cdot} + 2e^-$$

Here M represents the analyzed molecule and $M^{+\bullet}$ is its molecular ion which may be further fragmented depending on the energy.

Note: *Ionization potential is the energy required to remove the one electron from the molecule. When the transferred energy is equal to the ionisation potential of the molecule, it loses an electron and ionizes. For most elements, the Ionisation potential is in the range of 5 to 15 eV. It varies from 8 to 12 eV for organic compounds. When more energy is transferred to the molecule by the bombarding electron, a molecule M can undergo the various type of electron impact induced reactions, fragmentation of the molecule takes place as shown below. Generally, the spectrum is run at 70 eV (average energy of the electron beam).*

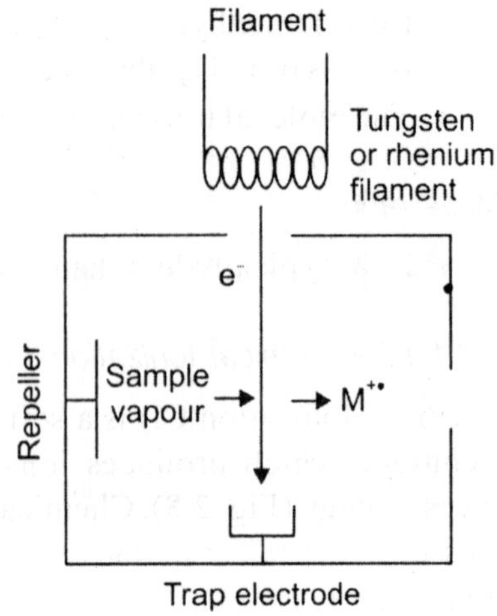

Fig 2.4. Electron impact ion source.

After the ions are produced, they are driven by a potential applied to an ion-repeller electrode, away from the ion source into the accelerating region of the mass spectrometer, where mass analysis takes place.

Most mass spectrometers use electrons with an energy of 70 electron volts (eV) for EI. Decreasing the electron energy can reduce fragmentation, but it also reduces the number of ions formed.

Sample introduction

- Heated batch inlet.
- Heated direct insertion probe.
- Gas chromatograph.
- Liquid chromatograph (particle-beam interface).

Benefits

- Well-understood.
- Can be applied to virtually all volatile compounds.
- Reproducible mass spectra.
- Fragmentation provides structural information due to more fragmentation (Hard source ionization).
- Libraries of mass spectra can be searched for EI mass spectral "fingerprint".

Limitations

- Sample must be thermally volatile and stable. To increase the volatility, chemical derivatives can be prepared. For example, Organic acids, fatty acids, etc. can be analysed by EI method with the formation of their methyl esters. Many chemical classes can be rendered volatile through the preparation of a variety of silylated products that enable mass and structural information to be obtained. Special chemical derivatives can be made that yield characteristic fragmentation properties, thereby aiding analysis. An example is the preparation of t-butyldimethylsilyl derivatives of steroids. These yield an abundant $[M\text{–}57]^+$ ion (generated by loss of C_4H_9) that is especially useful in quantitative measurements.

- The molecular ion may be weak or absent for many compounds.

Mass range

- Low Typically less than 1,000 Da.

2.2.1.1.2. Chemical Ionization

Chemical Ionization CI) is a soft" ionization technique which produces ions with little excess energy (Fig. 2.8). Chemical ionization uses ion-molecule reactions to produce ions from the analyte (M). Chemical Ionization (CI) is applied to samples similar to those analyzed by EI and is primarily used to enhance the abundance of the molecular ion.

The chemical ionization process begins when a reagent gas such as methane, isobutane, or ammonia is ionized by electron impact. A high reagent gas pressure (or long reaction time) results in ion-molecule reactions between the reagent gas ions and reagent gas neutrals. Some of the products of these ion-molecule reactions can react with the analyte molecules to produce analyte ions. For example, Chemical ionization involving methane is shown in Fig. 2.5.

A) EI of reagent gas to form ions:

$$CH_4 + e^- \longrightarrow CH_4^{+\bullet} + 2e^-$$

B) Reaction of reagent gas ions to form adducts:

$$CH_4 + CH_4^{+\bullet} \longrightarrow CH_3^{+\bullet} + CH_5^+$$

or

$$CH_4^+ \longrightarrow CH_3^+ + H^\bullet$$

$$CH_3^+ + CH_4 \longrightarrow C_2H_5^+ + H_2$$

C) Reaction of Reagent Gas Ions with analyte molecule (M):

$$CH_5^+ + M \longrightarrow CH_4 + MH^+\ (M+1)$$

$$C_2H_5^+ + M \longrightarrow C_2H_4 + MH^+(M+1)$$

$$CH_3^+ + M \longrightarrow CH_4 + (M\text{–}H)$$

Fig. 2.5. Chemical ionization reactions with methane gas.

In CI with the use of methane, the relevant peaks observed are MH^+, $[M + CH_5]^+$ and $[M + C_2H_5]^+$ but mainly MH^+.

Similarly, chemical ionization with isobutane and ammonia occurs. The Isobutane loses an electron upon EI and yields the corresponding radical cation, which will fragment mainly through the loss of hydrogen radical to yield a *t*-butyl cation, and to a lesser extent through the loss of a methyl radical:

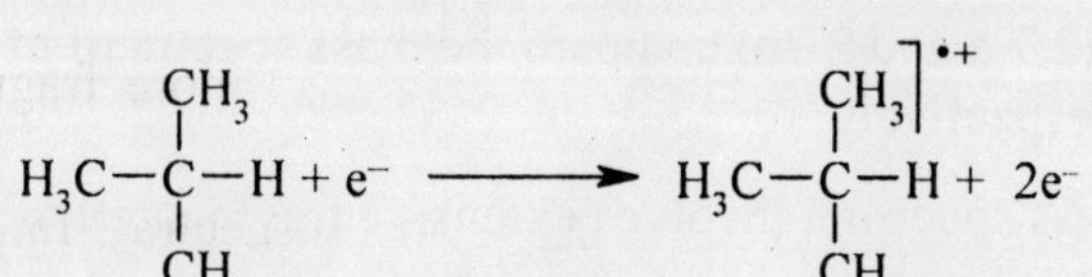

Isobutane

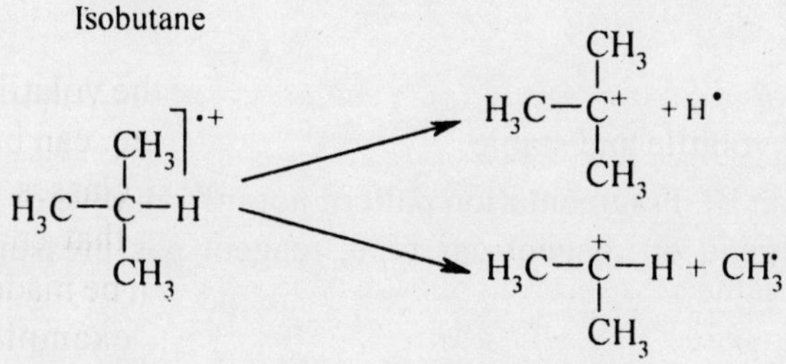

In isobutane positive ion CI, the main peak observed is MH^+.

$$M + C_4H_9^+ \longrightarrow (M + H)^+ + C_4H_8$$

With ammonia,

$$NH_3 + e^- \longrightarrow NH_3^{+\cdot} + 2e^-$$
$$NH_3 + NH_3^{+\cdot} \longrightarrow NH_4^+ + NH_2$$
$$NH_4^+ + NH_3 \longrightarrow N_2H_7^+$$
$$M + NH_4^+ \longrightarrow (M + H)^+ + NH_3$$

In this main peaks observed are MH^+ and $[M + NH_4]^+$.

Choice of reagent gas

Two factors determine the choice of the gas to be used:

- Proton affinity
- Energy transfer

The NH_3 is the most used reagent gas in CI because of low energy transfer of NH_4^+ compares to CH_5^+ for example.

Sample introduction

- Heated batch inlet.
- Heated direct insertion probe.
- Gas chromatograph.
- Liquid chromatograph (particle-beam interface).

Benefits

- Often gives molecular weight information through molecular-like ions such as [M+H]+, even when EI would not produce a molecular ion (CI gives the $[M + H]^+$ ion peak].
- Simple mass spectra, fragmentation reduced compared to EI method of ionization. The Figs. (2.6a and 2.6b) and (2.7 a and 2.7b) compare the mass spectra of m-nitrobenzyl alcohol and cyclophosphamide respectively.

The electron impact mass spectrum involves extensive fragmentation.

The chemical ionization spectrum is much simpler.

Limitations

Sample must be thermally volatile and stable.

Less fragmentation than EI. Fragmentation pattern not informative or reproducible enough for library search. Results depend on reagent gas type, reagent gas pressure or reaction time, and nature of sample.

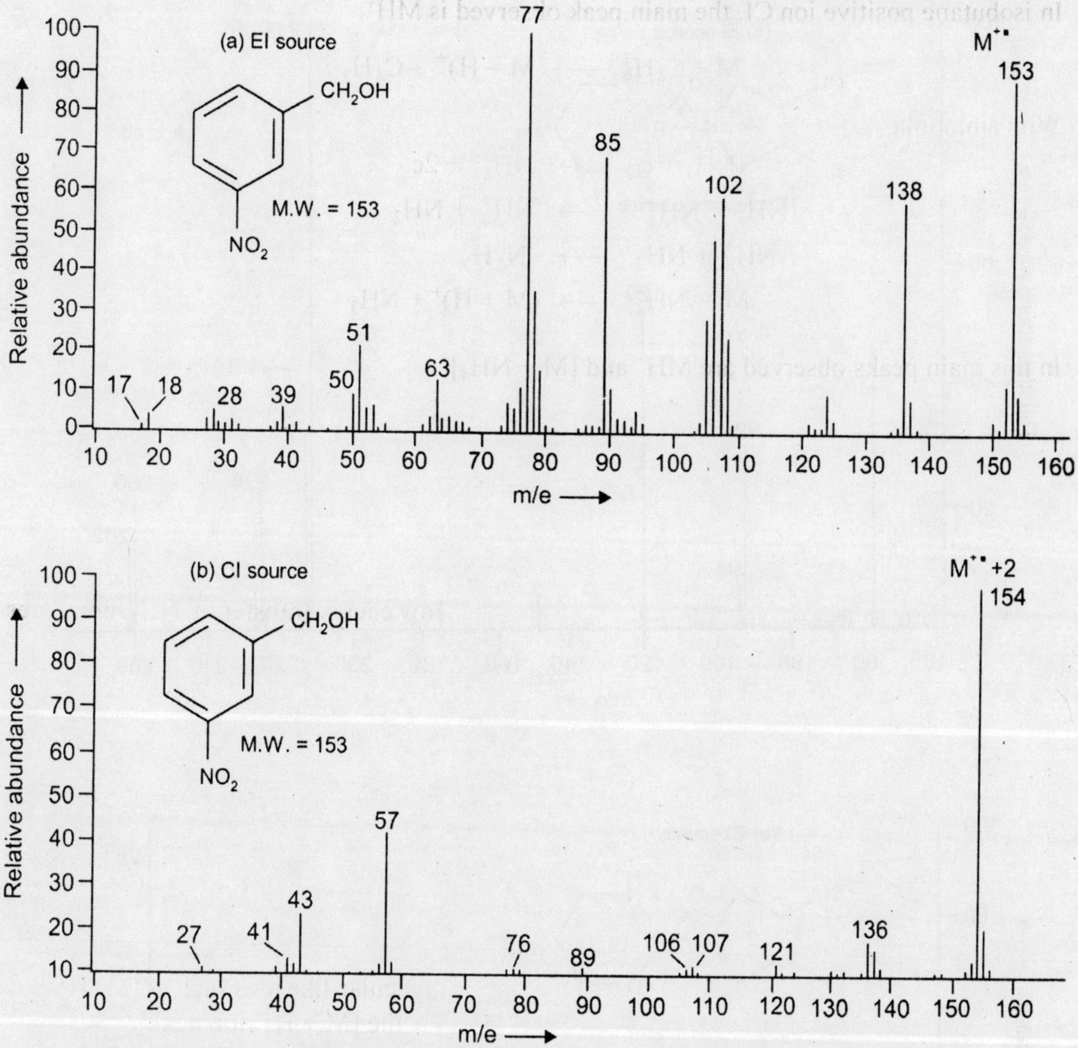

Fig. 2.6. Mass spectrum of m-Nitrobenzyl alcohol (a) EI source, (b) CI source.

Mass range

Low typically less than 1,000 Da.

Note: In order to rationalize the fragmentation of MH^+ ions, one must consider at which sites in the sample molecule the proton is attached. The spectrum may then be rationalised in terms of the fragmentation of the different types of MH^+ ions. In general, protonation occurs on hetero atoms having lone pairs of electrons, such as O, N and Cl. This frequently followed by charge-induced elimination of a molecule containing the hetero-atom. Other possible protonation sites are aromatic rings and regions of unsaturation.

Ephedrine ionised by methane CI, may protonate for example on the O atom of the OH group resulting in loss of water molecule.

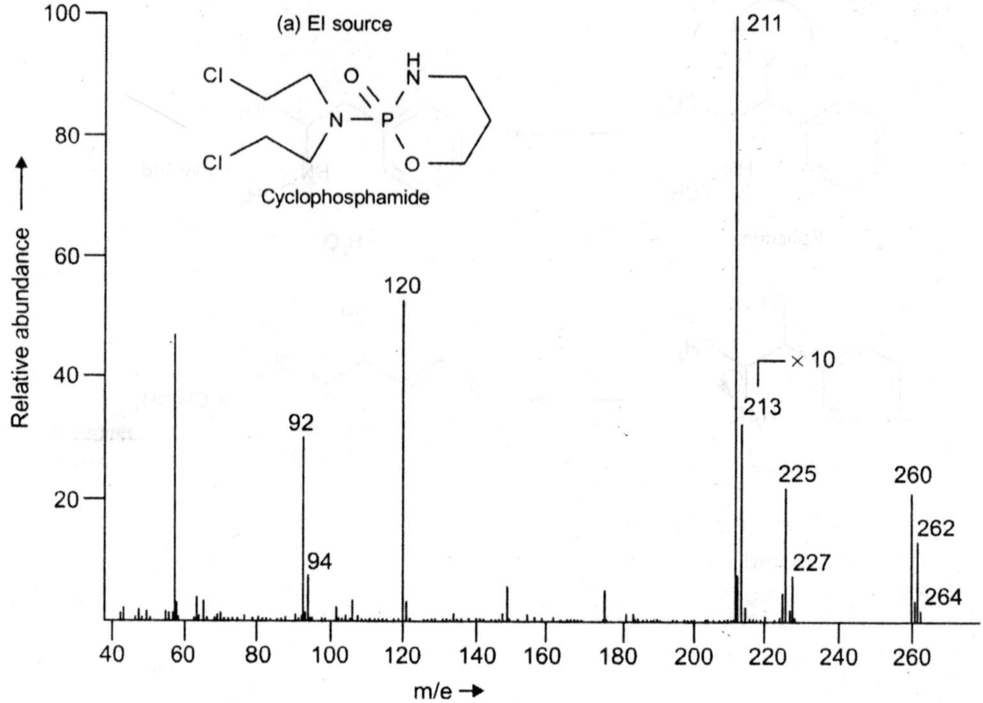

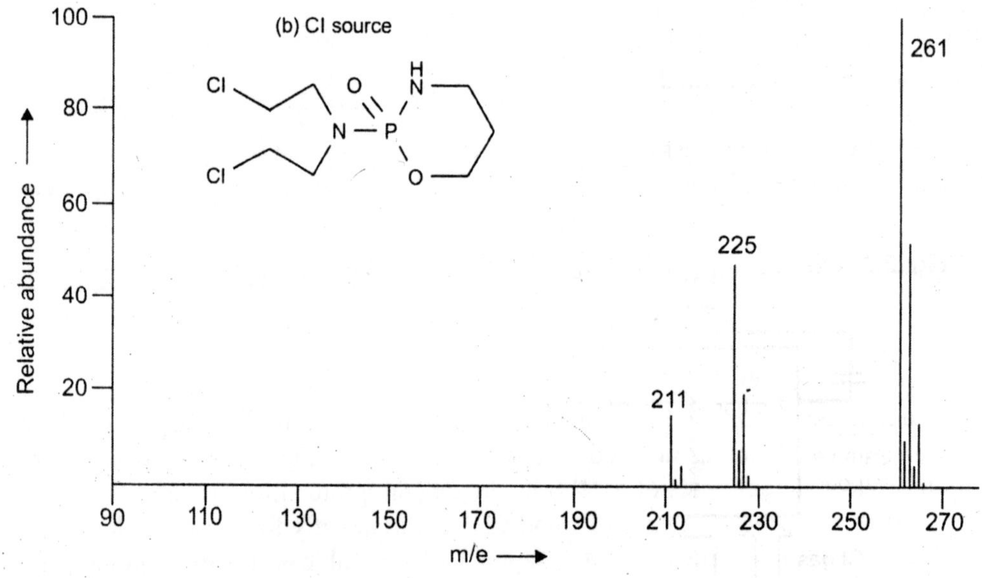

Fig. 2.7. Mass spectrum of Cyclophosphamide (a) EI source, (b) CI source.

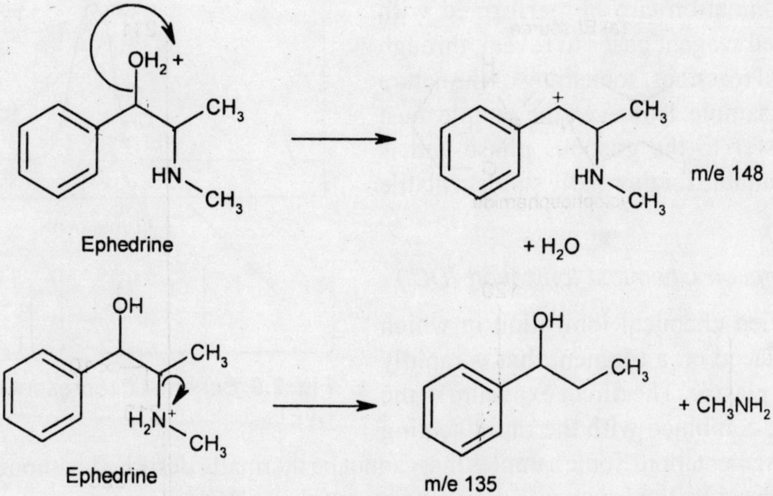

Protonation on the N atom leads to the loss of CH_3NH_2 by a similar mechanism, yielding an ion of m/e 135. Both m/e 148 and 135 are observed in the CI spectrum, indicating the presence of OH and $HNCH_3$ groups in the molecule.

Alternate CI-EI (A CE)

Electron and chemical ionization produce complementary information on volatilisable samples. This becomes particularly useful when analyzing compounds in complex mixtures by high-resolution capillary column gas chromatography. Although it is possible to run the same mixture twice, once by CI and once by EI, it can be difficult to replicate the chromatograms exactly. Furthermore, the time for each analysis is at least doubled. However, if the conditions in the source can be changed rapidly from EI to CI and back again during the elution time of the GC peak then the two spectra are known to be related and consecutive. ACE sources have a cycle time of around 1 second to record two spectra. If the GC peak is at least 4 seconds wide at the base it is possible to obtain two sets of data as the component of interest elutes (Fig. 2.9).

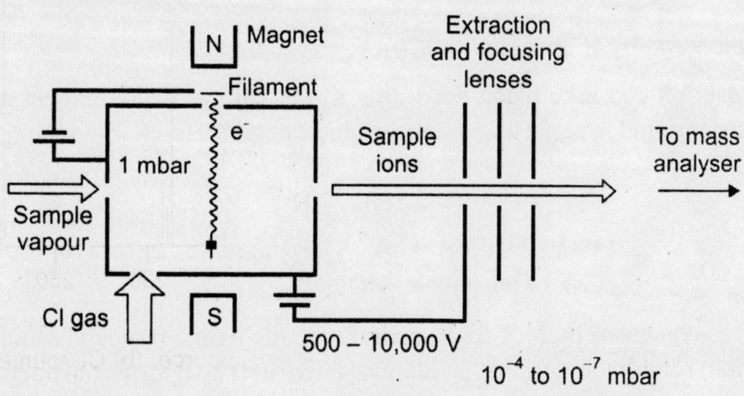

Fig. 2.8. Schematic diagram of chemical ion source.

Chemical ionization can be performed with carefully selected reagent gases to reveal, through specific chemical reactions, something of the nature of the unknown sample. However, the sample must withstand transfer to the gaseous phase and is therefore only suitable for thermally stable, volatile molecules.

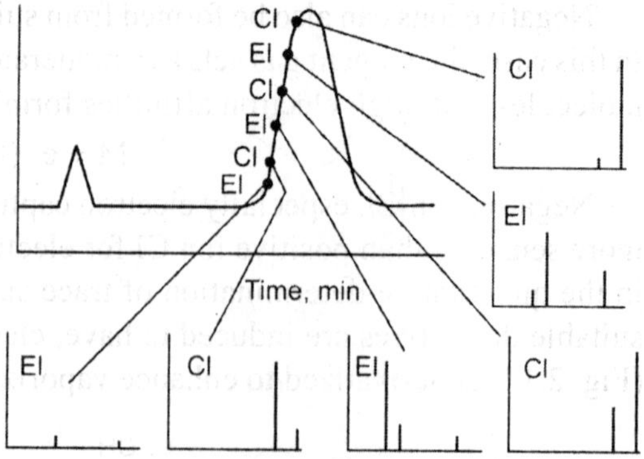

Fig. 2.9. Schematic representation of alternate CI/EI.

2.2.1.1.3. Desorption Chemical Ionization (DCI)

This is a modified chemical ionization in which the analyte is placed on a filament that is rapidly heated in the CI plasma. The direct exposure to the CI reagent ions, combined with the rapid heating acts to reduce fragmentation. Some samples that cannot be thermally desorbed without decomposition can be characterized by the fragments produced by pyrolysis DCI.

Sample introduction

- Sample deposited onto a filament wire.
- Filament rapidly heated inside the CI source.

Benefits

- Reduced thermal decomposition.
- Rapid analysis.
- Relatively simple equipment.

Limitations

- Not particularly reproducible.
- Rapid heating requires fast scan speeds. fails for large or labile compounds.

Mass range

Low Typically less than 1,500 Da.

2.2.1.1.4 Negative-ion chemical ionization (NCI)

Various types of reaction can take place according to the nature of the reagent gas used, e.g. a mixture of hydrocarbon and water (95:5) can produce negatively-charged sample ions by the following reactions:

$$H_2O + e^- \longrightarrow OH^- + H$$
$$AH + OH^- \longrightarrow A^- + H_2O$$
$$M + HO^- \longrightarrow MOH^-$$

Other possible reagent gases include hydrocarbon/organic halide/oxygen (which produces Cl^- and O^- attachment ions) and fluorocarbons yielding negative ions by hydride abstraction and fluorine attachment.

Negative ions can also be formed from suitable sample molecules by electron capture processes. In this case, the reagent gas acts as a moderator, generating thermal electrons that can then attach to molecules with high electron affinities forming negative radical ions.

$$M + e^{-} \text{ (thermal)} \longrightarrow M^{-\cdot}$$

Negative ion CI, especially electron capture ionisation, can be two to three orders of magnitude more sensitive than positive ion CI for electronegative molecules. It is therefore especially useful in the quantitative determination of trace substances that have, or that through the production of suitable derivatives are induced to have, electron-capturing properties. For example, testosterone (Fig. 2.10) is derivatized to enhance vaporization and ionization for NCI-GC/MS.

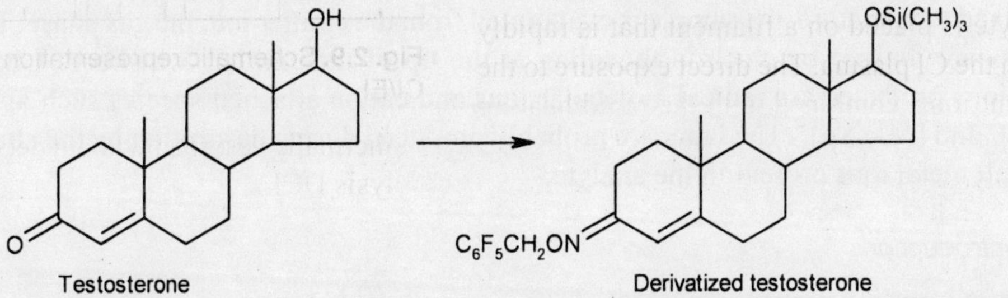

Fig. 2.10. The pentafluorobenzyl trimethyl silyl ether derivatives of steroids make them more amenable to high sensitivity measurements using negative chemical ionization.

Sample introduction

- Same as for CI,

Benefits

- Efficient ionization, high sensitivity.
- Less fragmentation than positive ion EI or CI.
- Greater selectivity for certain environmentally or biologically important compounds.

Limitations

- Not all volatile compounds produce negative ions.
- Poor reproducibility

Mass range

- Low Typically less than 1,000 Da.

2.2.1.2. Field Desorption ionization

These methods are based on electron tunneling from an emitter that is based at a high electrical potential. The emitter is a filament on which fine crystalline 'whiskers' are grown. When a high potential is applied to the emitter, a very high electric field exists near the tips of the whiskers.

There are two kinds of emitters used on JEOL mass spectrometers: carbon emitters and silicon emitters. Silicon emitters are robust, relatively inexpensive, and they can handle a higher current for field desorption. Carbon emitters are more expensive, but they can provide about an order of magnitude better sensitivity than silicon emitters.

Field desorption ionization method are soft ionization methods that tend to produce mass spectra with little or no fragment-ion content.

2.2.1.2.1 Field Desorption (FD)

This technique was developed by Beckly in 1969. The sample is deposited onto the emitter and the emitter is placed to a high potential (several kilovolts) and a current is passed through the emitter to heat up the filament. Mass spectra are acquired as the emitter current is gradually increased and at certain fixed temperature, the sample is evaporated from the emitter into the gas phase. The analyte molecules are ionized by electron tunneling at the tip of the emitter 'whiskers'. Characteristic positive ions produced are radical molecular ions and cation attached species such as $[M + H]^+$, $[M + Na]^+$ and $[M - Na]^+$. The latter are probably produced during desorption by the attachment of trace alkali metal ions present in the analyte.

Sample introduction

- Direct insertion probe.
- Sample is deposited onto the tip of the emitter by dipping the emitter into an analyte solution.
- Depositing the dissolved or suspended sample onto the emitter with a microsyringe.

Benefits

- Simple mass spectra, typically one molecular or molecular-like ionic species per compound.
- Little or no chemical background.
- Works well for non volatile molecules like proteins, carbohydrates, sugars and industrial polymers.

Limitations

- Sensitive to alkali metal contamination and sample overloading.
- Emitter is relatively fragile.
- Relatively slow analysis as the emitter current is increased.
- The sample must be thermally volatile to some extent to be desorbed.

Mass range

- Low-moderate, depends on the sample. Typically less than about 2000 to 3000 Da.
- some examples have been recorded from ions with masses beyond 10000 Da.

2.2.1.2.2. Field Ionization (FI)

The removal of electrons from any species by interaction with a high electrical field The sample is evaporated from a direct insertion probe, gas chromatograph, or gas inlet. As the gas molecules pass near the emitter, they are ionized by electron tunneling.

Sample introduction

- Heated direct insertion probe.
- Gas inlet.
- Gas chromatograph.

Benefits

- Simple mass spectra, typically one molecular or molecular-like ionic species per compound.
- Little or no chemical background.
- Works well for small organic molecules and some petrochemical fractions.

Limitations

- The sample must be thermally volatile. Samples are introduced in the same way as for electron ionization (EI).

Mass range

- Low Typically less than 1000 Da.

Comparison of Field ionization and Field desorption method

FI: sample is heated in a vacuum so as to volatilize it onto an ionization surface. FI is suited for use with volatile, thermally stable compounds. FI sources are arranged to function also as FD sources.

FD: the sample is placed directly on to the surface (dipping emitter in an analyte solution) before ionization but FD is needed for nonvolatile and/or thermally labile substances.

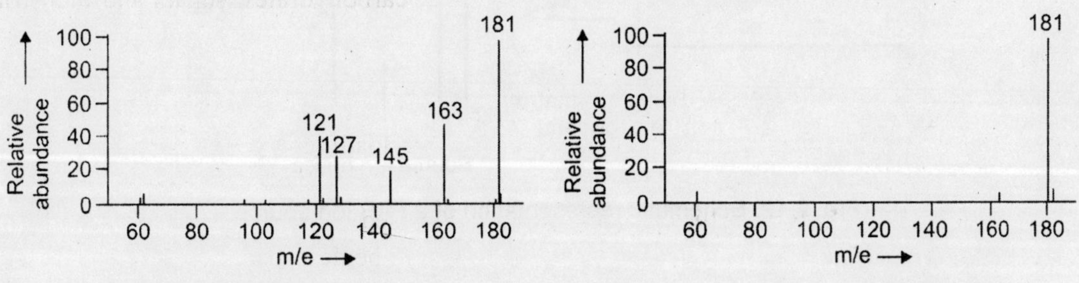

Fig. 2.11. (a) FI mass spectrum-D-glucose, (b) FD mass spectrum-D-glucose.

2.2.1.3 Particle Bombardment

In these methods, the sample is deposited on a target that is bombarded with atoms, neutrals, or ions. The most common approach for organic mass spectrometry is to dissolve the analyte in a liquid matrix with low volatility and to use a relatively high current of bombarding particles (FAB or dynamic SIMS). Other methods use a relatively low current of bombarding particles and no liquid matrix (static SIMS). The latter methods are more commonly used for surface analysis than for organic mass spectrometry.

The primary particle beam is the bombarding particle beam, while the secondary ions are the ions produced from bombardment of the target.

2.2.1.3.1. Fast Atom Bombardment (FAB)

FAB is a "soft" ionization method which overcomes many of the limitations of EI and CI. FAB works well for polar, thermally labile compounds. A FAB mass spectrum often contains a protonated molecule, $[M+H]^+$, and a few fragment ions. The analyte is dissolved in a liquid matrix such as glycerol, thioglycerol, m-nitrobenzyl alcohol, or diethanolamine and then a small amount (about 1 microliter) of it is placed on a target. The target is bombarded with a fast atom beam (for example, xenon atoms, accelerated through a potential difference of 5000–35 000 V; Xe atoms that are first ionized and then neutralized to give a neutral atom beam) that desorb molecular-like ions and fragments from the analyte (Fig. 2.12). Cluster ions from the liquid matrix are also desorbed and produce a chemical background that varies with the matrix used (Fig. 2.13).

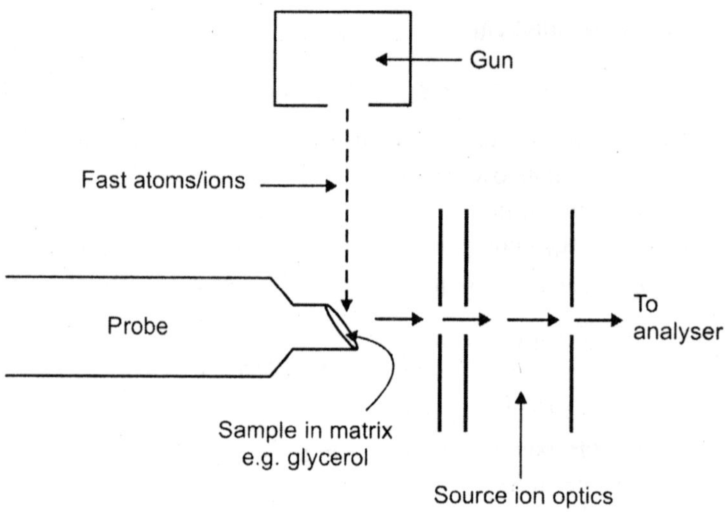

Fig. 2.12. Schematic representation of a FAB ion source.

Sample introduction

- Direct insertion probe.
- LC/MS (frit FAB or continuous-flow FAB).

Benefits

- Rapid and. simple.
- Relatively tolerant of variations in sampling.
- Good for a large variety of compounds.
- Strong ion currents — good for high-resolution measurements.

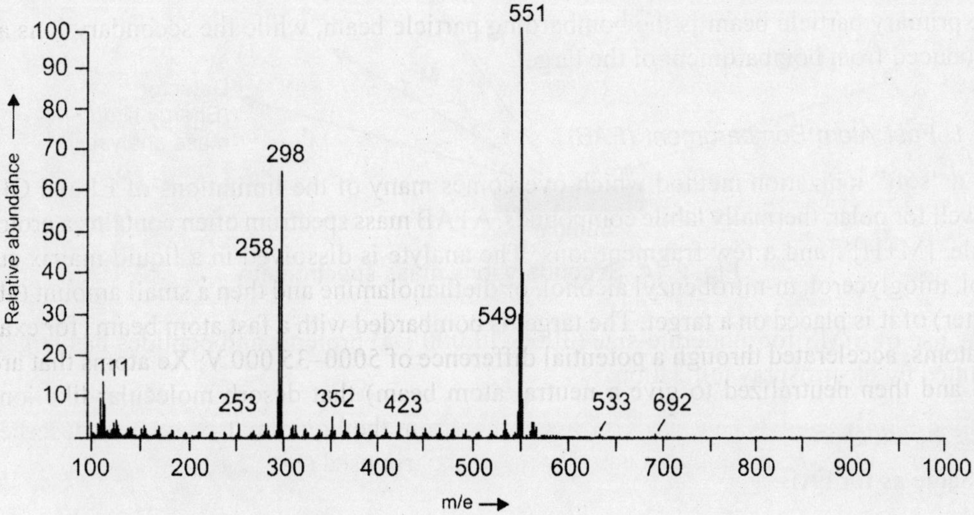

Fig. 2.13. FAB mass spectrum of unknown compound in m-Nitrobenzyl alcohol.

Limitations

- High chemical background decreases detection limits.
- May be difficult to distinguish low-molecular-weight compounds from chemical background
- analyte must be soluble in the liquid matrix
- no good for multiply charged compounds with more than double charges

Mass range

- Moderate Typically ~300 Da to about 6000 Da.

2.2.1.3.2 Secondary Ion Mass Spectrometry (SIMS)

SIMS is nearly identical to FAB except that the primary particle beam is an ion beam (e.g. cesium ions) rather than a neutral beam. In SIMS, the surface of the sample is subjected to bombardment by high energy ions - this leads to the ejection (or *sputtering*) of both neutral and charged (+/–) species from the surface. The ejected species may include atoms, clusters of atoms and molecular fragments.

In traditional SIMS it is only the positive ions that are mass analysed. This is primarily for practical ease but it does lead to problems with quantifying the compositional data since the positive ions are but a small, non-representative fraction of the total sputtered species. It should be further noted that the displaced ions have to be energy filtered before they are mass analysed (i.e. only ions with kinetic energies within a limited range are mass analyzed).

The most commonly employed incident ions (denoted by I^+ in the Fig. 2.14) used for bombarding the sample are argon ions (Ar^+) but other ions (e.g. alkali metal ions, Ga^+) are preferred for some applications. The mass analyzer is typically a quadrupole MS analyzer with unit mass resolution, but high specification time-of-flight (TOF) analyzers are also used and provide substantially higher sensitivity and a much greater mass range (at a higher cost).

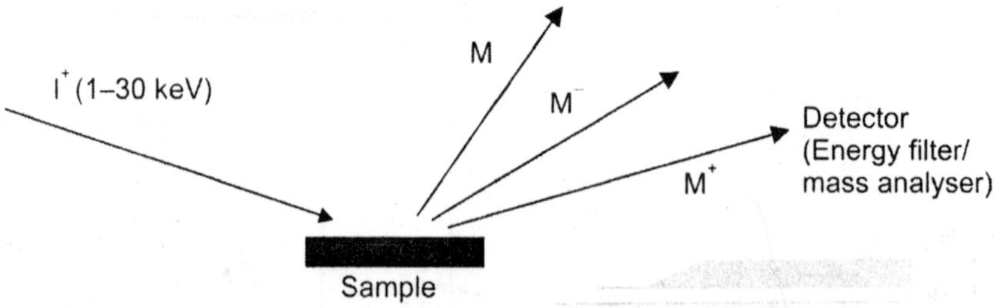

Fig. 2.14. Secondary ions mass spectrometry.

The use of SIMS for moderate-size (3000–13,000 Da) proteins and peptides has largely been supplanted by electrospray ionization.

Sample introduction

- Same as for FAB.

Benefits

- Same as for FAB, except sensitivity is improved for higher masses (3000 to 13,000 Da).

Limitations

Same as for FAB except.

- Target can get hotter than in FAB due to more energetic primary beam.
- High-voltage arcs more common than FAB.
- Ion source usually requires more maintenance than FAB.

Mass range

- Moderate typically 300 to 13,000 Da.

2.2.1.4. Atmospheric Pressure Ionization (Spray Methods)

As the name implies, APCI is a technique which creates ions at atmospheric pressure. A sample solution flows through a heated tube where it is volatilized and sprayed into a corona discharge with the aid of nitrogen nebulization. Ions are produced in the discharge and extracted into the mass spectrometer. APCI is best suited to relatively polar, semi-volatile samples. An APCI mass spectrum usually contains the quasi-molecular ion, $[M+H]^+$. These methods are well-suited for flow-injection and LC/MS techniques.

2.2.1.4.1. Electrospray Ionization (ESI)

ESI allows for large, non-volatile molecules to be analyzed directly from the liquid phase Large charged droplets are produced by 'pneumatic nebulization'; i.e. the forcing of the analyte solution through a needle at the end of which is applied a potential (Fig. 2.15). The potential used is sufficiently high to disperse the emerging solution into a very fine spray of charged droplets all at the same polarity. The solvent evaporates away, shrinking the droplet size and increasing the charge

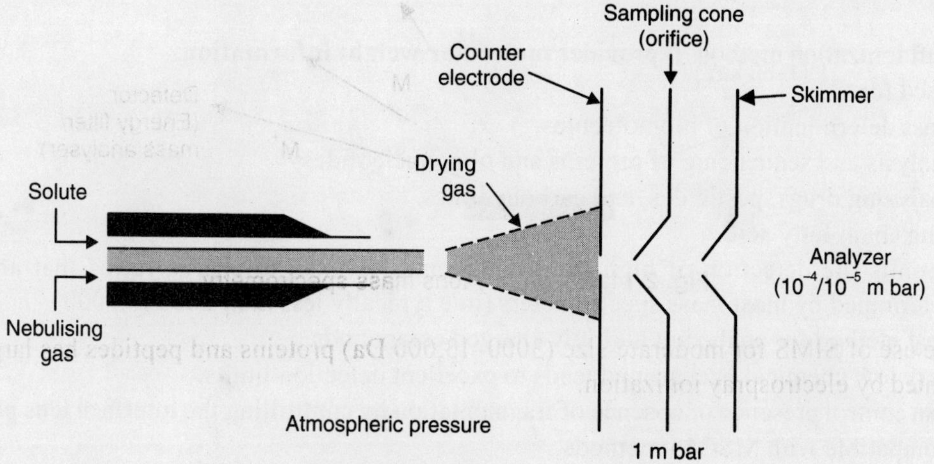

Fig. 2.15. Electrospary ionization source.

concentration at the droplet's surface. Eventually coulombic repulsion overcomes the droplet's surface tension and the droplet explodes. This 'Coulombic explosion' forms a series of smaller, lower charged droplets (Fig. 2.16). The process of shrinking followed by explosion is repeated until individually charged 'naked' analyte ions are formed. Increasing the rate of solvent evaporation, by introducing a drying gas flow counter current to the sprayed ions increases the extent of multiple-charging. Decreasing the capillary diameter and lowering the analyte solution flow rate i.e. in nanospray ionization, will create ions with higher m/e ratios (i.e. it is a softer ionization technique).

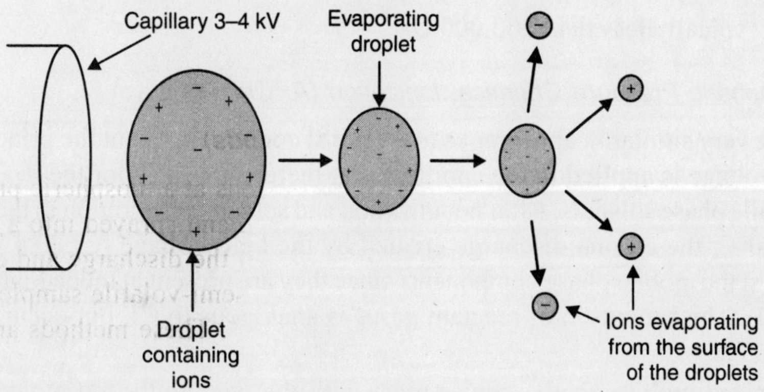

Fig 2.16. The electrospray ionisation process.

Sample introduction

- Flow injection.
- LC/MS.
- Typical flow rates are less than 1 microliter per minute up to about a milliliter per minute.

Benefits

- Soft ionization method, it provides **molecular weight information.**
- Used for:
  mass determination of biomolecules.
  analysis and sequencing of proteins and oligonucleotides.
  analyzing drugs, pesticides, and carbohydrates.
  long chain fatty acid.
- Permits the detection of high-mass compounds at mass-to-charge ratios that are easily determined by most mass spectrometers (m/e typically less than 2000 to 3000).
- Best method for analyzing multiply charged compounds.
- Very low chemical background leads to excellent detection limits.
- Can control presence or absence of fragmentation by controlling the interface lens potentials
- Compatible with MS/MS methods.

Limitations

- Multiply charged species require interpretation and mathematical transformation (can sometimes be difficult).
- Complementary to APCI. No good for uncharged, non-basic, low-polarity compounds (e.g. steroids).
- Very sensitive to contaminants such as alkali metals or basic compounds.
- Relatively low ion currents.
- Relatively complex hardware compared to other ion sources.

Mass range

- Low-high Typically less than 200,000 Da.

2.2.1.4.2. Atmospheric Pressure Chemical Ionization (APCI)

APCI sources are very similar in appearance to their ESI counterparts, but the principle is different. Unlike ESI, no voltage is applied to the capillary, but there is a heater for the evaporation of both analytes and mobile phase solvents. After nebulization and solvent evaporation in the heated chamber at about 300–500°C, the corona discharge created by the high voltage (ca. 3–4 kV) applied to a needle ionizes first the mobile phase components since they are present at much higher concentration than analytes (M). The formation of reactant gases is analogous to CI, but occurs at atmospheric pressure (Fig. 2.17).

Then, the ionized mobile phase species react with the analyte by ion-molecule reactions to generate analyte ions. As with ESI and other soft ionization techniques, mostly even-electron molecular adducts are formed, such as $[M+H]^+$, alkali metal adducts $[M + Na]^+$ and $[M + K]^+$ or $[M + NH_4]^+$ in case of the positive ion mode and mobile phase containing ammonium additives/buffers. In negative ion mode, $[M-H]^-$ is the predominate adduct ion. For example,

Ion primary formation:

$$N_2 + e^- \longrightarrow N_2^{+\bullet} + 2e^-$$

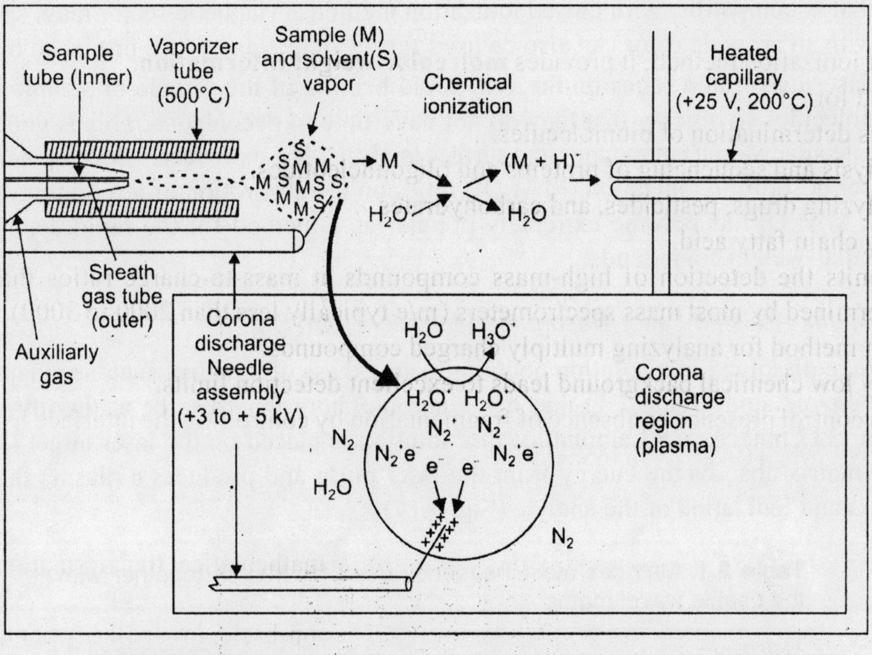

Fig. 2.17. Atmospheric pressure chemical ionization source.

Ion secondary formation:

$$N_2^{+\cdot} + H_2O \longrightarrow H_3O^+ + HO^\cdot$$

Proton transfer:

$$M + H_3O^+ \longrightarrow (M + H)^+ + H_2O$$

Sample introduction

- Same as for electrospray ionization.

Benefits

- Good for less-polar compounds.
- Excellent LC/MS interface.
- Compatible with MS/MS methods.

Limitations

- Complementary to ESI.

Mass range

- Low-moderate typically less than 2000 Da.

2.2.1.5. Laser Desorption

Laser desorption methods use a pulsed laser to desorb species from a target surface. Therefore, one must use a mass analyzer such as time-of-fight (TOF) or Fourier transform ion cyclotron resonance

(FT-ICR) that is compatible with pulsed ionization methods. Magnetic sector mass spectrometers equipped with an array detector can also be used for the detection of ions produced by MALDI.

Direct laser desorption relies on the very rapid heating of the sample or sample substrate to vaporize molecules so quickly that they do not have time to decompose. This is good for low to medium-molecular weight compounds and surface analysis. The more recent development of matrix-assisted laser desorption ionization (MALDI) relies on the absorption of laser energy by a matrix compound. MALDI has become extremely popular as a method for the rapid determination of high-molecular-weight compounds.

2.2.1.5.1. Matrix-Assisted Laser Desorption Ionization (MALDI)

The analyte is dissolved in a solution containing an excess of a matrix such as sinapinic acid or dihydroxybenzoic acid (Table 2.1) that has a chromophore that absorbs at the ultraviolet laser wavelength (337 nm). A small amount of this solution is placed on the laser target (probe) (Fig. 2.18). The matrix absorbs the energy from the laser pulse and produces a plasma that results in vaporization and ionization of the analyte (Fig. 2.19).

Table 2.1. Matrices most frequently used for MALDI together with the usable wavelengths

Matrix	*Wavelength (nm)*
Nicotinic acid	266, 220–290
Benzoic acid derivatives:	
2,5–Dihydroxybenzoic acid	266, 337, 355
Vanillic acid	266
2–Amino-benzoic acid	266, 337, 355
Pyrazine-carboxylic acid	266
3–Aminopyrazine–2–carboxylic acid	337
Cinnamic acid derivatives:	
Ferulic acid	266, 377, 355
Sinapinic acid	266, 337, 355
Caffeic acid	266, 337, 355
3–Nitrobenzyl alcohol	266

In MALDI-TOF MS the specific process is as follows:

Put the sample proteins into the solvent, i.e. matrix mixed with water. The sample proteins dissolve in the solvent. The matrix material also reacts with the proteins (analyte) to make the polymers become charged ions. No one really knows how this happens. Then, wait until the water in the solvent totally evaporates. When the water evaporates, the sample proteins are surrounded by the matrix, which forms a crystal lattice. Keep the sample proteins in some boxes which are formed by the matrix molecules (Table 2.1). Finally, put the target, i.e. proteins and 'boxes', into the source, using a beam of ultraviolet laser to fire it. This result in each protein picks up a proton and turns into gas phase ion.

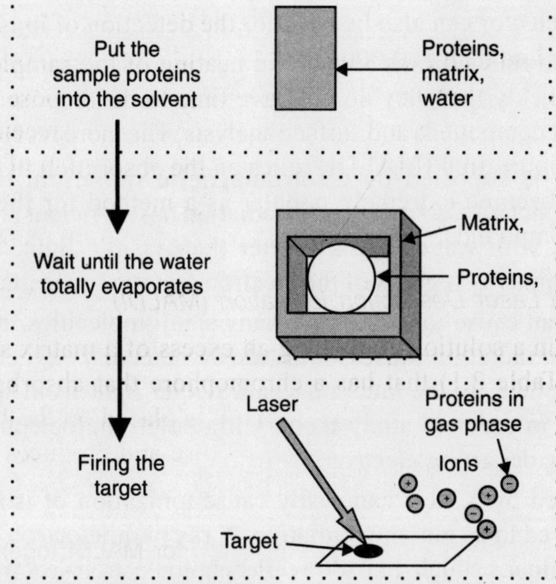

Fig 2.18. Process in the source.

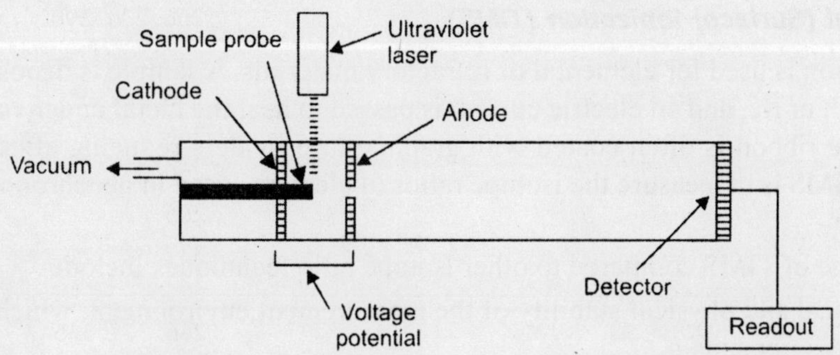

Fig 2.19. Schematic diagram of MALDI instrument.

Sample introduction

- Direct insertion probe.
- Continuous-ow introduction.

Benefits

- Rapid and convenient molecular weight determination.

Limitations

- MS/MS difficult.
- requires a mass analyzer that is compatible with pulsed ionization techniques.
- not easily compatible with LC/MS.

Mass range

- Very high Typically less than 500,000 Da.

2.2.1.6. Photoionization

If the ionization energy is supplied by electromagnetic radiation, the ionization is called photoionization. However, not all electromagnetic radiation has sufficient energy to cause ionization. Generally, only radiation with wavelengths shorter than visible light, 'that is, radiation in the ultraviolet, X ray, and gamma ray regions of the electromagnetic spectrum can produce ionization.

Ultraviolet radiation can cause ionization of many small molecules, including oxygen, O_2. In fact, short wavelength solar radiation causes ionization of molecular oxygen and molecular nitrogen found in the upper atmosphere. In the laboratory, ultraviolet light from special lamps or lasers is used to ionize molecules in order to study them. Ultraviolet photoelectron spectroscopy (UPS) measures the energy of the departing electron.

The high energy carried by X rays can easily cause ionization of isolated atoms. X rays are therefore frequently referred to as ionizing radiation. X ray photoelectron spectroscopy and Auger spectroscopy are two techniques which, like ultraviolet photoelectron spectroscopy, study the ejected electron to gain information about the atom from which it came.

2.2.1.7. Thermal (Surface) ionization (TIMS)

Thermal ionization is used for elemental or refractory materials. A sample is deposited on a metal ribbon, such as Pt or Re, and an electric current is passed to heat the metal under vacuum to a high temperature. The ribbon is often coated with graphite to provide a reducing effect. The primary application of TIMS is to measure the isotope ratios of elements used in geochronology and tracer studies.

The advantage of TIMS compared to other isotope ratio techniques include:

- The chemical and physical stability of the measurement environment, which lead to highly precise measurements,
- The ability to ionize and evaporate samples at different temperatures by using multiple filament assemblies,
- Near 100% transmission of ions from source to collector.

Limitations

The disadvantages include:

- not all elements are easily ionized, which restricts applications to elements with low ionization potentials;
- ionization is not equally efficient for all elements, and is generally less than 1%;

2.2.2 Mass Analyzers

Ions produced in the ionisation chamber are accelerated by the application of acceleration potential (2 to 8 kV). These ions enter in the mass analyser which differentiate them on the basis of mass to

Table 2.2. Comparison of ionization methods

Ionization Method	*Type of ion ion formed*	*Analytes*	*Sample intro*	*Mass limits*	*Method type*
EI	M^+, M^-	Small volatiles	GC, liquid or solid probe	10^3	Hard method structural information
CI	$[M + H]^+$, $[M + X]^+$	Small volatiles	GC, liquid or solid probe	10^3	Soft method
APCI	$[M + H]^+$, $[M + X]^+$ $[M - H]^-$	Small volatiles (less polar species)	LC or syringe	2×10^3	Soft method
FI/FD	$[M + H]^+$, $[M + X]+$	FI: volatiles FD: non volatile	GC, liquid or solid probe	2 × 103	Soft method
ES	$[M + nH]^{n+}$, $[M - nX]^{n-}$	Peptides, proteins nonvolatile	LC or syringe	2×10^5	Soft method multiply charged ion
FAB	$[M + H]^+$, $[M - H]^-$	Carbohydrates Organometallics peptides, nonvolatile	In viscous	6×10^3	Soft but harder than ESI or MALDI
MALDI	$[M + H]^+$, $[M + X]^+$	Peptides, proteins nucleotides	In solid matrix	5×10^5	Soft

charge ratio by magnetic and electric field. There are two main functions of a mass analyser (i) resolve the ion beam into its component ions and (ii) to maximise the resolved ions intensities (dispersive focussing).The efficiency of mass spectrometer depends on type of mass analyzer. Mass spectrometer can be classified into two types depending on efficiency- Low resolution and high resolution types. Two compounds, C_3H_6O and C_3H_8O have nominal masses of 58 and 60, and can be distinguished by low-res MS. But the compounds $C_2H_4O_2$ and C_3H_8O having the same nominal mass of 60 can not be differentiated by low resolution type mass spectrometer. It requires high-resolution mass spectrometer.

Molecular formula	Nomonal mass	Precise mass
$C_2H_4O_2$	60	60.02112
C_3H_8O	60	60.05754

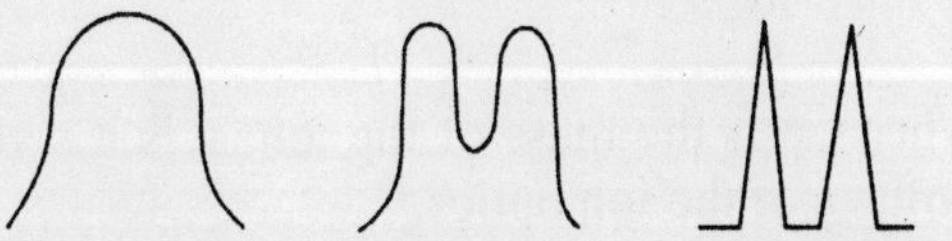

Fig. 2.20. Diagram showing three states of resolution.

In the low resolution mass spectrometer, the atomic weight of the most abundant isotopes are determined as a whole number, means $^1H = 1$; $^{16}O = 16$; $^{12}C = 12$; $^{14}N = 14$, etc.

Low resolution mass spectrometers cannot differentiates the CO, N_2, C_2H_4 as all will be recorded as whole number of which mass is 28.

From a physical point of view, only the atomic weight of most abundant isotope of carbon is equal to 12 exactly. The other atoms are not equal to whole numbers and their actual atomic weight can be determined to the sixth decimal place.

For example,

$^{1}H = 1.007825$	$^{16}O = 15.994915$
$^{12}C = 12.000000$	$^{19}F = 18.998405$
$^{14}N = 14.003074$	$^{32}S = 31.972074$

From these values, it can be observed that CO, C_2H_4 and N_2 show a significant difference in their actual masses.

$$CO = 27.994914,\ N_2 = 28.006158,\ C_2H_4 = 28.031299$$

The mass spectrometer with good resolving power can differentiate them. Resolving power can be calculated as :

$$\text{Resolving power (RP)} = \frac{m_1}{m_2 - m_1} = \frac{m_1}{\Delta m}$$

where m_1 and m_2 are the masses of two sample molecule.

For nitrogen and ethylene:

$$RP = \frac{28.006158}{28.031299 - 28.006158} = 1110$$

Hence, mass spectrometer possessing RP = 1110 can differentiate the masses of nitrogen and ethylene.

The different types of mass analyzers can be classified on the basis of their working principle as follows:

2.2.2.1 Mass analyzers involving magnetic field

To derive the fundamental equation of mass spectrometry, consider the electric and magnetic fields of mass spectrometer of magnetic deflection type.

In the electric field, the potential energy (eV) of an ion is equal to its kinetic energy (½ mv^2) after complete acceleration.

$$eV = \tfrac{1}{2} mv^2 \qquad \text{...2.1}$$

where m is the mass of the ion, v is it's velocity, e is the charge of the ion and V is the applied voltage of the ion optics.

The ions enter the flight tube between the poles of a magnet and are deflected by the magnetic field, H. Only ions of mass-to-charge ratio that have equal centrifugal and centripetal forces pass through the flight tube:

$$\frac{mv^2}{r} = Hev \qquad \text{...2.2}$$

centrifugal = centripetal forces.

where r is the radius of curvature of the ion path:

$$r = \frac{mv}{eH} \qquad \text{...2.3}$$

Substitute the value of v in equation 2.3:

$$r = \frac{m}{e.H}\sqrt{2V\frac{e}{m}} \quad ...2.4$$

On rearranging this equation:

$$\frac{m}{e} = \frac{H^2 r^2}{2V} \quad ...2.5$$

The equation 2.5 shows that the m/e of the ions that reach the detector can be varied by changing either H or V.

A. Single focusing mass analyzer

It is a directional focusing with the application of magnetic field. Hence, the instrument is defined as a 'direction' or 'single' focussing mass spectrometer (Fig. 2.21). Different ions are deflected by the magnetic field by different amounts. The amount of deflection depends on:

- The mass of the ion. Lighter ions are deflected more than heavier ones.
- The charge on the ion. Ions with 2 (or more) positive charges are deflected more than ones with only 1 positive charge.

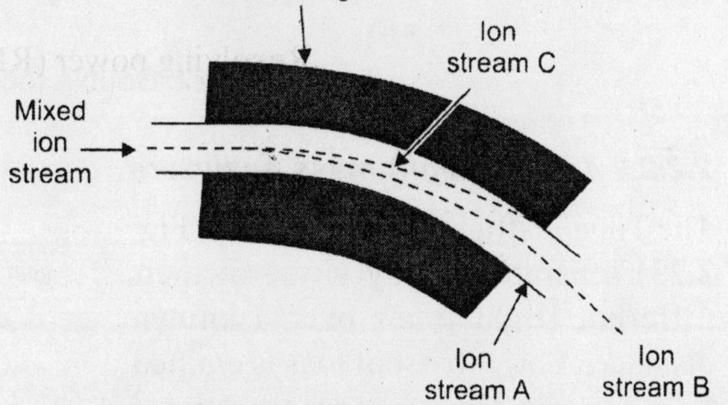

Fig 2.21. Magnetic sector mass analyzer.

These two factors are combined into the ***mass/charge ratio.*** Mass/charge ratio is given the symbol m/e (or sometimes m/z). For example, if an ion had a mass of 28 and a charge of 1+, its mass/charge ratio would be 28. An ion with a mass of 56 and a charge of 2+ would also have a mass/charge ratio of 28.

In the Fig. 2.18, ion stream A is most deflected - it will contain ions with the smallest mass/charge ratio. Ion stream C is the least deflected - it contains ions with the greatest mass/charge ratio. The mass spectrum is obtained when ions of different mass arrive at collector, one after the other. The time of arrival will be proportional to the square root of the m/e ratio. They have lower mass ranges.

B. Double Focussing mass analyzer

Double focusing mass spectrometers use a combination of magnetic and electrical fields to focus and sort ions. A common configuration for a sector instrument is the geometry shown in Fig. 2.22, in which a magnetic "sector" follows an electric "sector". The slit acts as a filter to select for a specific m/e value. The electric sector focuses the ions with respect to differences in kinetic energy that they may have as they exit the source region. "Double focusing," this combination of "angular" or "directional" focusing and energy focusing, provide mass resolution high enough to separate ions of the same nominal mass but different chemical formulae, such as C_2H_4, N_2 and CO at m/e 28. The so called "exact masses", more properly "high precision masses", of C_2H_4, N_2 and CO are 28.0313, 28.0061, and 27.9949 Daltons, respectively.

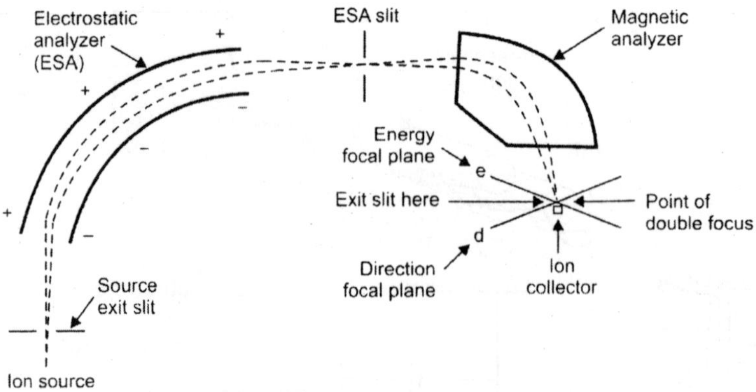

Fig. 2.22. Double focussing mass analyzer.

2.2.2.2 Time-of-flight mass analyzers

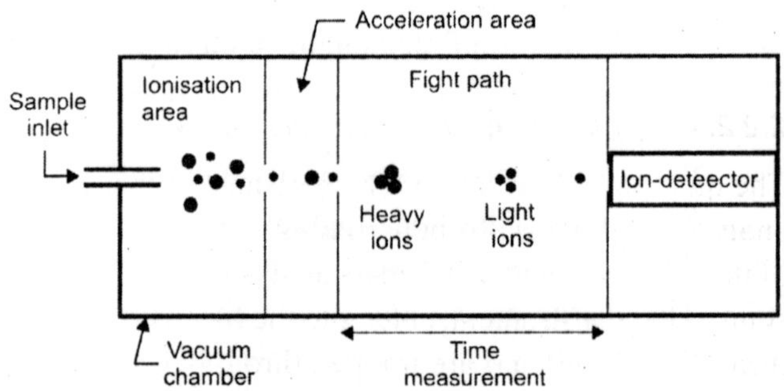

Fig 2.23. Time of Flight analyzer.

The Time-of-flight mass analyzers (Fig. 2.23) separate ions by virtue of their different flight times over a known distance. A brief burst of ions is emitted from a source. These ions are accelerated so that ions of like charge have equal kinetic energy and then are directed into a flight tube. Since kinetic energy is equal to $1/2\ mv^2$, where m is the mass of the ion and v is the ion velocity, the lower the ion's mass, the greater the velocity and shorter its flight time. The travel time from the ion source through the flight tube to the detector, measured in microseconds, can be transformed to the m/e value through the relationships described above. Because all ion masses are measured for each ion burst, TOF mass spectrometers offer high sensitivity as well as rapid scanning. They can provide mass data for very high-mass biomolecules.

2.2.2.3 Quadrupole mass analyzers

The **quadrupole(Q) mass spectrometer** consists of four precisely straight and parallel rods so arranged that the beam of ions from the ionization source of the spectrometer is directed axially between them (Fig. 2.24). A voltage comprising a DC component and a radio frequency component is applied between adjacent rods, opposite rods being electrically connected. Once inside the **quadrupole** the ions will oscillate in the (x) (y) direction as a result of the high frequency electric field. The oscillations are only stable for a certain function of frequency and the DC voltage otherwise the ions strike the rods and become dissipated. The mass range of the oscillating ions is scanned by changing the DC voltage and the frequency, keeping the ratio of the DC voltage to the frequency constant. Each mass is detected by an appropriate ion sensor. The resolution of the spectrometer can be increased by either employing **eight poles** or by connecting two or **three qaudupoles** in series.

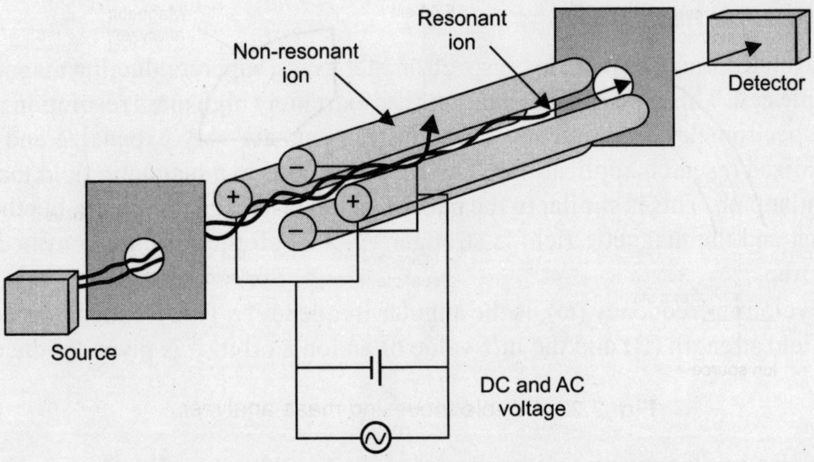

Fig. 2.24. Schematic diagram of quadrupole analyzer.

2.2.2.4. Quadrupole Ion Trap (QIT) mass analyzer

The quadrupole ion trap (QIT) mass analyser was developed in parallel with the quadrupole mass analyser by the third Nobel prize winning mass spectrometry pioneer, Wolfgang Paul. A schematic of the basic set up of a QIT mass analyzer is shown in Fig. 2.25. The ions, produced in the ionization source of the instrument, enter into the trap through the inlet and are trapped through action of the three hyperbolic electrodes: the ring electrode and the entrance and exit endcap electrodes. A combination of RF and DC voltages is applied to the electrodes to create a quadrupole electric field similar to the electric field for the quadrupole mass analyzer. This electric field traps ions in a potential energy well at the center of the analyzer. The mass spectrum is acquired by scanning the RF and DC fields to destabilize low mass to charge ions. These destabilized ions are ejected through a hole in one endcap electrode and strike a detector. The mass spectrum is generated by scanning the fields so that ions of increasing m/e value are ejected from the cell and detected. The trap is then refilled with a new batch of ions to acquire the next mass spectrum. The mass resolution of the ion trap is increased by adding a small amount 0.1 Pa (10 torr) of Helium as a bath gas. Collisions between the analyte ions and the inert bath gas dampen the motion of the ions and increases the trapping efficiency of the analyzer.

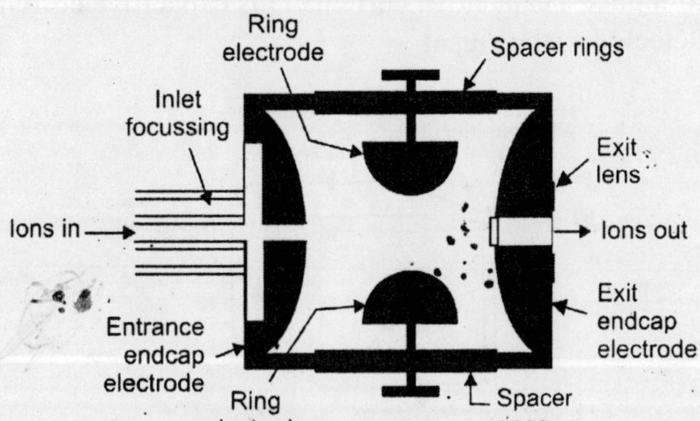

Fig. 2.25. A schematic (cutaway view) of a QIT mass analyzer.

The very nature of trapping and ejection makes a quadrupolar ion trap especially suited to performing experiments in structural elucidation studies.

2.2.2.5 Ion Cyclotron Resonance

The Ion Cyclotron Resonance (ICR) mass spectrometer uses a superconducting magnet to trap ions in a small sample cell. This type of mass analyzer has extremely high mass resolution and useful for tandem mass spectrometry experiments. These instruments are very expensive and are typically used for specialized research applications. The ICR traps ions in a magnetic field that causes ions travel in a circular path. This is similar to the path of an ion in a magnetic sector, but the ions are not traveling as fast and the magnetic field is stronger. As a result the ions are confined in the small volume of the trap.

The ion's cyclotron frequency (ω), is the angular frequency*. This frequency is determined by the magnetic field strength (B) and the m/z value of an ion's orbit. It is given by the expression:

$$\omega = \frac{B \times e}{m/z}$$

where e is a charge on electron and z is a charge on ion (which is usually taken as 1).

The relationship between the frequency and the mass shows that determining the mass in this case consists of determining the frequency. After ions are trapped in this cell they are detected by measuring the signal at this cyclotron frequency. This signal is measured by placing electrodes on each side of the ions circular orbit. An RF voltage is applied to the transmitter electrodes at the cyclotron frequency of the ion of interest. This RF energy moves ions at the applied frequency to a larger orbit. As these ions travel around the ICR cell they are close enough to the receiver electrodes to induce a capacitive current. This capacitive current oscillates at the cyclotron frequency and is detected as the signal.

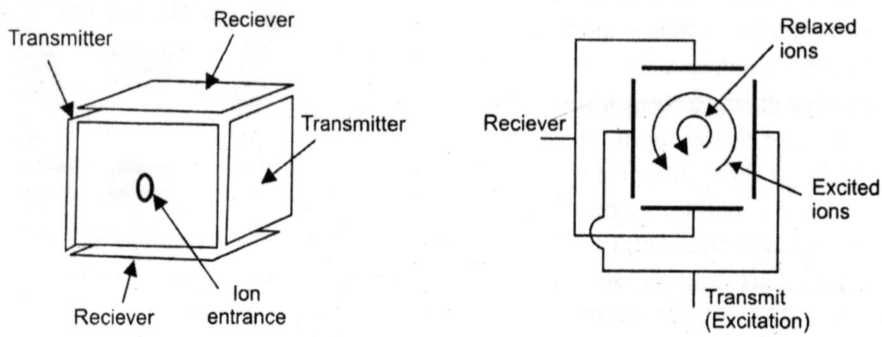

Fig 2.26. Schematic diagram of ICR, (A) Major components, (B) Ion motion within trap.

The ICR is also used as a Fourier Transform Mass Spectrometer (FT-MS). Instead of using a single excitation frequency, a fast RF pulse is applied to the transmitter electrodes. This simultaneously excites all the ions and produces a signal at the cyclotron frequency of each m/e ion present. This signal is similar to the Free Induction Decay (FID) produced in an FT-NMR experiment. A complete mass spectrum is obtained by using the Fourier transform to convert this signal from the time domain to the frequency domain.

* The angular frequency (ω) is in radians per second. The unit Hertz (Hz) is in cycles per second.

Table 2.3. Comparison of different mass analyzers

Analyzer	*System highlights*
Quadrupole	Unit mass resolution, fast scan, low cost
Sector (Magnetic and/or Electrostatic)	High resolution, exact mass
Time-of-Flight (TOF)	Theoretically, no limitation for m/e maximum, high throughput
Ion Cyclotron Resonance (ICR)	Very high resolution, exact mass; perform ion chemistry

2.2.3 Detectors

Several types of detectors are available for mass spectrometers. The choice of detector depends on the design of the instrument and the analytical applications that will be performed. Ion detectors can be divided into two classes. Some detectors are made to count ions of a single mass at a time and therefore they detect the arrival of all ions sequentially at one point (point ion collectors). Others detectors, such as photographic plates, image current detectors or array detectors, have the ability to count multiple masses and detect the arrival of all ions simultaneously along a plane (array collectors). The detector used for most routine experiments is the electron multiplier. Another type of detector is photographic plates coated with a silver bromide emulsion, it is sensitive to energetic ions. A photographic plate can give a higher resolution than an electrical detector.

2.2.3.1 Faraday cup

The Faraday cup is named after Michael Faraday who first theorized ions around 1830. A Faraday cup is made of a metal cup or cylinder with a small orifice. It is connected to the ground through a resistor, as illustrated in Fig. 2.27.

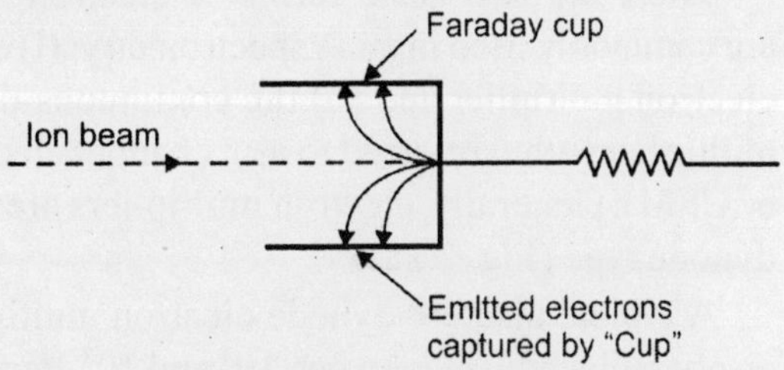

Fig. 2.27. Faraday cup.

When a beam or packet of ions hits the metal it gains a small net charge while the ions are neutralized by either accepting or donating electron. This leads to a current through the resistor. The discharge current is then amplified and detected. It provides a measure of ion abundance. Essentially the faraday cup is part of a circuit where ions are the charge carriers in vacuum and the faraday cup is the interface to the solid metal where electrons act as the charge carriers (as in most circuits). Because the charge associated with an electron leaving the wall of the detector is identical to the arrival of a positive ion at this detector, secondary electrons that are emitted when an ion strikes the wall of the detector are an important source of errors if they are not suppressed. In consequence, the accuracy of this detector can be improved by preventing the escape of reflected ions and ejected secondary electrons. Various devices have been used to capture ions efficiently and to minimize secondary electron losses. For instance, the cup is coated with carbon because it produces few secondary ions. The shape of the cup and the use of a weak magnetic field prevent also any secondary electrons produced inside to exit. The disadvantages of this simple and robust detector are its low sensitivity and its slow response time.

The Faraday cup was widely used in the beginning of mass spectrometry due to its accuracy because of the direct relation between the measured current and number of ions.

2.2.3.2 Electron multiplier

An electron multiplier is used to detect the presence of ions emerging from the mass analyzer of a mass spectrometer. It is essentially the "eyes" of the instrument .The task of the electron multiplier is to detect every ion of the selected mass passed by the mass analyzer. How efficiently the electron multiplier carries out this task represents a potentially limiting factor on the overall system sensitivity. Consequently, the performance of the electron multiplier can have a major influence on the overall performance of the mass spectrometer.

The basic physical process that allows an electron multiplier to operate is called secondary electron emission. When a charged particle (ion or electron) strikes a photoemmisive surface it causes secondary electrons to be released from atoms in the surface layer. The number of secondary electrons released depends on the type of incident primary particle, its energy and characteristic of the incident surface. Ultimately, the released electrons are collected at anode with the generation of current. The strength of current is proportional to number of electrons (or no of ions striking to photoemmissive surface).

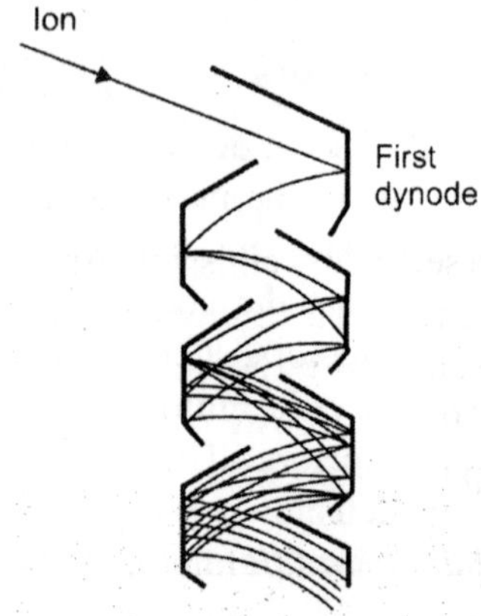

Fig. 2.28. Ion-optics of discrete-dynode electron multiplier showing the electron gain at each successive dynode. The electron cascading process results in gains up to 10^8 being achieved with ~21 dynodes.

There are two basic forms of electron multipliers that are commonly used in mass spectrometry: (i) discrete-dynode electron multiplier and (ii) the continuous-dynode electron multiplier (often referred to as a channel electron multiplier or CEM). Generally, electron multipliers are of the discrete-dynode type (Fig. 2.28).

A typical discrete-dynode electron multiplier has between 12 and 24 dynodes and is used with an operating gain of between 10^4 and 10^8, depending on the application. It has Cu/Be photoemmisive surface. These detectors have the advantage of being able to produce high output currents (in excess of 100 mA), but suffer from the disadvantage of being relatively unstable when repeatedly exposed to atmosphere.

In recent years, new structures have been fabricated based on aluminum dynodes, which are reportedly less susceptible to degradation but are bulky and relatively expensive.

The second type of multiplier is the continuous dynode multiplier. The vast majority of these is fabricated of glass, although some are constructed from coated ceramic materials or are a combination of glass and ceramic. These detectors are, in general, much more suitable for applications requiring frequent exposure to atmosphere. Most of these detectors are of the single channel type; however, microchannel plates (two dimensional arrays of single channels) have been used in applications involving simultaneous imaging of an entire mass spectrum and Time-of-Flight Mass Spectrometry.

Channeltron, Single Channel Electron Multipliers (CEMs) are durable and efficient detectors for positive and negative ions as well as electrons and photons. Fig. 2.29 illustrates the basic structure and operation of the Channeltron (CEM). A glass tube having an inner diameter of approximately 1 mm and an outer diameter of 2, 3, or 6 mm is constructed from a specially formulated lead silicate glass. When appropriately processed, this glass exhibits the properties of electrical conductivity

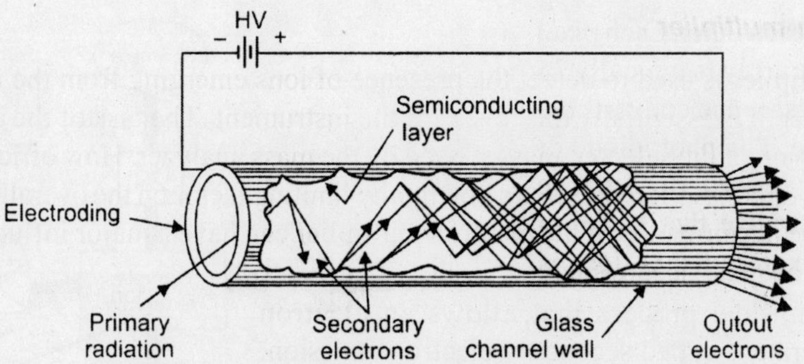

Fig. 2.29. Cutaway View of a CEM.

and secondary emission. An ion striking the input face of the device typically produces 2–3 secondary electrons. These electrons are accelerated down the channel by a positive bias. The electrons strike the channel walls, producing additional electrons (and so on) until, at the output end a pulse of 10^7 to 10^8 electrons emerges. Today, CEMs are the most widely used detector in quadrupole and ion trap mass spectrometers and find many applications in magnetic sector instruments as well.

2.2.3.3 Scintillator ('Daly' detector)

A fast ion causes electrons to be emitted and these are accelerated towards a second 'dynode'. In this case, the dynode consists of a substance (a scintillator) which emits photons (light). The emitted light is detected by a photomultiplier and is converted into an electric current. Since photon multipliers are very sensitive, high gain amplification of the arrival of a single ion is achieved. These detectors are also important in studies on metastable ions.

2.2.3.4 Array Detectors

Array detectors can attain very high sensitivities by collecting all the ions or ions over a large range of m/e ratios and determined simultaneously. This contrasts with conventional scanning methods using point detectors (e.g. electron multipliers) that collect only a small fraction of the ions in each mass channel as the spectrum is scanned. Photodiode arrays (PDA) are the most common form in which a microchannel plate detector is coupled to fibre optical channel via a phosphorescent screen (Fig. 2.30).

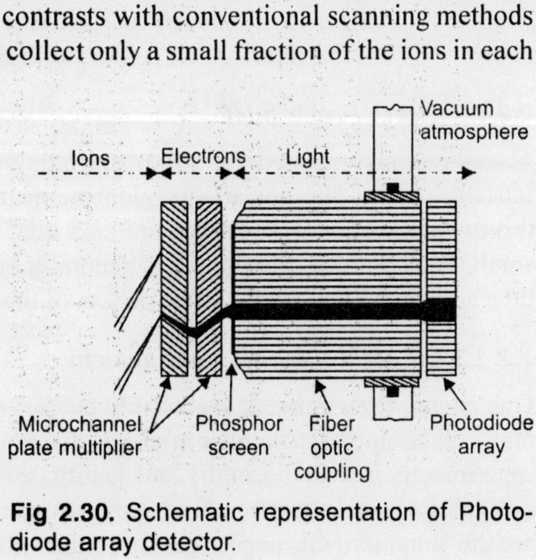

Fig 2.30. Schematic representation of Photodiode array detector.

Ions enter the microchannel plates and the electrons emitted strike the phosphorescent screen. The screen consists of a layer of aluminium coated with crystalline phosphor often composed of caesium iodide (CsI) and thallium (TI). This surface emits light in the form of photons that are transmitted down the fiber optic channels onto a charge or plasma-coupled, unlike the phosphor screen of the image intensifier, react independently of each other. Each pixel of the Photodiode array is typically 25 mm by 2.5 mm in size and converts the photons to charge. The photodiode of the CCD array record the charge necessary to neutralize that accumulated in each pixel and this data is integrated and stored.

2.2.4 Sample Inlet System

The sample has to pass from the atmosphere into the mass spectrometer under vacuum. To prevent interactions between the sample and residual molecules in the mass spectrometer, analysis has to be performed at a very low pressure. The inlet system has to control the flow of sample into the vacuum. This must happen at a relatively low flow rate to allow the vacuum pumps to maintain low pressure.

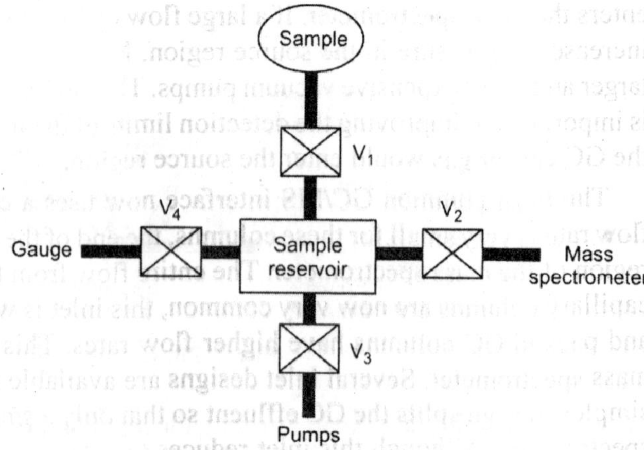

Fig. 2.31. Schematic representation of Batch inlet system.

Samples are introduced into mass spectrometer via some sample inlet system. The choice of inlet system depends upon nature of sample and method of ionization. Following are the different type of inlet system

2.2.4.1 Batch Inlet Systems

These systems are the simplest and simply involve the volatilization of the sample externally and then the gradual leakage of the volatilized sample into the evacuated ionization chamber (Fig. 2.31). For gases, the sample is introduced into the metering volume container and then expanded into the reservoir flask where it is then leaked into the ionization chamber. For liquids, a small quantity of sample is introduced into the reservoir and the pressure of the system is reduced to about 10^{-5} torr. The inlet system is lined with glass to avoid losses of polar analytes by adsorption.

2.2.4.2 Direct Probe Inlet

These systems are used for solids and non-volatile liquids and in these systems the sample is introduced into the ionization region by means of a sample holder, or probe, which is inserted through a vacuum lock. Probes are also used when the amount of the sample to be analyzed is small. With a probe, the sample is generally held on the surface of a glass or aluminum capillary tube and positioned within a few meters of the ionization source.

2.2.4.3 Chromatographic inlet system

Gas chromatography: It is probably the most common technique for introducing samples into a mass spectrometer. Complex mixtures are routinely separated by gas chromatography and mass spectrometry is used to identify and quantitate the individual component. Several different interface designs are used to connect these two instruments. The most significant characteristics of the inlets are the amount of GC carrier gas that enters the mass spectrometer and the amount of analyte that enters the mass spectrometer. If a large flow of GC carrier gas enters the mass spectrometer it will increase the pressure in the source region. Maintaining the required source pressure will require larger and more expensive vacuum pumps. The amount of analyte that enters the mass spectrometer is important for improving the detection limits of the instrument. Ideally all the analyte and none of the GC carrier gas would enter the source region.

The most common GC/MS interface now uses a capillary GC column. Since the carrier gas flow rate is very small for these columns, the end of the capillary is inserted directly into the source region of the mass spectrometer. The entire flow from the GC enters the mass spectrometer. Since capillary columns are now very common, this inlet is widely used. However, wide bore capillaries and packed GC columns have higher flow rates. This significantly increases the pressure in the mass spectrometer. Several inlet designs are available to reduce the gas flow into the source. The simplest design splits the GC effluent so that only a small portion of the total flow enters the mass spectrometer. Although this inlet reduces the gas load on the vacuum system, it also reduces the amount of analyte. Effusive separators and membrane inlets are more selective and transport a higher fraction of the analyte into the source region. Each of these methods has efficiency and resolution drawbacks but they are necessary for some experiments.

Liquid Chromatography: Liquid chromatography inlets are used to introduce thermally labile compounds not easily separated by gas chromatography. These inlets have undergone considerable development and are now fairly routine. Because these inlets are used for temperature sensitive compounds, the sample is ionized directly from the condensed phase.

2.2.5 Vacuum System

All mass spectrometers operate at very low pressure (high vacuum). This reduces the chance of ions colliding with other molecules in the mass analyzer. Any collision can cause the ions to react, neutralize, scatter, or fragment. All these processes will interfere with the mass spectrum. To minimize collisions, experiments are conducted under high vacuum conditions, typically 10^{-2} to 10^{-5} Pa (10^{-4} to 10^{-7} torr) (1 Pa = 133.32 torr) depending upon the geometry of the instrument. This high vacuum requires two pumping stages. The first stage is a mechanical pump that provides rough vacuum down to 0.1 Pa (10^{-3} torr). The second stage uses diffusion pumps or turbomolecular pumps to provide high vacuum. ICR instruments have even higher vacuum requirements and often include a cryogenic pump for a third pumping stage. The pumping system is an important part of any mass spectrometer but a detailed discussion is beyond the scope of this chapter.

2.2.6 Data System

The final component of a mass spectrometer is the data system. It is the heart of the mass spectrometry instrument. Without it, it is difficult to deal vast number of informations from mass spectrometric analysis. This part of the instrument has undergone revolutionary changes in the past twenty years. It has evolved from photographic plates and strip chart recorders to data systems that control the instrument, acquire hundreds of spectra in a minute and search tens of thousands of reference spectra to identify an unknown. Because these systems are evolving so rapidly, a through discussion is not included in this paper. Interested readers should study the manuals for their instrument.

CHAPTER 3

Types of Ions

The ions which form in ionization chamber of mass spectrometer are molecular ions, isotopic ions, fragment ions, rearrangement ions, multiple charged ions, negative ions and ions formed by ion molecule interaction.

3.1 MOLECULAR ION

It is an ion formed by the removal from (positive ions) or addition to (negative ions) a molecule of one or more electrons without fragmentation of the molecular structure. The mass of this ion corresponds to the sum of the masses of the most abundant naturally occurring isotopes of the various atoms that make up the molecule (with a correction for the masses of the electron(s) lost or gained). For example, the mass of the molecular ion of ethyl bromide $C_2H_5\,^{79}Br$ (Fig. 3.1) will be 2×12 plus 5×1.0078246 plus 78.91839 minus the mass of the electron (m_e). This is equal to 107.95751 u – m_e, u being the unified atomic mass unit based on the standard that the mass of the isotope ^{12}C = 12 u exactly.

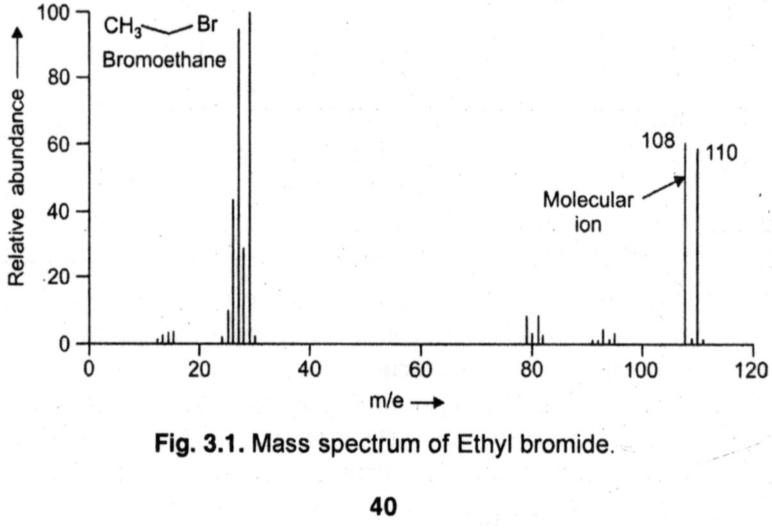

Fig. 3.1. Mass spectrum of Ethyl bromide.

If the molecular ion appears, it is the highest mass in an EI spectrum (except for isotope peaks discussed below). This peak represents the molecular weight of the compound. Its appearance depends on the stability of the compound. Double bonds, cyclic structures and aromatic rings stabilize the molecular ion and increase the probability of its appearance. Many molecules with especially labile protons do not display molecular ions; an example of this is alcohols, where the highest molecular weight peak occurs at m/e one less than the molecular ion (M–1). The molecular ion is often given the symbol M^+ or $M^{\dagger}$ – the dot in this second version represents the fact that somewhere in the ion there will be a single unpaired electron. It is also called parent ion. It is the precursor of other ions appeared in the mass spectrum. It means that other type of ions are formed from the molecular ions.

3.2 ISOTOPIC IONS

Many elements in their natural states contain heavier isotopes, because mass spectrometer measures mass to charge ratio, hence these isotopes also appear in the mass spectrum as isotopic ion peak. These peaks appear in the mass spectrum in the last region of mass spectrum just after molecular ion peak. The most abundant isotope of carbon is ^{12}C but natural carbon also contains ^{13}C and ^{14}C. Although as natural beta emitter, the latter is extremely valuable for radiotracer work, its natural abundance is so low as to make it almost inconsequential to mass spectrometry. This case is not exist for ^{13}C because its natural abundance is 1.08 percent in carbon. Hence the mass spectrum of methane (Fig. 3.2) shows molecular ion peak at m/e 16 due to $^{12}CH_4$ but also contain isotopic ion peak at m/e17 due to $^{13}CH_4$, the two ions are having relative abundance of 99:1. As the number of carbon atom in a compound increases so also do the chances of incorporating one ^{13}C atom into the molecule rather than ^{12}C atom. A compound with ten carbon atoms would yield a molecular ion, M^+, and isotopic ion one unit greater $(M + 1)^+$, which would be about $10 \times 1.08 = 10.8$ percent of the abundance of M^+. The chance of finding two ^{13}C atoms in the same molecule increase with the increasing number of carbon atoms so that $(M + 2)^+$ start to become more prominent. The chance of finding more than two ^{13}C atoms are very small except with large number of carbon atoms and $(M + 3)^+$ can safely ignored. For a compound of ten carbon atoms, the approximate relative height of

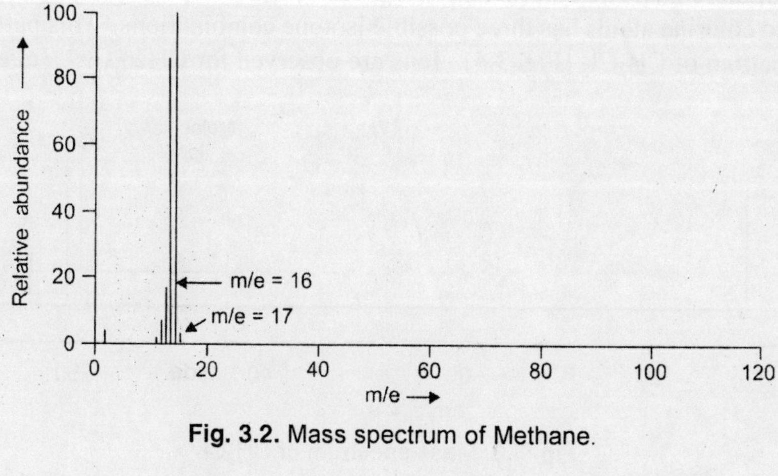

Fig. 3.2. Mass spectrum of Methane.

M^+, $(M+1)^+$, $(M+2)^+$ and $(M+3)^+$ are 100:10:0.45:0.01 from which it can be seen how unimportant are peaks greater than $(M+2)^+$. Tables are available giving the relative heights of M^+, $(M+1)^+$ and $(M+2)^+$ peaks for various elemental compositions (Beynon and Williams 1963). All the carbon compounds contain molecular and fragment ion accompanied by isotopic ion one and two unit greater, making the appearance of mass spectrum complex. Table 3.1 gives, for some elements commonly met in mass spectrometry, the approximate natural abundances of most significant isotopes. From the table, it should be noted that bromine, chlorine and sulphur have particularly abundant isotopes separated by two mass units. For this reasons, the bromine and chlorine containing compounds especially recognized by mass spectrometry and by examining the isotopic ion pattern in the molecular ion region, the number of bromine and chlorine atom can be determined in a original molecule.

Table 3.1. Natural abundance of some elements

Element	*Isotope*	*Relative abundance*	*Isotope*	*Relative abundance*	*Isotope*	*Relative abundance*
Carbon	^{12}C	100	^{13}C	1.11		
Hydrogen	^{1}H	100	^{2}H	0.016		
Nitrogen	^{14}N	100	^{15}N	0.38		
Oxygen	^{16}O	100	^{17}O	0.04	^{18}O	0.20
Sulfur	^{32}S	100	^{33}S	0.78	^{34}S	4.40
Chlorine	^{35}Cl	100			^{37}Cl	32.5
Bromine	^{79}Br	100			^{81}Br	98.0

Chlorine is an excellent example of how isotope distributions are useful for determining the presence of chlorine atom in a molecule. The molecular weight of chlorine is 35.45 u. This is calculated from the natural abundance of ^{35}Cl (75%) and ^{37}Cl (25%). The natural abundance of these two isotopes is observed in the mass spectrum as two peaks separated by m/e-2 with a relative intensity of 3:1. The mass spectrum of CH_3Cl (Fig. 3.3) clearly shows two peaks with the isotope distribution pattern for an ion with a single chlorine atom. $CH_3\,^{35}Cl$ (m/e 50) and $CH_3\,^{37}Cl$ (m/e 52) are separated by m/e 2 and have the 3:1 abundance ratio characteristic of an ion with a single chlorine atom. If more than one chlorine atom is present, the isotope abundance is more complex. An ion with two chlorine atoms has three possible isotope combinations. This pattern is apparent in the mass spectrum of CH_2Cl_2 (Fig. 3.4). Ions are observed for $CH2^{35}Cl^{2+}$ (m/e 84), CH2 ^{35}Cl

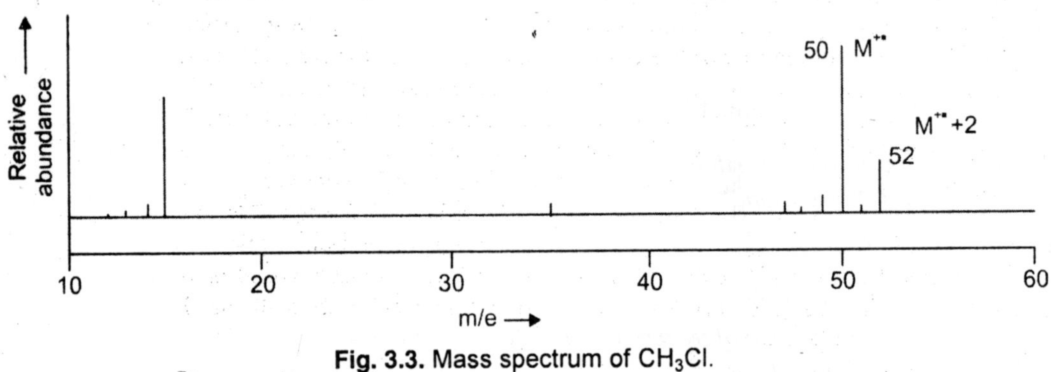

Fig. 3.3. Mass spectrum of CH_3Cl.

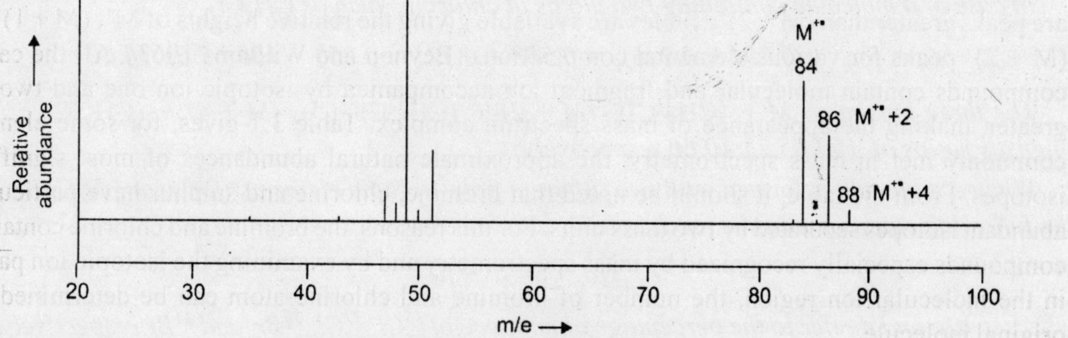

Fig. 3.4. The mass spectrum of CH_2Cl_2.

$^{37}Cl^+$ (m/e 86), and CH $^{37}Cl_2$ (m/e 88). Based upon the probability of each combination of isotopes, the relative intensity of these peaks is 10:6:1. The 3:1 isotope ratio for an ion with a single chlorine atom is observed at m/e 49 and m/e 51. This corresponds to $CH_2{}^{35}Cl$ and $CH_2{}^{37}Cl$ fragments formed by loss of Cl from the molecular ion. Careful examination of the spectrum also shows ions produced by loss of H$^{\cdot}$ and H_2.

Similarly, the mass spectrum of propyl bromide (Fig. 3.5) has two prominent peaks of equal intensity at 122 (M^+) and 124 $(M + 2)^+$ and then two more at 79 and 81 belonging to the bromine fragment. The relative height of the peaks at 122 and 124 is almost equal due to their isotopes ^{79}Br (100%) and ^{81}Br(98%).

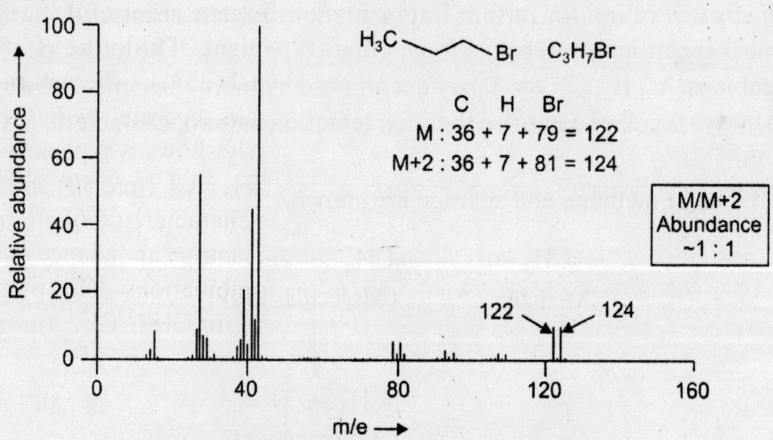

Fig. 3.5. Mass spectrum of Propyl bromide.

Note: *In general, the contribution of various isotopes of different elements can be calculated from the following expression.*

$$(a + b)^n$$

where

a = *% natural abundance of the lighter isotope*
b = *% natural abundance of the heavy isotope*
n = *number of atoms of the element present in a molecule*

In case of a molecule containing two atoms of chlorine, such as CH_2Cl_2,

$$(a + b)n = (0.754 + 0.246)_2 = 0.568 + 0.371 + 0.060 = 100:65.65:10.60$$

The three ions-mass M + ($CH_2^{35}Cl$), (M + 2) + ($CH_2^{35}Cl^{37}Cl$), (M + 4) + ($CH_2^{37}Cl_2$) have intensity ratios of 100:65.25:10.60 respectively.

When a molecule is formed with two different poly-isotopic elements (for example Cl and Br) the following equation must be used.

$$(a + b)^n (c + d)^r$$

where a, b, c and d refer to the percentage abundance of ^{35}Cl, ^{37}Cl, ^{79}Br, and ^{81}Br respectively, and n and r are the number of atoms of chlorine and bromine respectively.

3.3 FRAGMENT IONS

When a molecule is ionized by removal of an electron, a moleculer ion ($M^{+\bullet}$, a cation radical) is produced. This molecular ion may contain sufficient excess internal energy to fragment by ejection of neutral particle (N) with the formation of fragment ion ($A^{+\bullet}$ or A^+). A neutral molecule gives a radical cation as the molecular ion, and the fragment ion may be either a radical cation or cation. The ejected neutral particle (N) may a radical or neutral molecule.

If the fragment ion ($A^{+\bullet}$) has sufficient excess of internal energy, the further decomposition may occur with the formation of new fragment ions(B^+, C^+, etc.) until there is insufficient excess of internal energy in any one of ion for further fragmentation. Such a series of decomposition when elucidated from mass spectrum is refered as fragmentation pathway. The molecular ion ($M^{+\bullet}$) and any of the fragment ions(A^+, B^+, C^+, etc.) may decompose by more than one pathway. The various fragmentation pathways together comprise the fragmentation pattern, characteristic of a compound under investigation.

Here, fragment ions of methane and acetone are shown.

$$\underset{\text{Methane}}{CH_4} + e^- \longrightarrow \underset{\text{(Molecular ion)}}{CH_4^{+\bullet}} + 2e$$

$$\downarrow$$

$$\underset{\text{(Fragment ion)}}{CH_3^+} + H^\bullet$$

$$\underset{\text{Acetone}}{CH_3COCH_3} + e^- \longrightarrow \underset{\text{(Molecular ion)}}{CH_3COCH_3^{+\bullet}} + 2e^-$$

$$\downarrow$$

$$\underset{\text{(Fragment ion)}}{CH_3C{\equiv}O^+} + CH_3^\bullet$$

3.4 REARRANGEMENT IONS

Rearrangement ions are fragments whose origin cannot be described by simple cleavage of bonds in the molecular ion, but are a result of intramolecular atomic rearrangement during fragmentation. Rearrangements involving migration of hydrogen atoms in molecules that contain a heteroatom are especially common. One important example is Mclafferty rearrangement:

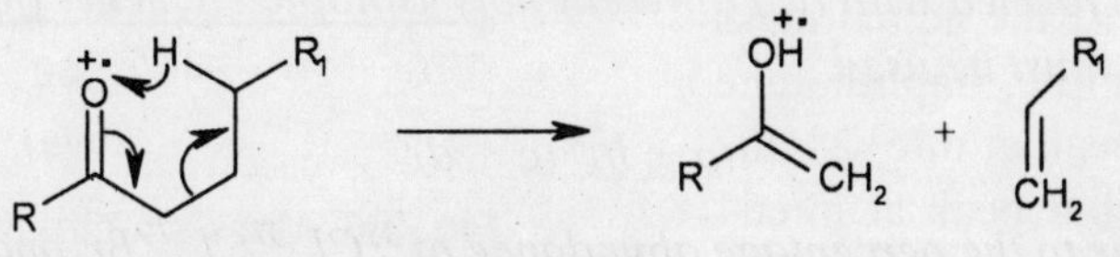

R may be H, alkyl group, O alkyl, NH_2, Cl, OH etc.

To undergo Mclafferty rearrangement, a molecule must possess; an appropriately located heteroatom (e.g. O), a π-system (usually a double bond) and an abstractable hydrogen γ to the C=O system. Such rearrangements often account for prominent characteristic peaks and are consequently very useful for our purpose. They can frequently be rationalized on the basis of low-energy transitions and increased stability of the products. Rearrangements resulting in elimination of stable neutral molecule are common (e.g. the olefin product in the McLafferty rearrangement). Rearrangement peaks can be recognized by considering the mass (m/e) number for fragment ions and for their corresponding molecular ions. A simple (no rearrangement) cleavage of an even-numbered molecular ion gives an odd numbered fragment ion and simple cleavage of an odd-numbered molecular ion gives an even-numbered fragment. Observation of a fragment ion mass different by 1 unit from that expected for a fragment resulting from simple cleavage (e.g., an even-numbered fragment mass from an even-numbered molecular ion mass) indicates rearrangement of hydrogen has accompanied fragmentation. Rearrangement peaks may be recognized by considering the corollary to the "nitrogen rule". Thus even-numbered peak derived from an even-numbered molecular ion is a result of two cleavages, which may involve a rearrangement.

In some compounds, structural features also promote double McLafferty rearrangements (MR) as shown below.

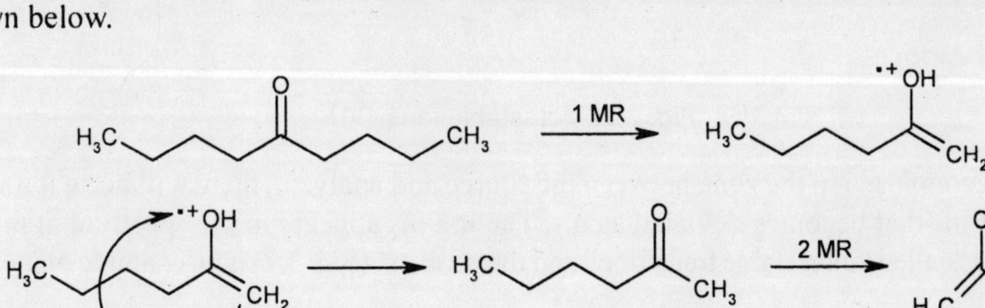

3.5 MULTIPLE CHARGED IONS

In mass spectrometry, the formation of ions carrying single positive charge is most probable process. The formation of multiply charged (M^{n+}) ions is least probable process. Hence, these are generally of no importance in mass spectrometry. However, sometimes doubly or triply charged ions are observed and may be useful for the interpretation of mass spectra. The removal of two or more electrons from a molecule without fragmentation is possible in case of organic compounds with aromatic rings and heteroaromatic compounds. Double and triple charged ions are formed by removal of two or more electrons respectively and they appear at 1/2 and 1/3 of the actual mass respectively. For example, naphthalene shows molecular ion peak at m/e128 due to singly charged ion but peak at m/e64 appears due to doubly charged (M^{2+}) (Fig. 3.6) (half value of molecular mass of naphthalene). The doubly charged ion undergoes fragmentation to give doubly charged ions which are recorded at m/e values numerically equal to one-half of their actual mass numbers.

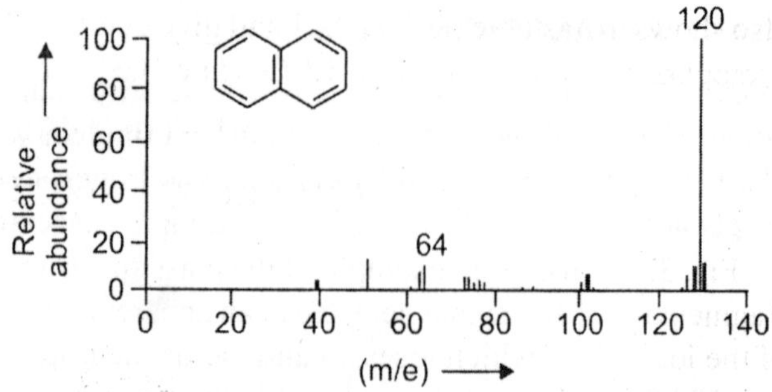

Fig. 3.6. Mass spectrum of Naphthalene.

3.6 METASTABLE IONS

These ions are formed with sufficient excitation to dissociate spontaneously during its flight from the ion source to the detector. The presence of metastable ion is indicated by broad peaks, called "metastable peak", that do not usually appear at whole mass numbers.

If the average life time of ion (m1) is >5 × 10^{-6} secs, the ion is accelerated, deviated and recorded as m_1. If the average life time of ion m_1 <5 × 10^{-6} secs, it fragment before acceleration to give a new ion of mass m_2.

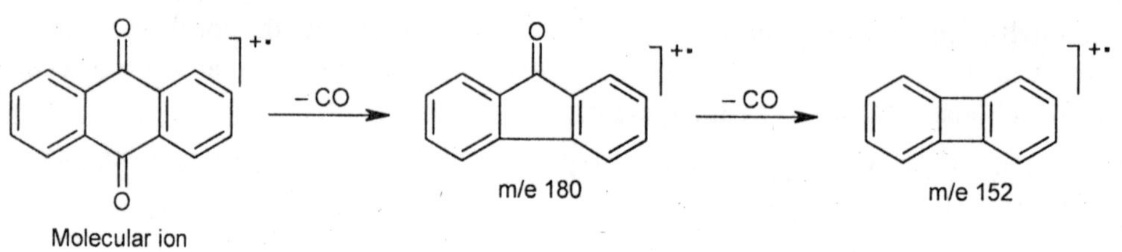

Fig. 3.7. Metastable ions.

If the ion decomposed in the zone between the source and analyzer, there will be an ion with the acceleration of m_1 that becomes deviated as m_2. The ion m_2 appears in the spectrum at m*. Such decomposition is called "metastable transition" and the peak m* (Fig. 3.7) is an example of metastable transition.

The numerical value of m* is given by

$$m^* = (m_2)^2/m_1$$

where m_1, m_2,and m* are the masses(strictly m/e) of the ions m_2^{+}, m_2^{+} and m* respectively and $m_1 > m_2$. For example, toluene shows intense peak at m/e91(C_7H_{7+}) amd m/e65 (C_5H_{5+}) and appearance of a broad peak at 46.4 (= $65^2/91$) indicates that atleast some of the ions at m/e 65 arise through ejection of C_2H_2 (26 mass unit) from the ions at m/e 91. The mass spectrum of acetophenone also shows metastable peak at 92.1 and give evidence for the decomposition of the molecular ion of acetophenone (m /e 120) to $C_6H_5CO^+$ (m/e 105) in one step because the predicted mass:

$$m^* = (105)^2/120 = 91.88$$

$$C_6H_5COCH_3^{+\cdot} \longrightarrow C_6H_5CO^+ + {}^\cdot CH_3$$

Fig. 3.8 shows as an example of the mass spectrum of theobromine, which shows the metastable fragmentation. The signal detected at an apparent m/e 87.9 comes from the metastable fragmentation of the ion at 137, which loses 28 and yields the fragment, m/e109. Similarly, the signal at apparent m/e 104.3 comes from the metastable fragmentation 180→137.

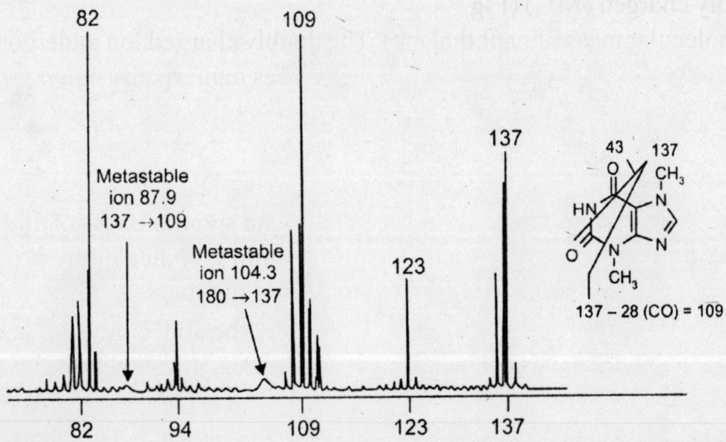

Fig. 3.8. Mass spectrum of theobromine showing metastable peaks.

3.7 NEGATIVE IONS

Ion source that operates at pressure of up to 1 Torr (133 Pa) produce high concentration of low energy electrons which may react directly with suitable molecules to form negative ion and fragment ions. Alternatively a reagent gas may be used to generate negative chemical ionization.

Negative ions formed in the ion source are less abundant than positive ions by a factor of 10^{-4}. These are formed from a neutral molecule(AB) by three mechanisms:

(i) Poduction of a couple of ions

$$AB + e^- \longrightarrow A^+ + B^- + e$$

(ii) Capture of an electron with dissociation

$$AB + e^- \longrightarrow A + B^-$$

(iii) Capture of electron

$$AB + e^- \longrightarrow AB^-$$

The suitability of electron attachment may be very high for compounds containing electronegative elements and it may be enhanced for other compound by making the use of fluorinated derivatives.

3.8 IONS FORMED BY ION MOLECULE INTERACTION

The percentage of molecules of a compound ionized to the vapor in ionization chamber is very low. Therefore, there is possibility of collision between molecular ion and neutral molecule. In such a collision, the molecular ion can subtract an atom from the neutral molecule, forming a heavier ion. The simplest example is the protonation of the molecular ion, resulting in the formation of M + 1 peak. This peak can be differentiated from the isotopic peak with the help of high resolution data. This reaction occurs when the sample pressure is high.

CHAPTER 4

Determination of Molecular Formula

It is difficult to get the exact molecular formula solely on the basis of mass spectral data. A mass spectrum can only give the idea about the probable molecular formula. It needs the confirmation from the other spectral (IR and NMR) data.

The prime step to determine the molecular formula is determination of molecular ion peak. If the molecular ion appears, it will be the highest mass in an EI spectrum (except for isotope peaks discussed earlier). This peak will represent the molecular weight of the compound. Its appearance depends on the stability of the compound. Double bonds, cyclic structures and aromatic rings stabilize the molecular ion and increase the probability of its appearance and thus increase its abundance. There are two situations in which the identification of the molecular ion peak may be difficult.

(a) The molecular ion does not appear or is very weak. The obvious remedy in most cases is to run the spectrum at maximum sensitivity (and accept the resulting loss in resolution) and to use a larger sample. (Sometimes a large sample exaggerates the M + 1 peak) Still the molecular ion may not be evident and then other sources of information may be useful. The type of compound may be known, and the molecular mass may be deduced from the breakdown pattern. For example, alcohol usually give a very weak parent molecular ion peak but often show a pronounced peak resulting from loss of water (M–18).

(b) The molecular ion is present but is one of several peaks which may also be as prominent. In this situation, the question is that of purity. If the compound can be assumed to be pure, the usual problem is to distinguish the molecular ion peak from a more prominent M–1 peak. One good test is to reduce the energy of the bombarding electron beam to near the appearance potential. This will reduce the intensities of all peaks, but will increase the intensity of the molecular ion relative to other peaks, including fragmentation peaks (but not molecular ion peaks) of impurities. Another test frequently used is to increase the size of the sample, or increase the time the sample spends in the ionization chamber by decreasing the ion repeller voltage. In either case the net effect is to increase the opportunity for bimolecular collisions to occur in the ion chamber. The most common result of the bimolecular collision of a molecular ion containing a heteroatom (O, N or S) is a contribution to the M + 1 peak (i.e., the net effect is the transfer of a hydrogen atom from a neutral molecule to the molecular ion). Thus an increase in peak size relative to other peaks, as sample size is increased or the repeller voltage is decreased, designates that peak as the M + 1 peak and affords an indirect identification of the molecular ion. Of course the dependance of the M + 1 on a sample size must be kept in mind when the peak is used to establish a molecular formula of a compound containing a heteroatom. Many peaks can be ruled out as possible molecular ions simply on grounds of following reasonable structure requirements:

(i) **Nitrogen rule** is often helpful identifying the molecular ion peak. It states that a molecule of even-numbered molecular weight must contain no nitrogen or an even number of nitrogen atoms; an odd-numbered molecular weight requires an odd number of nitrogen atoms. This rule holds for all compounds containing carbon, hydrogen, oxygen, nitrogen, sulfur, and the halogens, as well as many of the less usual atoms such as phosphorous, boron, silicon, arsenic, and the alkaline earths.

Molecule :	NH_3	H_2NNH_2	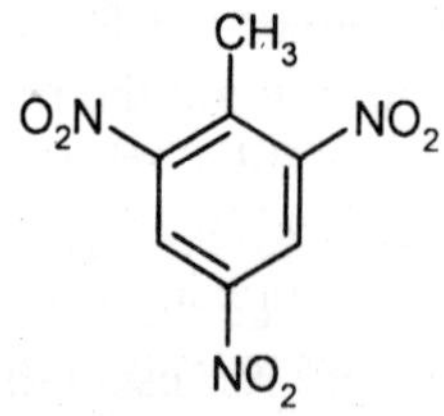	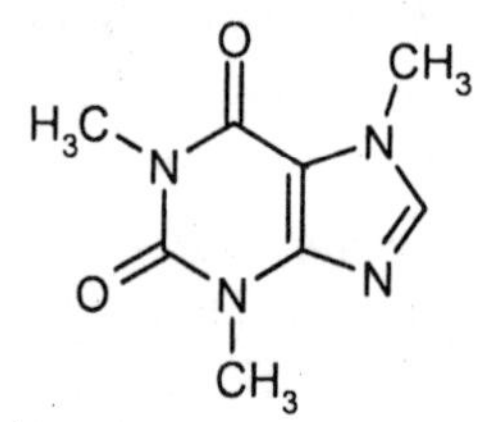
Formula :	NH_3	N_2H_4	$C_7H_5N_3O_6$	$C_8H_{10}N_4O_2$
m/e for M (amu) :	17	32	227	194

This distinction is also illustrated nicely by the following two examples (Figs. 4.1 and 4.2). The unsaturated ketone, 4–methyl–3–pentene–2–one, below has no nitrogen so the mass of the molecular ion (m/e = 98) is an even number. Most of the fragment ions have odd-numbered masses. Diethylmethylamine, on the other hand, has one nitrogen and its molecular mass (m/e = 87) is an odd number. A majority of the fragment ions have even-numbered masses (ions at m/e = 30, 42, 56 & 58 are not labeled). The weak even-electron ions at m/e = 15 and 29 are due to methyl and ethyl cations (no nitrogen atoms).

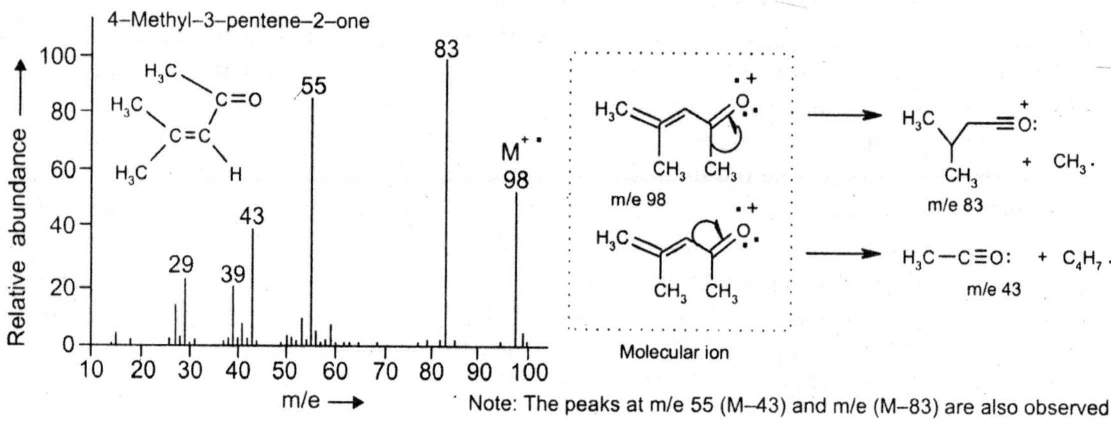

Note: The peaks at m/e 55 (M–43) and m/e (M–83) are also observed

Fig. 4.1. Mass spectrum of 4–Methyl–3–pentene–2–one.

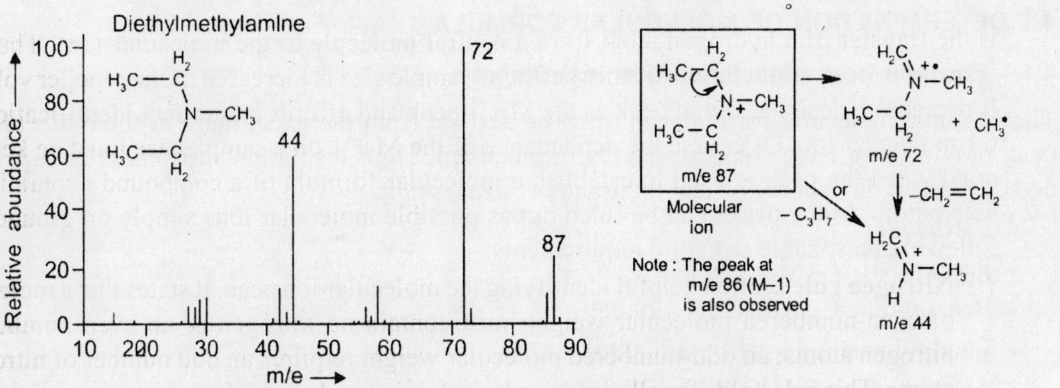

Fig. 4.2. Mass spectrum of Diethylmethyl amine.

(ii) A useful corollary states that fragmentation at a single bond gives an odd-numbered ion fragment from an even-numbered molecular ion, and an even-numbered ion fragment from an odd numbered molecular ion. For this corollary to hold, the fragment must contain all nitrogen(if any) of the molecular ion.

(iii) Consideration of the breakdown pattern coupled with other information also assists in identifying molecular ions. It should be kept in mind that; the intensity of the molecular ion peak depends on the stability of the molecular ion. The most stable molecular ions are those of purely aromatic systems. If substituents that have a favourable mode of cleavage are present, the molecular ion peak will be less intense, and the fragment peaks relatively more intense. In general the following group of compounds will, in order of decreasing ability, **give prominent molecular ion peaks:** aromatic compounds > conjugated alkenes > cyclic compounds > organic sulphides > short, normal alkanes.

Recognizable molecular ions are usually produced for these compounds in order of decreasing ability: Ketones > amines > esters > carboxylic acids-aldehydes-amides-halides. The **molecular ion is frequently not detectable** in aliphatic alcohol, nitrites, nitrates, nitro compounds, nitriles and in high.

The presence of M–15 peak (loss of CH_3) or an M–18 peak (loss of H_2O) or an M–31 Peak (loss of OCH_3 from methyl esters), etc., is taken as confirmation of the molecular ion peak. An M–1 peak is common and occasionally an M–2 peak (loss of H_2 by either fragmentation or thermolysis or even a rare M–3 peak (from alcohol) is reasonable. Peaks in the range of M–3 to M–14, however, indicate that contaminants may be present or that the presumed molecular ion peak is actually a fragment ion peak. Loss of fragments of masses 19 to 25 are also unlikely (except for the loss of F = 19 or HF = 20 from flourinated compounds). Loss of 16 (O), 17(OH), or 18 (H_2O) are likely only if an oxygen atom is in the molecule.

Another way of confirming a molecular ion is that all fragments in the spectrum (other than impurities) should come from the assigned molecular ion with logical loss of neutral fragments. If a fragment or two do not comply this will mean either the assigned molecular ion is not really the molecular ion but a fragment ion or the fragment does not belong to the compound but to a background contaminant.

4.1 DETERMINATION OF MOLECULAR FORMULA

4.1.1 Formula from high resolution instrument

The probable molecular formula can often be derived from the exact mass of the molecular ion peak provided we have some structures in our mind. High resolution instrument is capable of detecting mass differences of few thousands of a mass unit.

For example:

- Purine $C_5H_4N_4$ (M = 120.044)
- Benzimidine $C_7H_8N_2$ (M = 120.069)
- Ethyl toluene C_9H_{12} (M = 120.096)
- Acetophenonone C_7H_8O (M = 120.058)

If the measured mass of molecular ion peak is 120.070 ($\pm$0.005), then all except $C_7H_8N_2$ are excluded as possible formula.

4.1.2 Formula from isotope ratios

Low resolution instrument can discriminate between ions differing in mass by whole mass number. It can also yield useful information about the formula of a compound provided only that the molecular ion peak is sufficiently intense ion peak that its height and the height of the ($M^{+\bullet}$ + 1) and ($M^{+\bullet}$ + 2) isotope can be determined accurately.

For example:

- $C_6H_4N_2O_4$ (dinitrobenzene)
- $C_{12}H_{24}$ (Olefin)

Both has molecular weight ~ 168 but calculation of $M^{+\bullet}$ + 1/$M^{+\bullet}$ ratio give the possibility of appropriate molecular formula.

$C_6H_4N_2O_4$

^{13}C $6 \times 1.08 = 6.48\%$

^{2}H $4 \times 0.015 = 0.060\%$

^{15}N $2 \times 0.37 = 0.74\%$

^{17}O $4 \times 0.04 = \mathbf{0.16\%}$

$$\frac{M^{+\bullet}+1}{M^{+\bullet}} = 7.44\%$$

$C_{12}H_{24}$

^{13}C $12 \times 1.08 = 12.96\%$

^{2}H $24 \times 0.015 = \mathbf{0.36\%}$

$$\frac{M^{+\bullet}+1}{M^{+\bullet}} = 13.32\%$$

In an approximate but rapid manner, ratios $M^{+\bullet}$ + 1/$M^{+\bullet}$ and $M^{+\bullet}$ + 2/$M^{+\bullet}$ can be determined in the following ways :

$$M^{+} + 1/M^{+} = (1.1\% \times \text{No. of carbon atom}) + 0.36\% \times \text{No. of nitrogen atoms} + 0.2\% \times \text{No. of nitrogen atoms}$$

$$\frac{M^{+\bullet}+2}{M^{+\bullet}} = \frac{(1.1\% \times \text{No. of carbon atom})^2}{200}$$

4.1.3 Molecular formula from Beynon table

Generally, position of the molecular ion and isotopic ion peak along with their intensities are mentioned in mass spectral data. For example, in a compound following mass spectral data are recorded:

150 ($M^{+\bullet}$)	100%
151 ($M^{+\bullet} + 1$)	9.9%
152 ($M^{+\bullet} + 2$)	0.9%

To know the molecular formula of this compound, we select all the compounds of molecular weight – 150 possessing the nearly same $M^{+} + 1$ and $M^{+} + 2$ peak intensities from Beynon Table:

	$M^{+\bullet} + 1$	$M^{+\bullet} + 2$
(i) $C_7H_{10}N_4$	9.25	0.38
(ii) $C_8H_8NO_2$	9.23	0.78
(iii) $C_8H_{10}N_2O$	9.61	0.61
(iv) $C_8H_{12}N_3$	9.98	0.45
(v) $C_9H_{10}O_2$	9.96	0.84
(vi) $C_9H_{12}NO$	10.34	0.68
(vii) $C_9H_{14}N_2$	10.71	0.52

There are seven molecular formula at the molecular weight – 150 possessing same or nearly same $M^{+\bullet} + 1$ and $M^{+\bullet} + 2$ (intensities peak). According to nitrogen rule, molecular formulas, (ii), (iv) and (vi) are rule out (compound possessing even numbered molecular weight should possess even number nitrogen or no nitrogen atoms). Then, it is observed that molecular formula $C_9H_{10}O_2$ (V) possess the more close $M^{+\bullet} + 1$ (9.96) and $M^{+} + 2$ (0.84) values. Hence, it is the possible molecular formula of the compound which should be further verified from the IR, NMR and mass fragmentation pattern.

How the M + 2 (and possibly M + 4) peak arises, and its use in showing the presence of chlorine or bromine in a compound.

4.1.4 Molecular formula from molecular and isotopic ion peaks

Mass → Formula

Example 1

Molecular ion	*m/e*	*Relative abundance*	*Conclusions*
M	102	100%	Mass = 102 Even number of nitrogens
M + 1	103	6.9	6.9 ÷ 1.1 = 6.3, Six carbons
M + 2	104	0.38	S, Cl or Br atom absent Oxygen atom?

$M - C_6 = 102 - (6 \times 12) = 30$ amu for oxygen, nitrogen, hydrogen

Oxygens	*Nitrogens*	*30 – O – N = H*	*Formula notes*
0	0	30 – 0 – 0 = 30	C_6H_{30} Violates hydrogen rule
1	0	30 – 16 – 0 = 14	$C_6H_{14}O$ reasonable
2	0	30 – 32 – 0 = –2	Not possible
0	2	30 – 0 – 28 = 2	$C_6H_2N_2$ Reasonable

Two molecular formula are possible and one formula can be selected/ruled out on the basis of other spectral data.

Example 2

Molecular ion	*m/e*	*Relative abundance*	*Conclusions*
M	157	100%	Mass = 157 Odd number of nitrogens
M + 1	158	9.39	9.39 ÷ 1.1 = 8.5 Eight or nine carbons
M + 2	159	34	One chlorine; no bromine; # of sulfur?

$M - C_8 - N - Cl = 157 - (8 \times 12) - 14 - 35 = 12$ amu for oxygen, nitrogen, hydrogen
Not enough for amu for oxygen or another nitrogen
Probable molecular formula = $C_8H_{12}NCl$

Example 3

Molecular ion	*m/e*	*Relative abundance*	*Conclusions*
M	148	100%	Mass = 148 Zero or even number of nitrogens
M + 1	149	11.25	11.25 ÷ 1.1 = 1..23 Ten carbons
M + 2	159	34	One chlorine; no bromine; # of sulfur?

148 – 120 (C_{10}) = 28 amu (atomic mass units) for oxygen, nitrogen and hydrogen.

Oxygens	*Nitrogens*	*28– O– N = H formula*	*Comments*
None	None	28 – 0 – 0 = 28	$C_{10}H_{28}$ Violates hydrogen rule
One	None	28 – 16 – 0 = 12	$C_{10}H_{12}O$ Reasonable
None	Two	28 – 0 – 28 = 0	$C_{10}N_2$ Reasonable

Index of Hydrogen Deficiency (IHD)

It indicates the sum of the number of rings and pi bonds in a molecule. Once the formula is known, it is possible to calculate the hydrogen deficiency of the molecule. For instance, for a saturated hydrocarbon without rings, the formula is C_nH_{2n+2}. The difference between the number of hydrogens in the formula and 2m + 2 divided by two is the hydrogen deficiency or a sum of the number of bonds and rings.

Each multiple bond and each ring contributes 1 degree of hydrogen deficiency to a compound:

Structural unit	*Contribution to index of hydrogen deficiency*
Double bond	1
Triple bond	2
Ring	1

The hydrogen deficiency in molecules containing C, H, N, O, Cl, Br, or I for the molecule $C_cH_hN_nO_oX_x$ (where X represents any halogen and c, h, n and x represents the total number of carbon, hydrogen, nitrogen and halogen atoms respectively) can be calculated from the equation:

$$\text{Index of hydrogen deficiency (U)} = \frac{(2c + 2 - h + n - x)}{2}$$

Where does this equation come from?

- The **maximum number of hydrogen *atoms for*** "c" carbon atoms is 2c + 2 (for example, saturated hydrocarbon, methane has one cárbon atom, $2 \times 1 + 2 = 4$)
- From this number, subtract the "h" hydrogens that you have.
- Since, like hydrogen, a halogen only forms one bond, then they can be treated as if they are hydrogens, so subtract them as well.
- Oxygen forms two bonds, therefore it has **no impact** (compare H count for methane, CH_4, and methanol, CH_3OH). Both has same index of hydrogen deficiency.
- Nitrogen forms three bonds. This means for "n" nitrogens, "n" extra hydrogen atoms are needed (compare the H count for methane, CH_4, and methyl amine, CH_3NH_2), therefore, add "n". Both has zero index of hydrogen deficiency.
- The factor of 0.5 accounts for us counting H ***atoms***, but adding hydrogen, H_2, ***molecules***.

Example 1

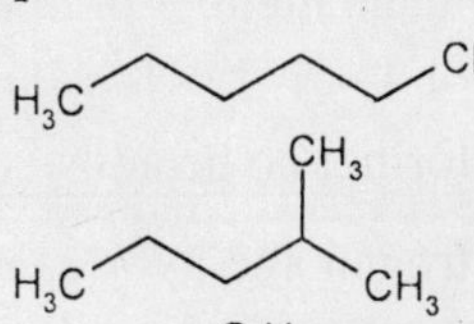

C_6H_{14}
IHD = 0

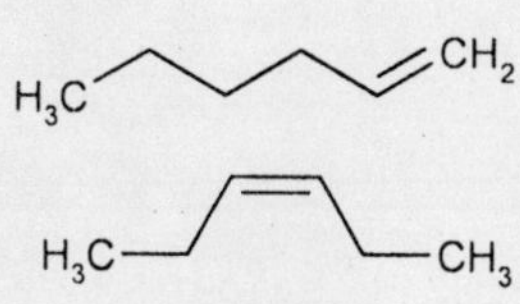

C_6H_{12}
IHD = 1

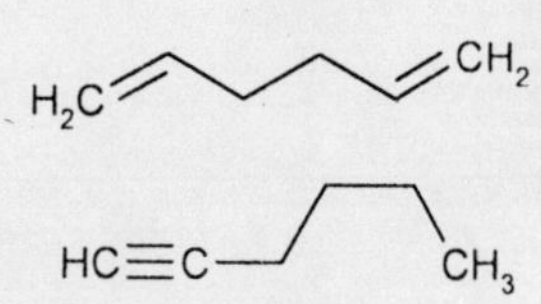

C_6H_{10}
IHD = 2

Example 2

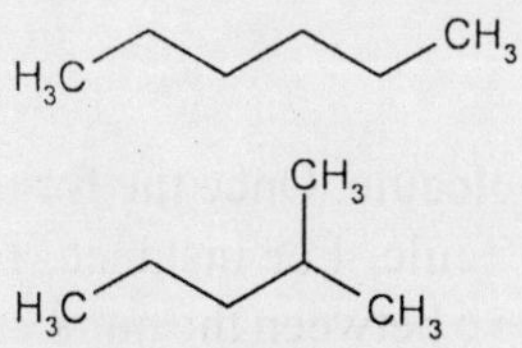

C_6H_{14}
IHD = 0

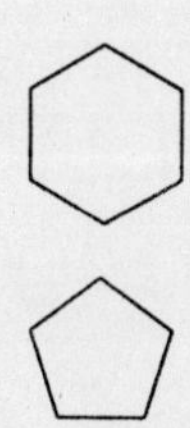

C_6H_{12}
IHD = 1
(Confirm the presence of one ring

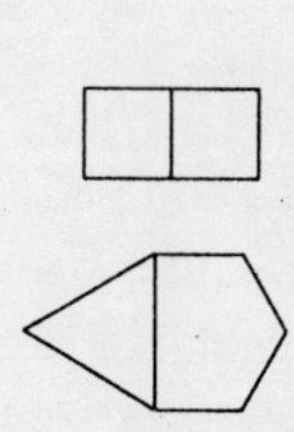

C_6H_{10}
IHD = 2
(Confirm the presence of two rings)

Example 3

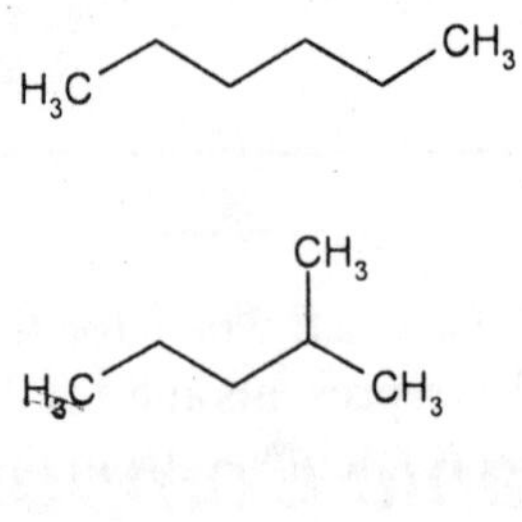

C_6H_{14}
IHD = 0

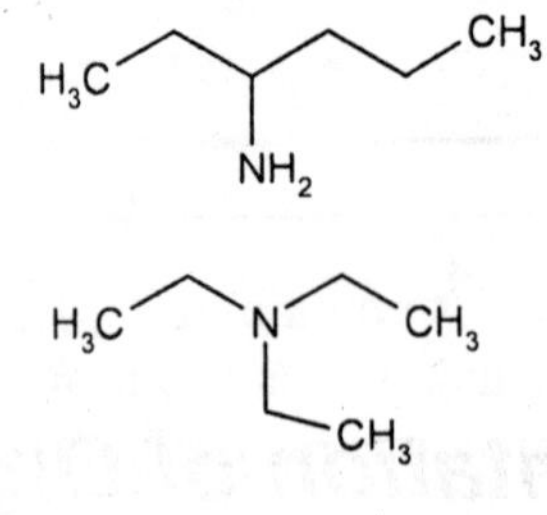

$C_6H_{15}N$
IHD = 0

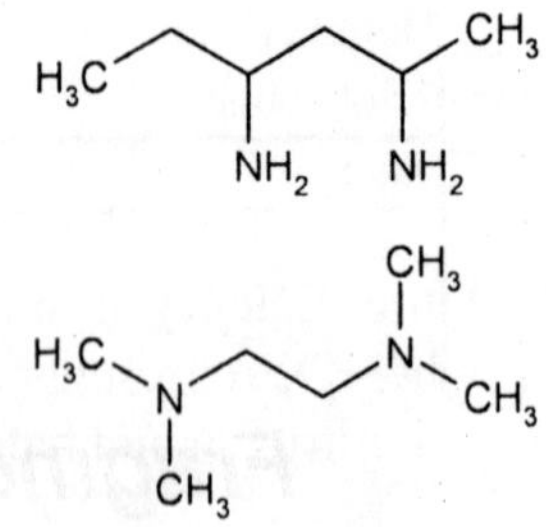

$C_6H_{16}N_2$
IHD = 0

CHAPTER

5 Fragmentation of Organic Compounds

5.1 INTRODUCTION

Fragment ions are formed from the molecule (M) during Ionization Process as:

$$M \xrightarrow[70\ eV]{IE} M^{+\bullet} \xrightarrow{\text{Excess energy}} \text{Fragment ion}^{+\bullet} + \text{Neutral radicals}$$

Molecular ion

Electron will be removed from orbital having the lowest ionization potential (IP). In general non bonding (n) electrons possess lowest and the sigma (a) have highest while pia (p) lies in between the sigma and non bonding.

$$\text{Ionization potential (IP): } n < \pi < \alpha$$

For example, methane has the high energy requirement in comparison to ethylene and methyl amine indicated by Ionization potential.

Molecule	*Ionization potential*
CH_4	12.6 eV
C_2H_4	10.52 eV
CH_3NH_2	10.3 eV

Ionization mechanism

$$H_3C \cdot\cdot CH_3 \xrightarrow[IE]{e^-} H_3C \cdot + CH_3 \ + 2e^-$$

a two-electron sigma bond → a one-electron bond;

$$H_2C \overset{\cdot\cdot}{—} CH_3 \xrightarrow[IE]{e^-} H_2C \overset{\cdot +}{—} CH_2 \ + 2e^-$$

a two-electron pi bond → a one-electron pi bond

$$H_3C - \ddot{\underset{\cdot\cdot}{O}}H \xrightarrow[IE]{e^-} H_3C - \overset{\cdot +}{\underset{\cdot\cdot}{C}}H_2 + 2e^-$$

a lone pair
electron removed

The products of the ionization process are called Molecular (M^+) Ions. They are radical cations. It is the radical cations that fragment to give a cation, the observed species in the mass spectrum, and a neutral radical. Fragmentation occurs via homolytic cleavage, heterolytic cleavage, alpha cleavage, beta cleavage and rearrangement process depending on structural features of organic compound. This will be elucidated in the coming text.

5.2 STEVENSON'S RULE

Fragmentation often produces both a radical and a cation. This can be represented by the following equation:

$$R—R_1 + e^- \longrightarrow R—R_1^{+\cdot} \begin{cases} R^{\cdot} + R_1^+ & \text{Radical} \quad \text{Cation} \\ R^+ + R_1^{\cdot} & \text{Cation} \quad \text{Radical} \end{cases}$$

Molecular ion
(Radical cation)
$+ 2e^-$

The factor that determines which of the fragments is a radical or a cation can be emphasized as a competition between two cations to capture the electron:

$$R^+ \ldots\ldots\ldots e^- \ldots\ldots\ldots R_1$$

According to ***Stevenson's rule***, if two charged fragments are in competition to produce a neutral radical by electron attachment, the radical having the highest ionization energy will be produced. The other ion, whose corresponding neutral radical has lower ionization energy, will hold its charge and will thus be the observed fragment. Indeed, this reaction can be considered as a competition between two cations to carry away the electron:

$$R^+ \ldots\ldots\ldots e^- \ldots\ldots\ldots R_1$$

5.3 IONS WITH ODD OR EVEN NUMBERS OF ELECTRONS

Organic molecules, without exception, are species with an even number of electrons. Because ionization occurs by the removal of an electron, the molecular ion can be identified with radical-ion that possesses an odd number of electrons, or rather, an unpaired. A molecular ion, or any ion, with an odd number of electrons (i.o.e) can decompose by homolytic or heterolytic processes. The homolytic cleavage occurs by the use transfer of a single electron, and this is indicated by the use of an arrow with one hook $\frown$.

$$CH_3—\overset{\frown}{CH_2}—CH^+—\dot{C}H_2 \longrightarrow \dot{C}H_3 + CH_2{=}CH—CH_2^+ \longleftrightarrow {}^+CH_2—CH{=}CH_2$$

The heterolytic cleavage occurs by the transfer of a pair of electrons and indicated by a conventional arrow ↷.

$$CH_3CH_2{-}Br^{+\bullet} \longrightarrow CH_3CH_2^+ + Br^-$$

In both cases, an ion with an even number of electrons (i.e.e.) is obtained by the elimination of an uncharged fragment with an odd number of electrons (radical, r).

When there are two consecutive or simultaneous fragmentation of an ion with an odd number of electrons, an ion with an odd number of electrons (i.o.e.) and a neutral molecule with an even number of electrons (n.e.e.) are formed by either type of cleavage (homolytic or heterolytic).

$$R{-}\underset{H}{\underset{|}{CH}}{-}\underset{OH}{\underset{|}{CH_2}} \longrightarrow R{-}CH^{\bullet}{-}CH_2^+ + H_2O$$

The majority of ions in a spectrum have an even number of electrons. Either they decompose by loss of a non-charged fragment or a neutral molecule with an even number of electrons to give an ion with an even number of electrons, or they decompose by loss of a radical to give an ion with an odd number of electrons. The latter fragmentation is very rare.

$$CH_3{-}CH_2CH_2^+ \longrightarrow {}^+CH_3 + CH_2{=}CH_2$$

$$CH_3{-}CH_2CH_2^+ \longrightarrow {}^{\bullet}CH_3 + CH_2{-}{}^+CH_2$$

The ions with an even number of electrons give rise to a significant series of peaks for many types of compounds, particularly in the lower part of mass spectrum. The aliphatic hydrocarbons form two series of alkyl ions, $C_nH_{2n}^+$, $C_nH_{2n+1}^+$, the aliphatic amines a series of $C_nH_{2n+2}N^+$, the alcohol a series of $C_nH_{2n+1}O^+$, the ketones a series of $C_nH_{2n}O^+$. In all cases the series are useful for recognizing the class to which a substance belongs.

The concepts expressed above are summarized in Table 5.1.

Table 5.1.

i.o.e. ⟶ i.e.e + r.	simple homo- and heterolytic cleavage
i.o.e. ⟶ i.o.e + n.e.e.	double cleavage
i.e.e. ⟶ i.e.e + n.e.e.	simple heterolytic cleavage
i.e.e. ⟶ i.o.e + r.	simple homolytic cleavage

5.4 FACTORS INFLUENCING THE FRAGMENTATION

The mass spectrum of a molecule shows the numerous peaks, some of them are intense whereas others are weak or scarcely visible. The formation of fragment ions depends on the (i) preferential breakage of some bonds in comparison to others, and (ii) on the stability of some fragments because of their structure. In conclusion, the formation of ions depends on three factors:

1. The relative strength of the bonds.

2. The stability of the fragmentation products. These may be neutral molecule, radicals and positive ions.
3. The relative spatial rearrangements of the atoms or groups.

5.4.1 Relative strength of the bonds

The energies of the most common bonds of an organic molecule are shown in Table 5.2. The weakest bond (C–I, C–Br, C–Cl) are preferentially broken in comparison to other. Similarly, breakage of single bond requires less energy in preference to double or triple bond.

Table 5.2. Energy profile of some bonds present in organic compounds (kCal/mole)

Bond	*Energy*	*Bond*	*Energy*	*Bond*	*Energy*
C–H	97.8	C = N	147	C–F	116
C–C	82.6	C–O	85.5	C–Cl	81
C = C	145.1	C = O	179	C–Br	68
C ≡ C	199.6	C–S	65	C–I	51
C–N	72.8	C = S	128	O–H	110.6

5.4.2 Stability of the fragments

Fragment ions are established by following under mentioned process.

5.4.2.1 Inductive effect

The formation of tertiary cations is favored with respect to secondary or primary ions. For example, in the mass spectra of *n*–butyl alcohol and *t*–butyl alcohol, the fragment ions $C_4H_9^+$ are formed in both cases but more abundant in the case of t-butanol- because tertiary butyl ion is stabilized by the inductive effect of the alkyl groups attached to carbon atom, carrying the positive charge. To some extent, it is also stabilized by hyperconjugation effect, that is delocalisation of the electron of a C–H bond to form a p bond with an adjacent carbon atom having an empty orbital.

$$CH_3CH_2CH_2CH_2-\overset{\bullet+}{O}H \longrightarrow CH_3CH_2CH_2CH_2^+ + {}^{\bullet}OH$$

n-Butyl alcohol

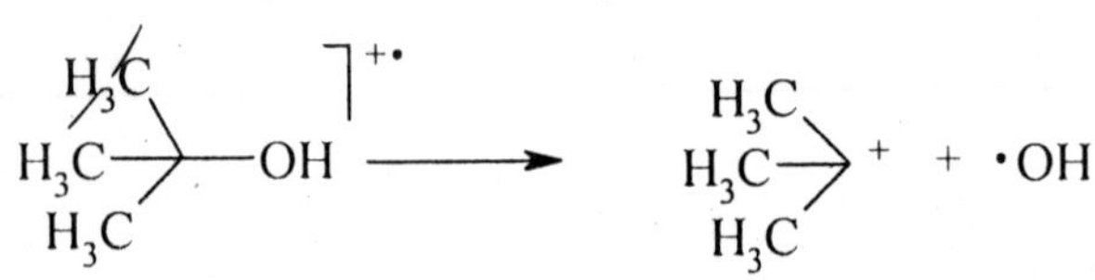

t-Butyl alcohol

In the straight chain paraffins, the rupture of the alkyl chain takes place in one C–C bonds. In branched paraffin's, the fragmentation occurs at the most substituted carbon atom to give the most stability to the ion thus formed. For example, in isopentane, the fragmentation occurs at the bonds of the carbon atom at the C–2 position and the ions have the following order of stability:

$$\underset{\substack{\text{Isopentane}\\\text{(Molecular ion)}}}{CH_3-CH_2-\overset{\overset{\large CH_3}{|}}{C}H-CH_3} \longrightarrow CH_3-CH_2-\overset{\overset{\large CH_3}{|}}{\underset{+}{C}}H > \overset{\overset{\large CH_3}{|}}{\underset{+}{C}}H-CH_3 > CH_3\underset{+}{C}H_2 > \underset{+}{C}H_3$$

The inductive effect also has an influence on the breaking of a bond. In a compound R–X in which X can be Cl, Br, O, S or N, the electronegativity of hetero atom lowers the electron density of the R–X bond. Formation of an alkyl ion occurs according to below mentioned reaction:

$$R\text{–}Cl \longrightarrow R^+ + {}^{\bullet}Cl$$

$$R\text{–}O\text{–}R \longrightarrow R^+ + {}^{\bullet}OR$$

The order of electron attraction is Cl > Br, O, S > I > N, C, H.

The unsaturated functional groups, such as carbonyl group, have a similar effect.

$$R\text{–}\overset{\overset{\large O}{\|}}{C}\text{–}R \longrightarrow R\text{–}CO^{\bullet} + R^+$$

The above three fragmentations are heterocyclic fragmentation directed by the ionic center present on the heteroatom.

5.4.2.2 Neighboring electron participation

The carbonyl compounds, such as ketones, aldehydes, esters, amides and the corresponding sulphur derivatives, give rise to ions of $C^+ = X^-$ stabilized in the canonical form $-C{\equiv}X^+$. For example, acetone shows the presence of fragment, CH_3CO^+ in its mass spectrum.

$$CH_3\text{–}\overset{\overset{\large O^{+\bullet}}{\|}}{C}\text{–}CH_3 \longrightarrow CH_3\text{–}C\equiv O^+ + {}^{\bullet}CH_3$$

The canonical form is stabilized by heteroatom which possesses at least a couple of electrons not used in bonding. The fragmentation reaction can be represented by the homolytic cleavage directed by the radical center present on oxygen.

The non bonding electrons of an atom can also stabilize a positive charge on carbon atom, as in the case of $C_4H_8Br^+$ and $C_4H_8Cl^+$ which are formed from the halide.

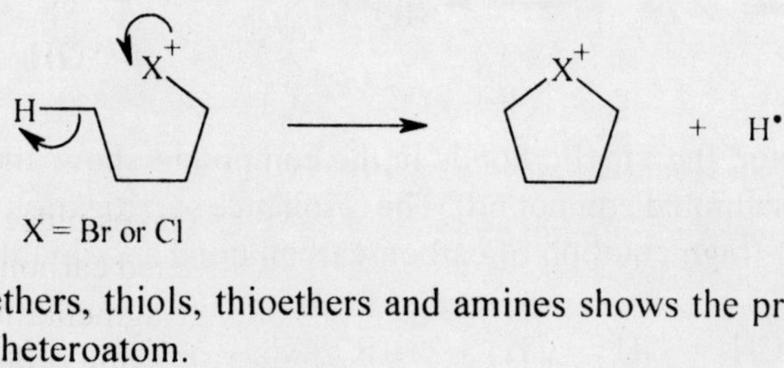

X = Br or Cl

Similarly, alcohol, ethers, thiols, thioethers and amines shows the presence of fragment ions which are stabilized by heteroatom.

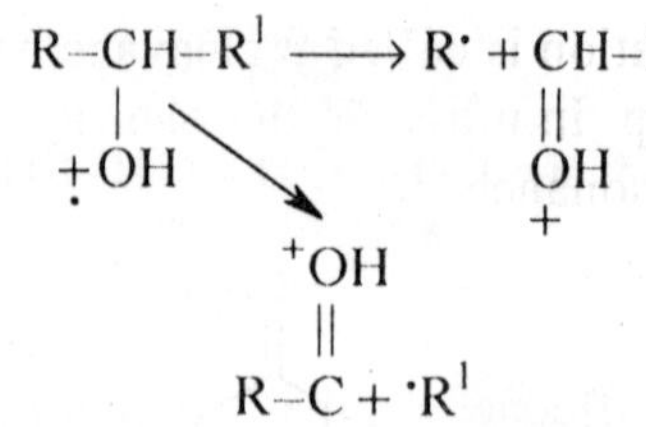

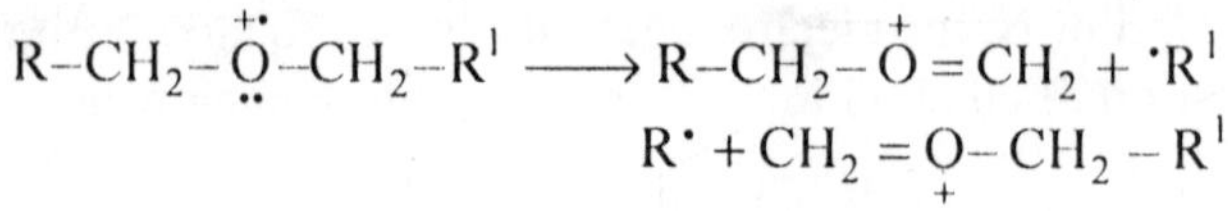

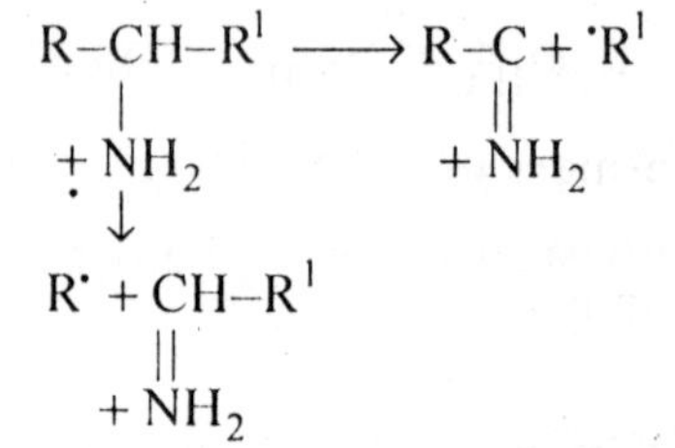

The fragmentaticn reaction is represented as a **homolytic reaction** directed by the radical center present on the heteroatom. It is indicated by an **alpha cleavage** because the bond is adjacent to that alpha carbon and the heteroatom.

The capacity of a heteroatom to stabilize an adjacent positive charge is very high for nitrogen atom and decrease gradually, passing through S, O and the halogen for which is very low. In the following given example, the stabilizing capacity of various atoms, in the same molecule is compared. The numerical values indicated below the formulae represent the percentage abundance of the CH_2X ions.

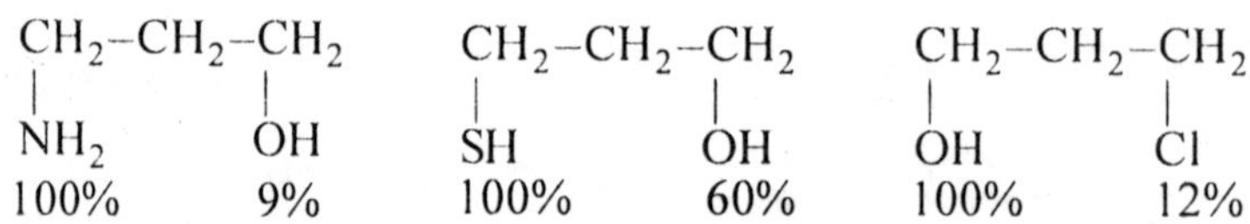

5.4.2.3 Resonance effect

Vinyl chloride and allyl chloride behave differently toward solvolysis. The first is extremely resistant to nucleophilic reagent whereas the second reacts by the SN_1 mechanism to form ionic intermediate stabilized by resonance.

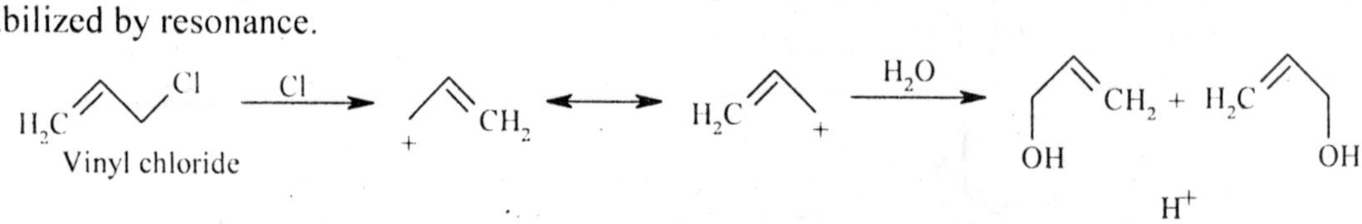

In the mass spectrometer, the vinylic bonds in the compound show allylic cleavage(favored fragmentation mode in unsaturated compound). The resonance stabilization of an allyl cation leads to increased probability of fragmentation of carbon-carbon bond a to double bonds.

$$\left[R{-}CH_2{-}CH{=}CH_2\right]^{+\cdot} \longrightarrow R^{\cdot} + CH_2 \overset{...}{=} \underset{+}{C}H \overset{...}{=} CH_2$$

This homolytic type of fragmentation is called β cleavage because there is rupture of β bond with respect to the functional group. In mircene, the cleavage of the central allylic bond gives $C_5H_9^+$ ion at m/e 69 stabilized by resonance.

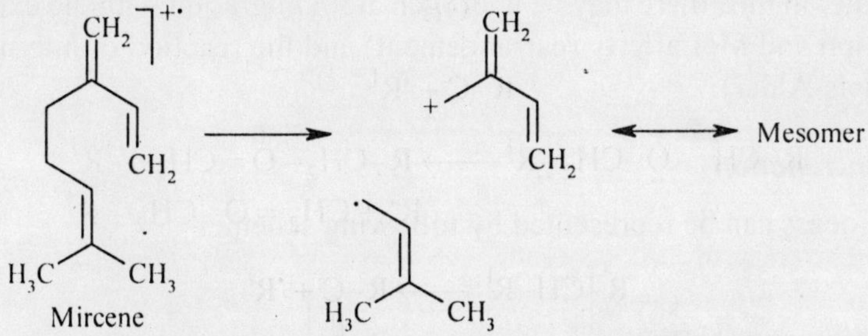

The β **cleavage** is one of the most characteristic fragmentation pathways for aromatic hydrocarbons with an alkyl side chain. The ion that is formed is represented by tropylium structure because all the carbon- atoms are equivalent.

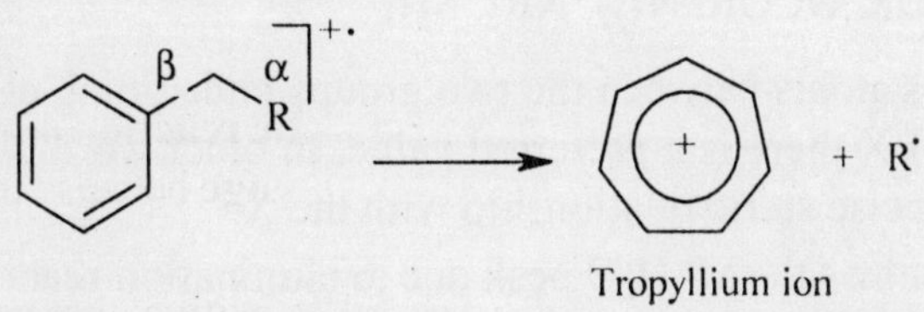

The β **cleavage** is also characteristic for five member aromatic heterocyclic compounds with an alkyl side chain in the α or β position.

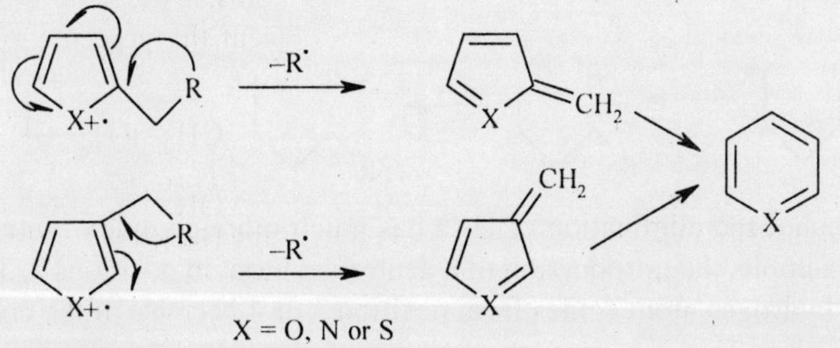

In the case of acetophenone, benzophenone, benzoic acid and substituted benzoates, the abundance of acyl ion, formed as in reaction decreases if the substituent X is an electron donor whereas it increases if X ia an electron acceptor.

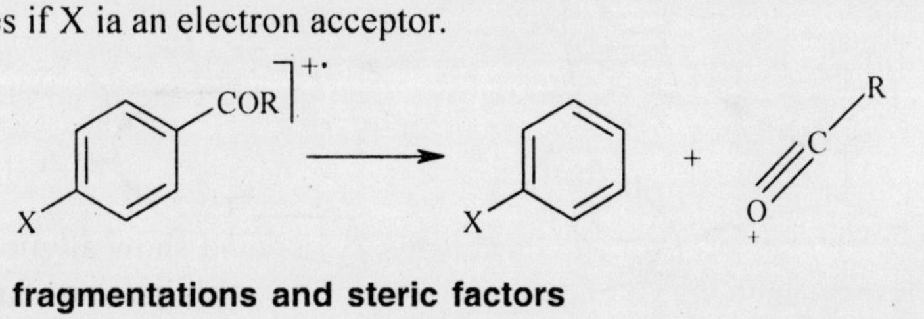

5.4.3 Multi-center fragmentations and steric factors

The fragmentation so far observed involve the cleavage of only one bond. In a complex molecule, the interaction of various functional groups can give a complicated fragmentation reaction that involves the rupture of more than one bond. This is called a multi-center fragmentation.

A multi-center fragmentation is governed by a number of factors: The center involved in the fragmentation must have a suitable arrangement in space; the formation of a stable neutral molecule is the driving force of the process; and the fragmentation occurs by an energetically favorable cyclic transition state. In this, there may be hydrogen atom migration with the expulsion of neutral fragment (elimination and McLafferty rearrangement) and the reaction of internal rearrangement of bonds (Retro Diels-Alder).

5.4.3.1 Elimination reaction

This elimination process can be represented by following scheme:

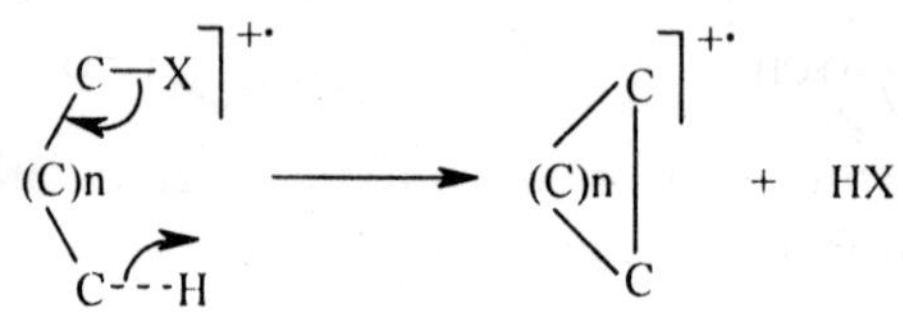

where X = Cl, Br, I, OH, OR, OCOR, NH_2, NR_2, SH.

The number of carbons atoms between the two groups undergoing elimination (H and X) can vary but for every atom of X there is a preferred value. In other word, the hydrogen atom that is eliminated must have a precise steric relationship with the X.

For example, alcohol shows the M–H_2O peak due to elimination-reaction. The present reaction shows 1,4-elimination reaction to exhibit the loss of water.

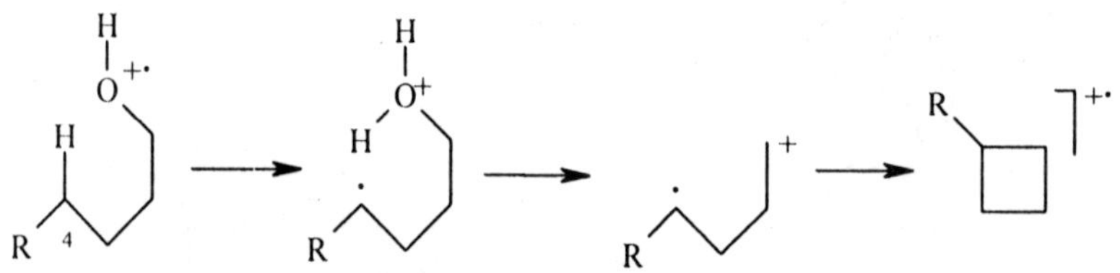

In the cyclic alcohol the elimination of H_2O has much more complex route. In cyclohexanol (Scheme 5.1), for example, the introduction of a deuterium atom in positions 2, 3 or 4 demonstrate that the eliminated hydrogen atom comes from position 3 or 4 because of the conformation of the ring.

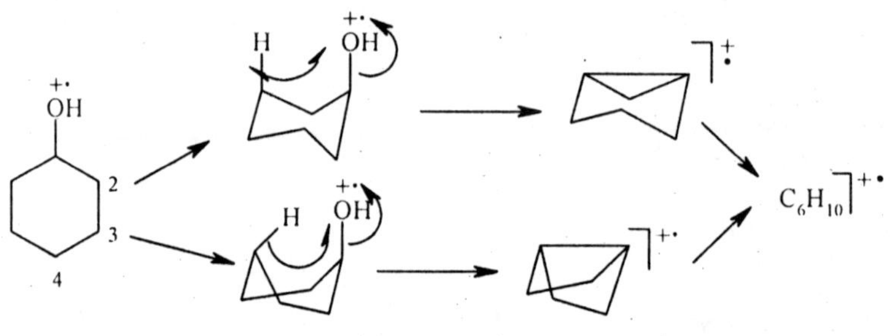

Scheme 5.1. Fragmentation pathway in cyclohexanol.

Similarly, there is elimination of hydrogen chloride/bromide in alkyl chloride/bromide.

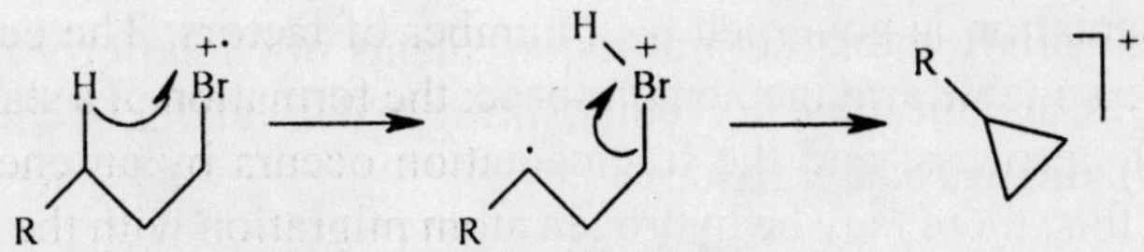

5.4.3.2 Ortho effect

Ortho disubstituted aromatic system or cis olefins can give rise to the specific migration of a hydrogen atom onto an atom or group that is eliminated in a form of neutral molecule.

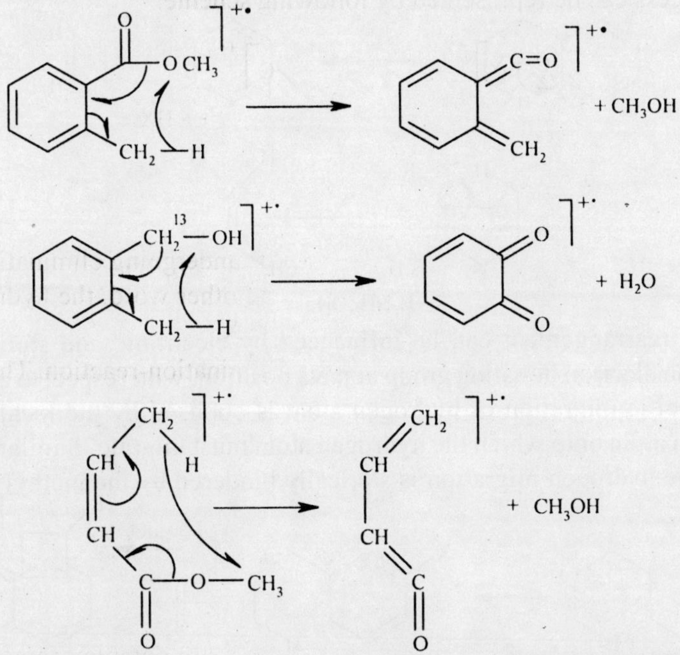

It is useful to distinguish between cis and trans compounds and o, m and p-isomers.

5.4.3.3 MacLafferty rearrangement

This fragmentation mode is characteristic of ketones, aldehydes, acids, esters, amides.

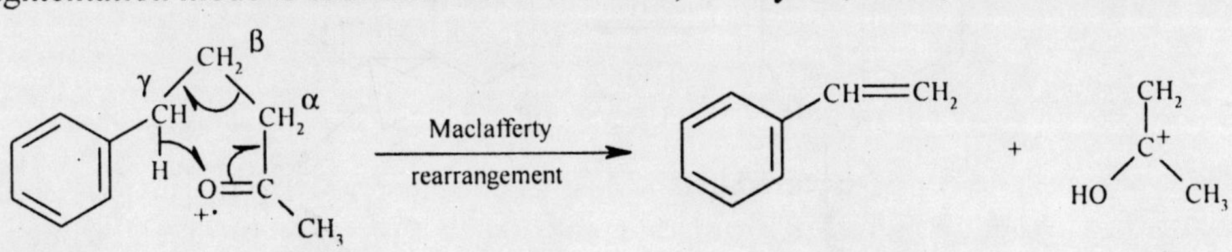

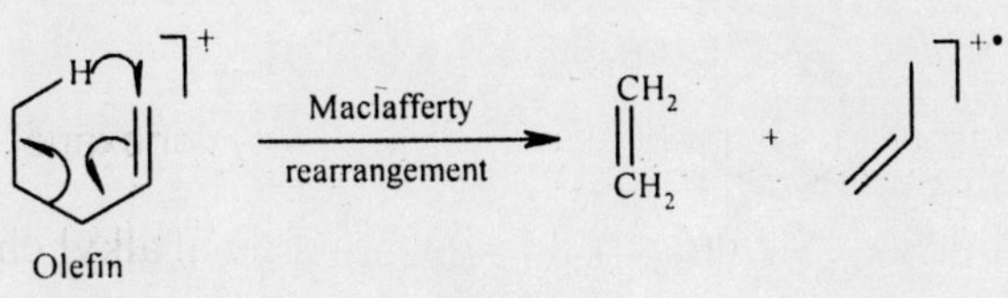

Other molecules that satisfy the structural requirements of Mclafferty rearrangement are the olefins, the alkyl benzenes, and the alkyl aryl ether, nitrogen derivatives of carbonyl group (oximes, hydrazones, and imines), nitriles and epoxides.

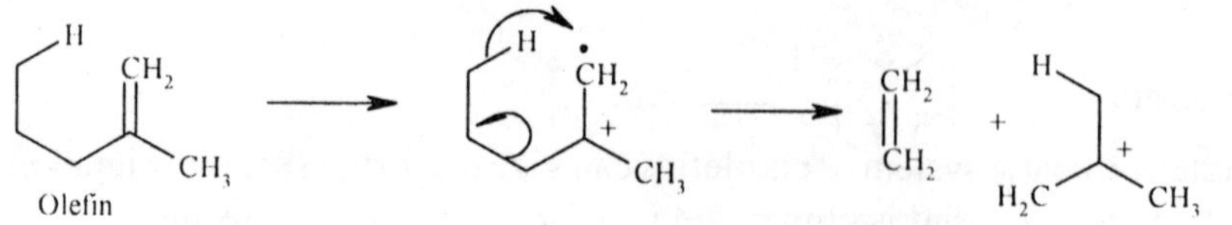

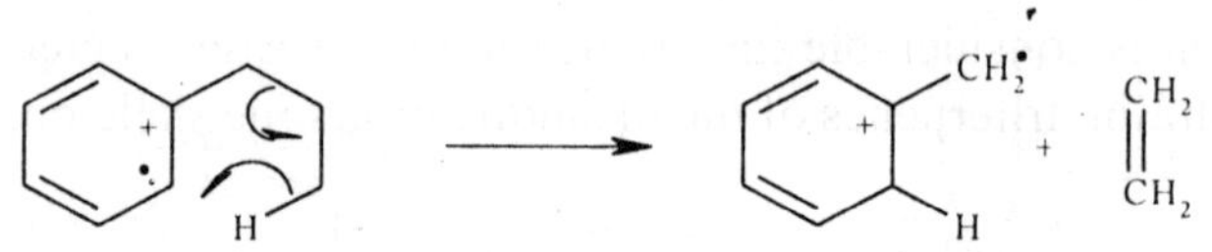

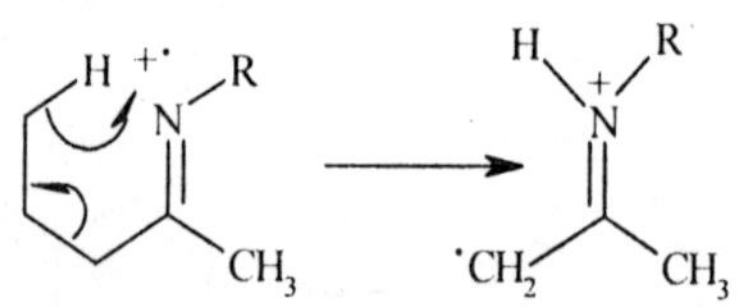

R = H, NH_2, OH

The McLafferty rearrangement can be influenced by electronic and steric factors. In alkyl benzenes that have an electron donating group at meta position, with respect to alkyl side chain, the tendency of the specific migration of hydrogen atom is opposed by the localization of positive charge on the carbon atom onto which the hydrogen atom must migrate. Similarly ,in a compound, in which R=CH_3, the hydrogen migration is sterically hindered by the methyl group in the ortho position.

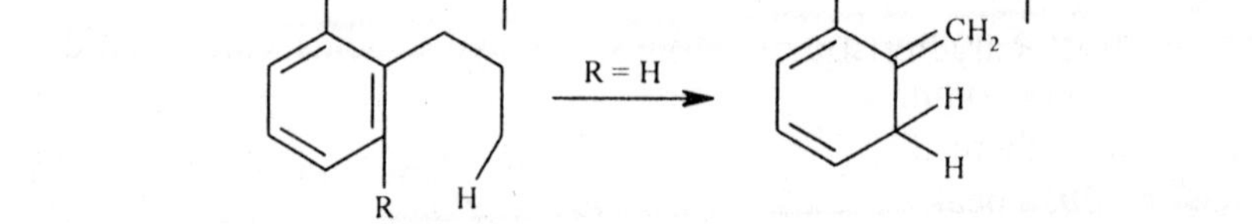

X = Electron donor

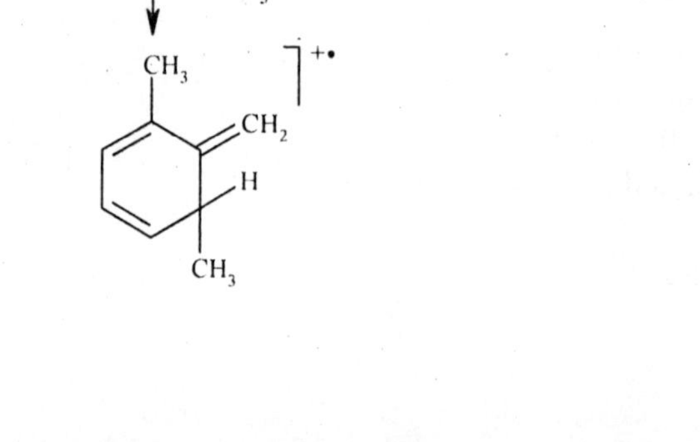

5.4.3.4 Retro Diels-Alder reaction

This multi centre fragmentation is very common in mass spectrum of cyclic olefins. Usually, a positively charged, diene fragment and a neutral olefinic fragment are formed.

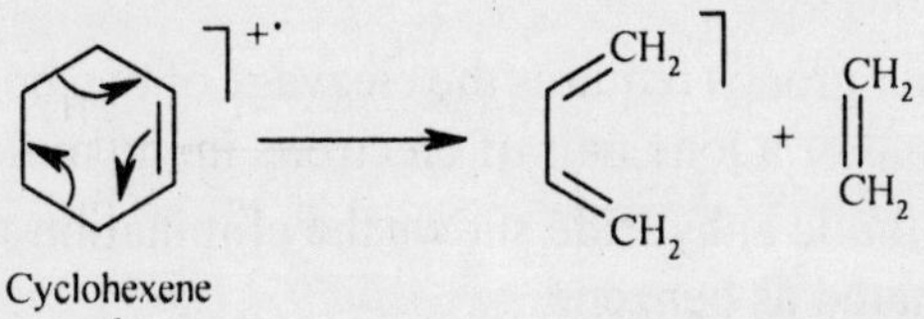

Cyclohexene

This type of reaction is considerable importance in the structural-determination of numerous compounds, such as tetralin, triterpenes of the oleanolic or ursolic skeleton.

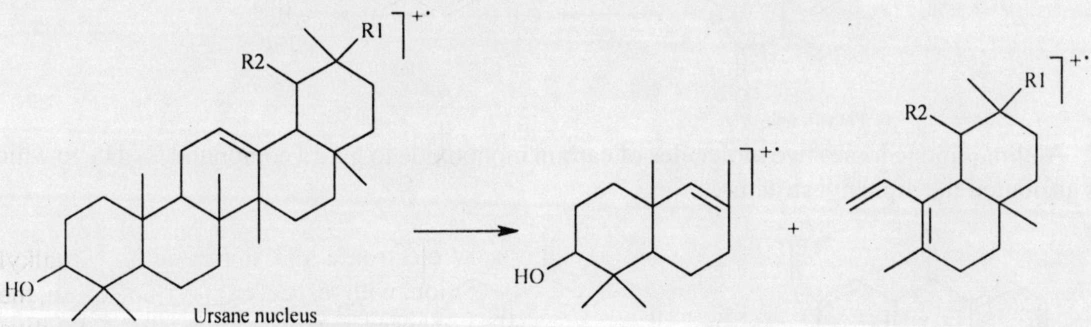

Ursane nucleus

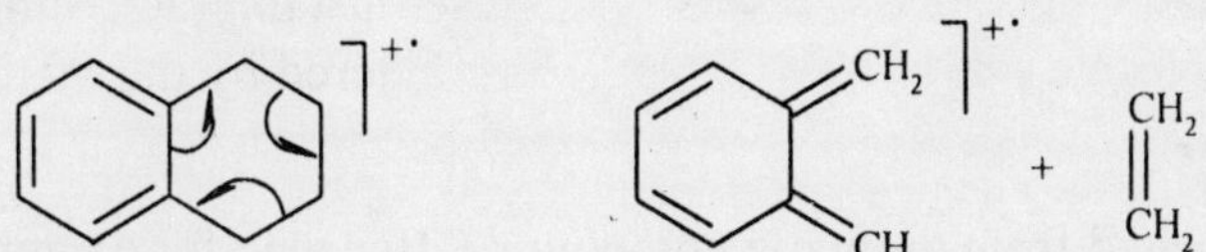

Tetralin

5.4.3.5 Hydrogen migration

The MacLafferty rearrangement and the elimination of HX are the examples of the specific migration of hydrogen atoms or groups of atoms with the expulsion of a neutral molecule.

In the mass spectrum of a complex molecule, the migration of a different type from those mentioned above is also a very common fragmentation process. Some processes are not specific, as in saturated hydrocarbons where there is complete randomization of hydrogen. The spectrum neopentane shows at m/e 29, a peak attributed to an ethyl group that is not present in the molecule.

5.4.3.6 Expulsion of a stable neutral molecule

Expulsion of neutral molecules like CO, CO_2, N_2, SO_2, $CH_2 = C{=}O$, $CH_2 = CH_2$ and $CH \equiv CH$ has a considerable importance in the course of a fragmentation. The expulsion of ketene and ethylene occurs in general through the hydrogen migration reaction, as already shown in McLafferty rearrangement for ethylene, and as indicated in the following reaction of an acetate to alcohol and to form ketene.

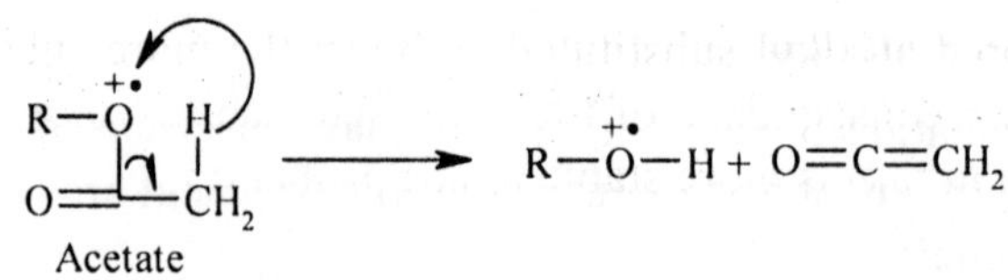

The elimination of the other groups requires the cleavage of two bonds without hydrogen transfer and the formation of new bond or a lone pair of electrons in the molecule that is eliminated.

The mass spectrum of phthalic anhydride shows the elimination first of CO_2 and then of CO to give an ion at m/e 76, designated as benzene.

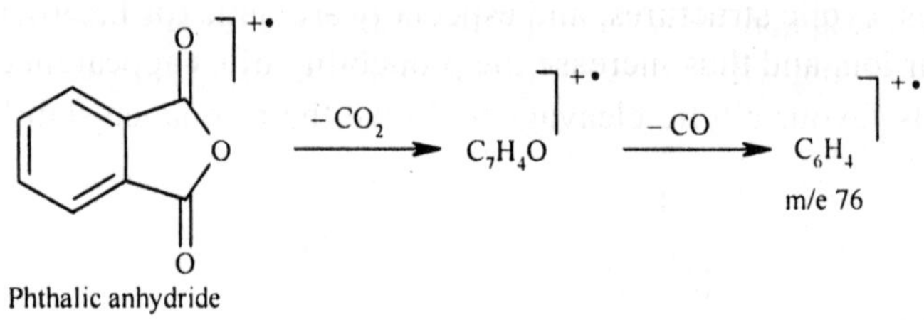

Anthraquinone losses two molecules of carbon monooxide to give a compound $C_{12}H_{10}$ to which is attributed the diphenyl structure.

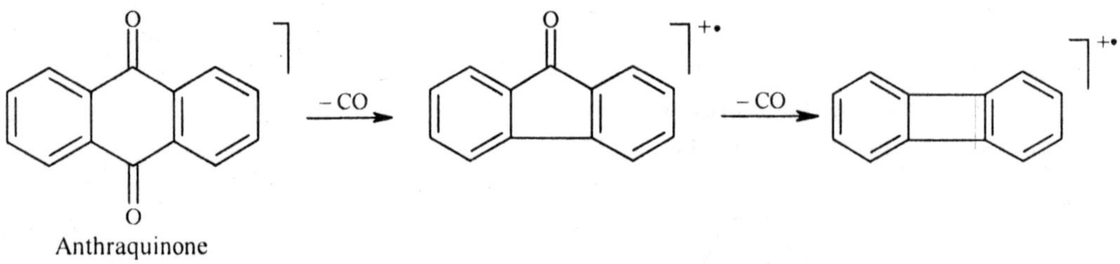

Acetylene is eliminated from aromatic compounds. Benzene for example, loses a molecule of acetylene, but it is not possible to assign a reliable mechanism from this reaction. It seems that the molecular ion of benzene should be represented by the open chain form and not the cyclic form.

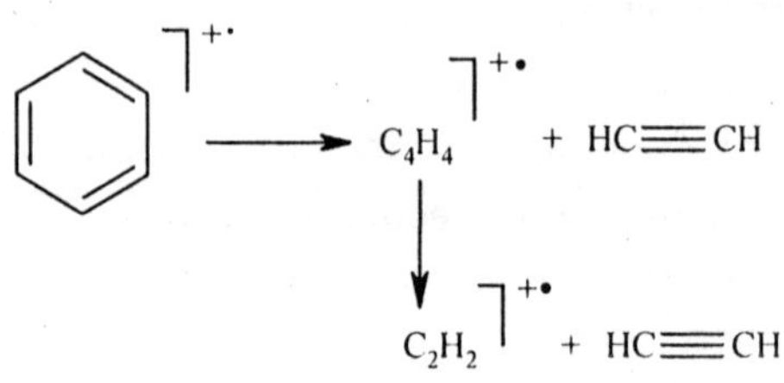

5.5 HANDY RULES OF FRAGMENTATION

A number of general rules for predicting prominent peaks in electron- impact spectra can be written and rationalized by using standard concepts of physical organic chemistry:

1. The relative height of the molecular ion peak is greatest for the straight-chain compound and decreases as the degree of branching increases (See Rule 3).
2. The relative height of the molecular ion peak usually decreases with increasing molecular weight in a homologous series. Fatty esters appear to be an exception.

3. Cleavage is favored at alkyl substituted carbons; the more substituted, the more likely is cleavage. This is a consequence of the increased stability of a tertiary carbocation over a secondary, which in turn is more stable than a primary:

   Cation stability order:

$$CH_3^+ < RCH_2^+ < R_2CH^+ < R_3C^+$$

   Generally, the largest substituent at a branch is eliminated most readily as a radical, presumably because a long-chain radical can achieve some stability by delocalization of the lone electron.
4. Double bonds, cyclic structures, and especially aromatic (or heteroaromatic) rings stabilize the molecular ion, and thus increase the probability of its appearance.
5. Double bonds favour allylic cleavage and give the resonance-stabilized allylic carbonium ion.

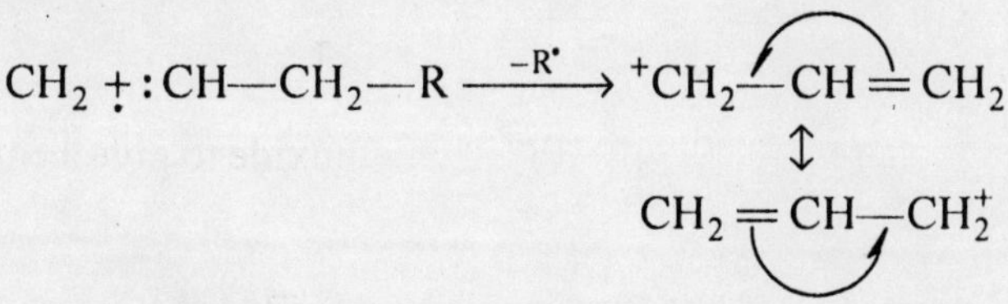

6. Saturated rings tend to lose side chains at the a-bond. This is merely a special case of branching (Rule 3). The positive-charge tends to stay with the ring fragment. Unsaturated rings can undergo a *retro*-Diels-Alder reaction:

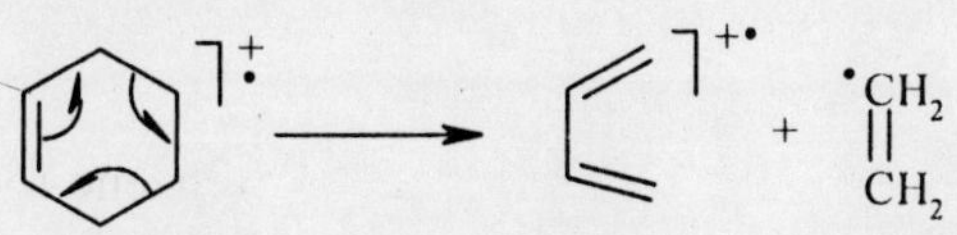

7. In alkyl-substituted aromatic compounds, cleavage is very probable at the bond beta to the ring, giving the resonance-stabilized benzyl ion or, more likely, the tropylium ion:

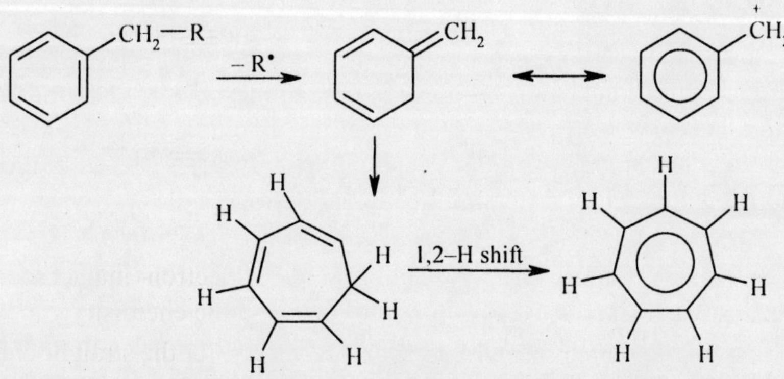

8. C–C bonds next to a heteroatom (Y) are frequently cleaved, leaving the charge on the fragment containing the heteroatom whose nonbonding electrons provide resonance stabilization.

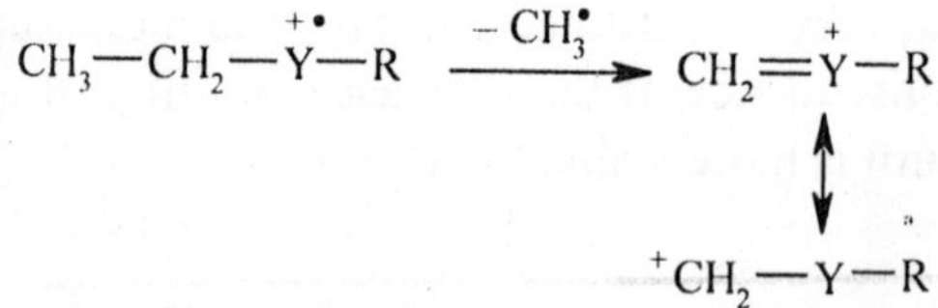

Y = O, N or S

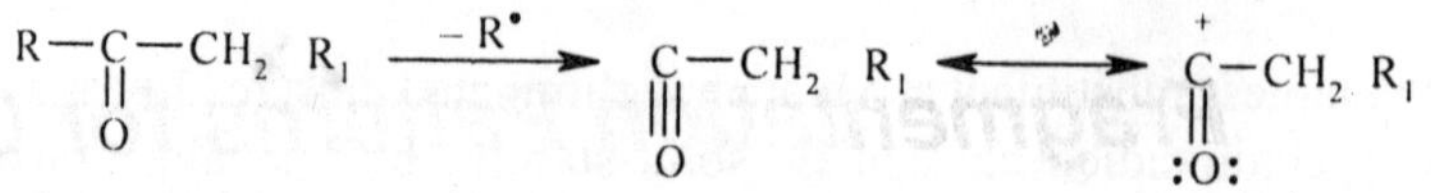

9. Cleavage is often associated with elimination of small stable neutral molecules, such as carbon monoxide, olefins, water, ammonia, hydrogen sulphide, hydrogen cyanide, mercaptans, ketene, or alcohols.

CHAPTER

6

Fragmentation Patterns for Organic Functional Groups

Organic molecules fragment in very specific ways depending upon the functional groups present in the molecule. These fragments (if positively charged) are detected in mass spectrometry. The presence or absence of various mass peaks in the spectrum can be used to deduce the structure of the compound in question. This chapter illustrates fragmentation pathways for the major classes of organic functional groups. On the basis of these fragmentation pathways, a great deal of structural informations from the mass spectrum can be deduced.

6.1 HYDROCARBON

6.1.1 Saturated hydrocarbon

The mass spectrum of saturated hydrocarbons (Fig. 6.1, hexane) shows detectable molecular ion peak. The spectrum generally consists of a number of even-electron fragment ions formed by expulsion of a radical (often a methyl group) from the molecular ion, followed by loss of ethene due to the fission process shown Scheme 6.1

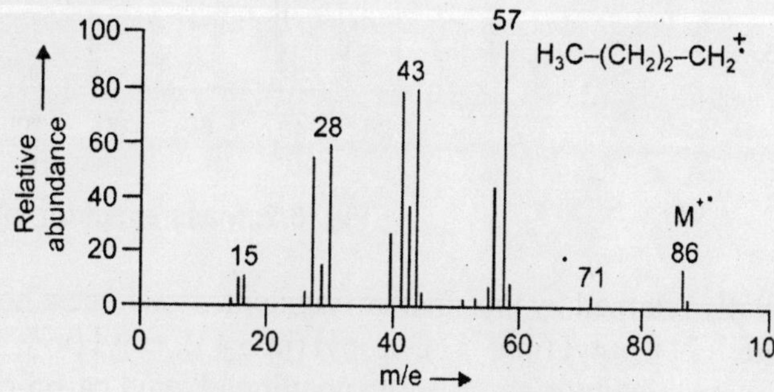

Fig. 6.1. Mass spectrum of Hexane.

This example also serves to demonstrate the *Even Electron Rule* for fragmentation of cations and cation-radicals; odd electron ions decompose by loss of radicals or even electron molecules, while even-electron ions decompose by loss of even-electron molecules.

The mass spectrum of dodecane (Fig. 6.2) illustrates the behavior of a long chain aliphatic hydrocarbon. The molecular ion peak of this straight long chain hydrocarbon is always present, though of low intensity in comparison to hexane. Since there is no heteroatom in this molecule, there are no non-bonding valence shell electrons. Consequently, the radical cation character of the molecular ion (m/e 170) is delocalized over all the covalent bonds. Fragmentation of C-C bonds will take place to produce a mixture of alkyl radicals and alkyl cations. The positive charge is

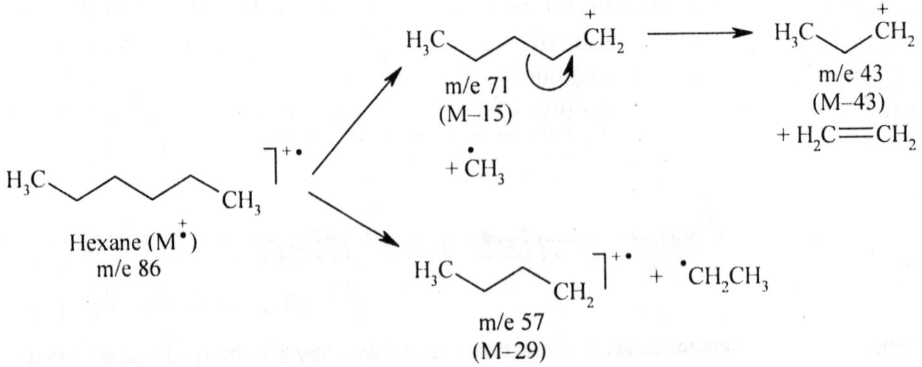

Scheme 6.1. Fragmentation pattern for Hexane.

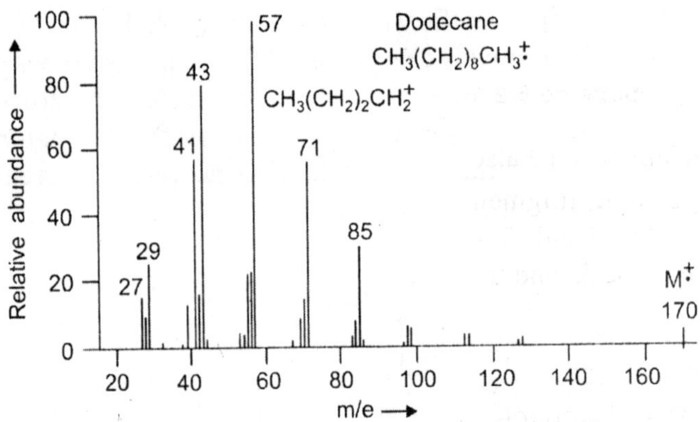

Fig. 6.2. Mass spectrum of Dodecane.

usually retained by the smaller fragment, so we see a homologous series of hexyl (m/e 85), pentyl (m/e = 71), butyl (m/e 57), propyl (m/e 43), ethyl (m/e 29) and methyl (m/e 15) cations. These are accompanied by a set of corresponding alkenyl carbo-cations (e.g. m/e 55, 41 and 27) formed by loss of 2 H. In most alkane spectra the propyl (C3) and butyl (C4) ions are the most abundant.

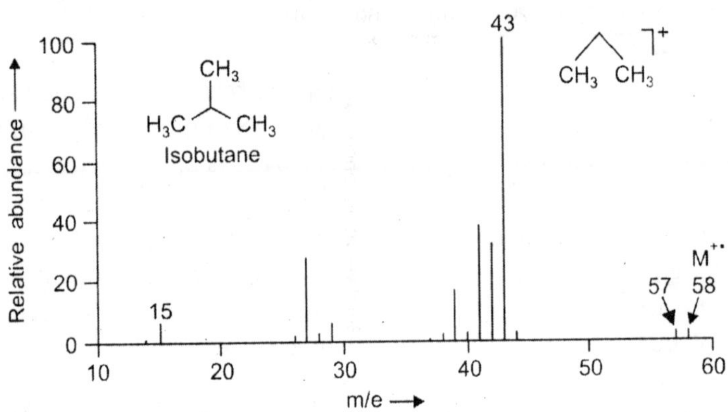

Fig. 6.3. Mass spectrum of Isobutane.

6.1.2 Branched Hydrocarbon

Spectra of branched saturated hydrocarbons are generally similar to those of straight-chain compounds, but the smooth curve of decreasing intensities is broken by the preferred fragmentation at each branch. This is due to the formation of stable secondary and tertiary carbocations. For this reason, the molecular ion is much less abundant than for straight-chain alkanes. The most important mode of fragmentation in branched alkanes usually occurs at the branch point. In the mass spectrum of isobutane (Fig. 6.3), there is reduced intensity of the molecular ion peak (m/e 58). The Scheme 6.2 below shows the mechanism of fragmentation of isobutane.

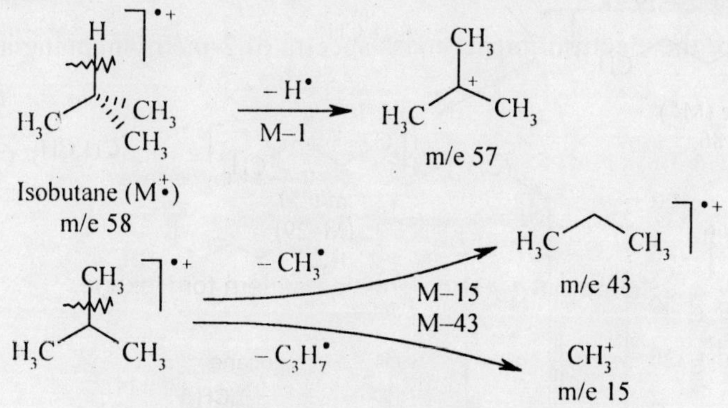

Scheme 6.2. Fragmentation pattern for Isobutane

The effect of branching can be also shown with the example of isomeric hexanes (Fig. 6.4).

Hexane shows the same fragmentation pattern as other unbranched alkanes. Thus, alkyl carbocations at m/e 15, 29, 43 and 57 provide the dominant peaks in the spectrum. The m/e 57 butyl cation (M-29) is the base peak, and the m/e 43 and 29 ions are also abundant.

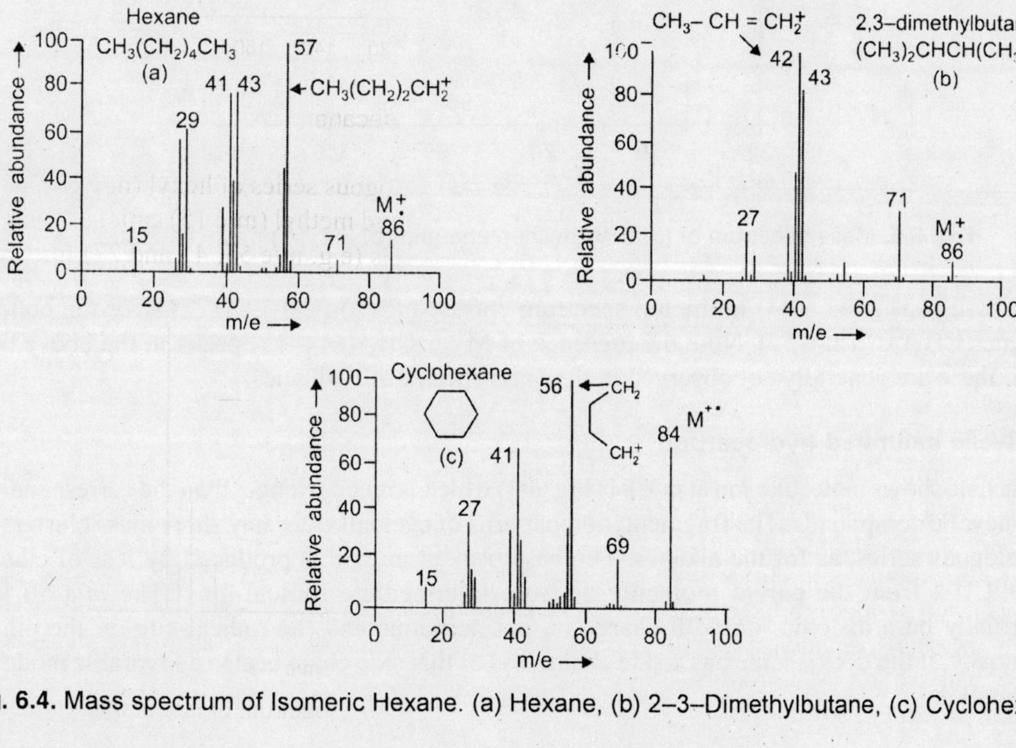

Fig. 6.4. Mass spectrum of Isomeric Hexane. (a) Hexane, (b) 2–3–Dimethylbutane, (c) Cyclohexane.

Chain branching clearly influences the fragmentation of this isomeric hexane. The molecular ion at m/e 86 is weaker than that for hexane itself and the M-15 ion at m/e 71 is stronger. The m/e 57 ion is almost absent (try to find a simple cleavage that gives a butyl group). An isopropyl cation (m/e 43) is very strong, and the corresponding propene radical-cation at m/e 42, produced by loss of propane, gives the base peak.

Similarly, compare the electron impact mass spectra of 2-methylheptane and 2,2,3-trimethylpentane (Fig. 6.5).

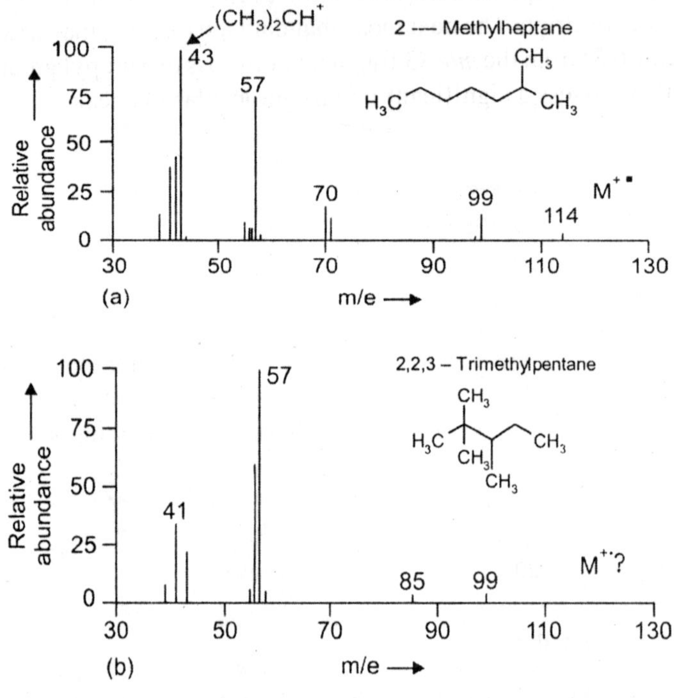

Fig. 6.5. Mass spectrum of (a) 2-Methylheptane and (b) 2,2,3-Trimethylpentane.

The base peak (m/e = 43) in the top spectrum corresponds to $(CH_3)_2CH^+$ and for the bottom spectrum, $(CH_3)_3C^+$ (m/e 57). Note the presence of $M^{+\bullet} - CH_3^{\bullet}$ (M – 15) peaks in the above two spectra: these are generally not observed in the mass spectra of *n*-alkanes.

6.1.3 Cyclic saturated hydrocarbon

Cyclohexane shows molecular ion at m/e 84 (Fig. 6.4) which is much stronger than the corresponding ions in acyclic compounds. The fragmentation patterns of cycloalkenes may show mass clusters in a homologous series, as for the alkanes. The base peak at m/e 56 is produced by loss of ethene ($CH_2 = CH_2$) from the parent molecule or from intermediate radical-ions. The *m/e* 56 ion may initially be a distonic ion with charge on one terminus and the radical site on the other. Additionally, if the cycloalkane has a side chain, loss of that side chain is also a favorable mode of fragmentation.

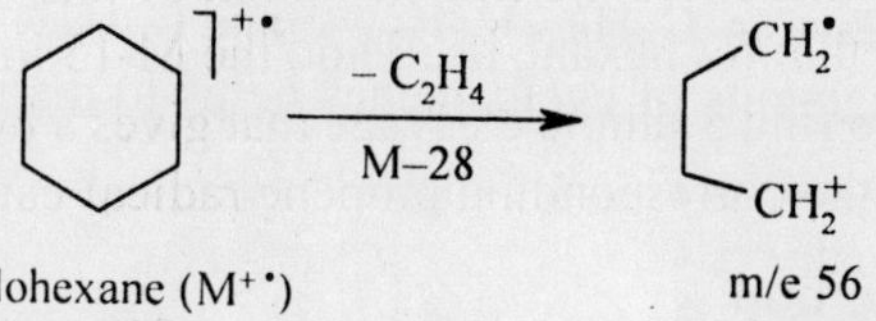

The Fig. 6.6 contains the mass spectrum of methyl cyclohexane. Note that the loss of the methyl side chain is perhaps the most important fragmentation event, and the M–15 ion of *m/e* 83 gives the most intense signal in the spectrum. The next most abundant ion (*m/e* 55) may arise by the subsequent loss of ethylene (Scheme 6.3) from the *m/e* 83 fragment or by loss of a propyl group via rearrangement but it is not clear. It also possess a significant intense molecular ion peak.

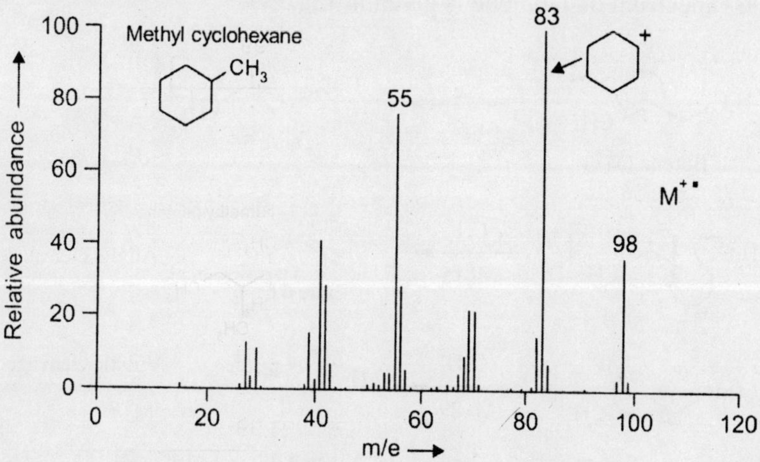

Fig. 6.6. Mass spectrum of Methyl cyclohexane.

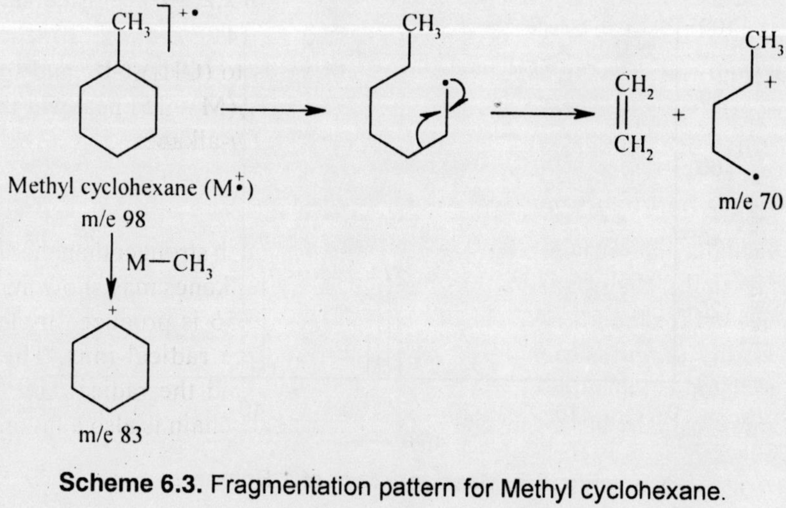

Scheme 6.3. Fragmentation pattern for Methyl cyclohexane.

Cycloalkanes tend to cleave in $C_nH_{2n}^+$, $C_nH_{2n-1}^+$, and $C_nH_{2n-2}^+$ fragments. The larger number of even numbered mass fragments of cycloalkenes helps to distinguish this class of compounds from the acyclic alkanes.

6.1.4 Unsaturated hydrocarbon

6.1.4.1 Alkene

The mass spectra of most alkenes show distinct molecular ions. This is probably due to the loss of a π-bonding electron, leaving the carbon skeleton relatively undisturbed. The most important fragmentation events for alkenes involve cleavage of the allylic (favored) and vinylic (less favored) carbon-carbon bonds. For terminal alkenes, allylic fragmentation forms an allylic carbocation of *m/e* 41. The fragmentation mechanism for 1-butene shown in Scheme 6.4 illustrates these points. The complete mass spectrum of 1-butene is given in Fig. 6.7.

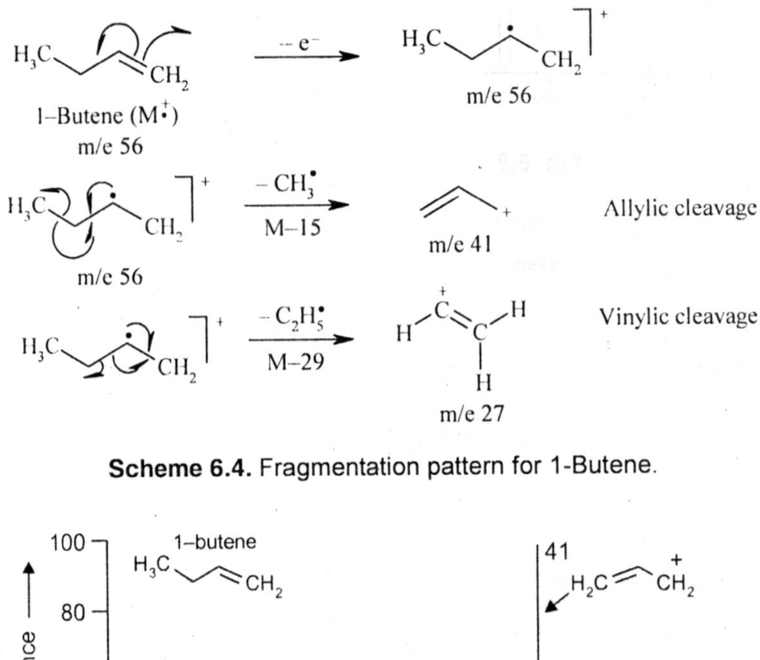

Scheme 6.4. Fragmentation pattern for 1-Butene.

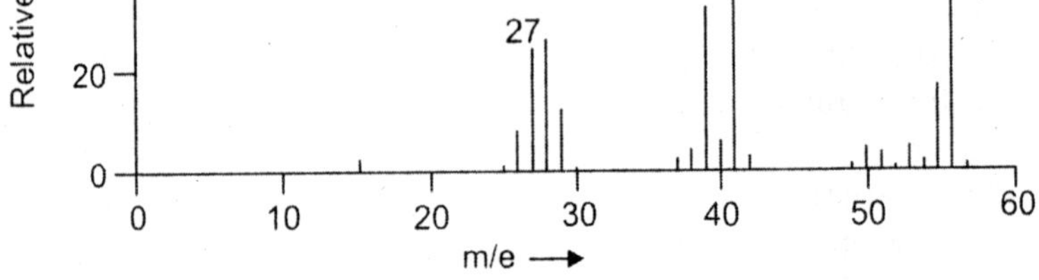

Fig. 6.7. Mass spectrum of 1-Butene

Alkenes usually form fragments corresponding to $C_nH_{2n+1}^+$, $C_nH_{2n}^{+\cdot}$, and $C_nH_{2n-1}^+$ (the latter two fragment ion series are more abundant). It is very difficult to locate the position of the double bond in an alkene because of the easy migration of the double bond by hydride and hydrogen atom shifts. For this reason, the mass spectra of alkene isomers are nearly identical and almost impossible to distinguish, as is illustrated in Fig. 6.8 and 6.9, which contains the mass spectra for 2- and 3-heptene, respectively.

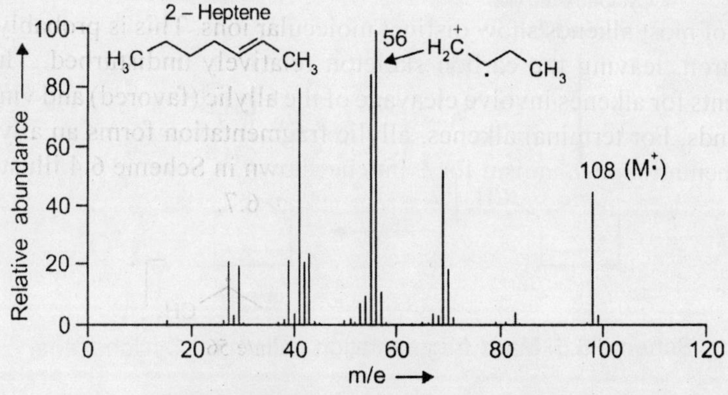

Fig. 6.8. Mass spectrum of 2-heptene

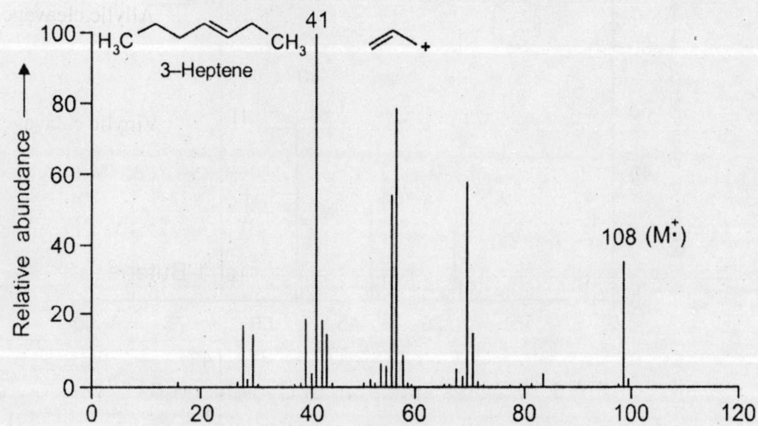

Fig. 6.9. Mass spectra of 3-Heptene.

6.1.4.2 Cyclic alkene

The mass spectra of cyclic alkenes show distinct molecular ions. It may be impossible to locate the position of a double bond due to migration. The mechanism of fragmentation for cyclic alkenes is virtually the same as for straight chain alkenes. One noteworthy characteristic is the fragmentation of cyclic hexene to undergo a reverse Diels-Alder reaction as indicated in Scheme 6.5 This rearrangement is characteristic of many isoprenoid natural products and of tetralin derivatives, and is useful for assigning structure and distinguishing isomers. Here, product ion enthalpy governs the dissociation pathway. The fragment with the lowest ionization energy (IE) will preferentially take the charge. The difference in activation energy equals the difference in IE. The complete mass spectrum of cyclohexene is given in Fig 6.10.

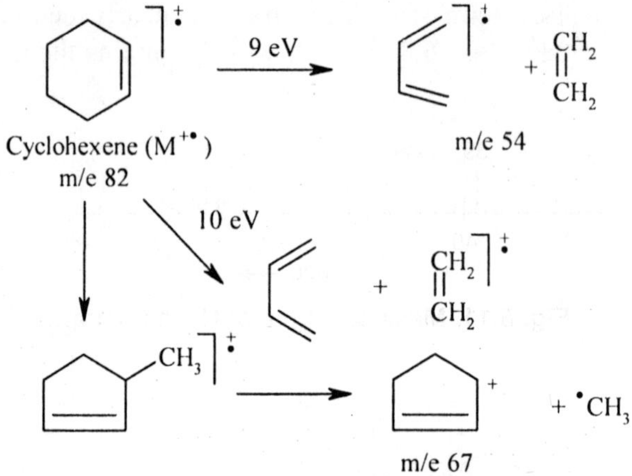

Scheme 6.5. Mass fragmentation pattern for Cyclohexene.

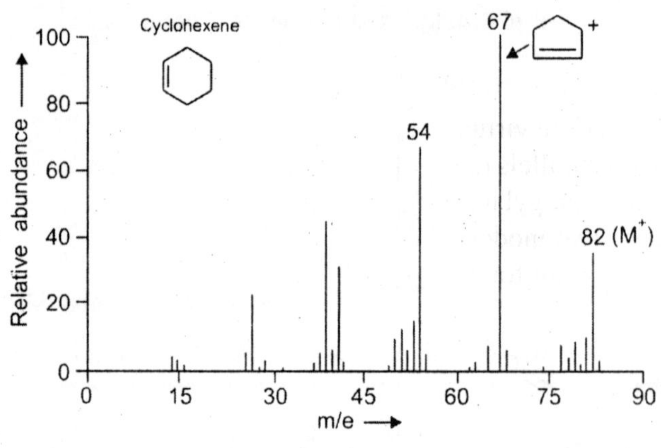

Fig 6.10. Mass spectrum of Cyclohexene

Similarly, Methyl cyclohexene shows the fragmentation as per Scheme 6.6.

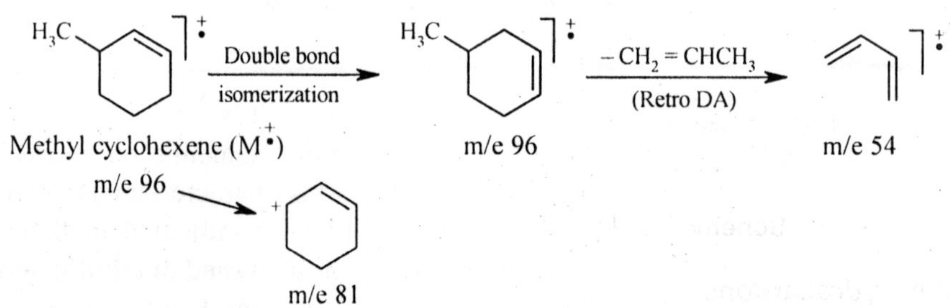

Scheme 6.6. Fragmentation pattern for Methyl cyclohexene.

Norbornene (Fig 6.11) also shows the formation of diene with the release of olefin.

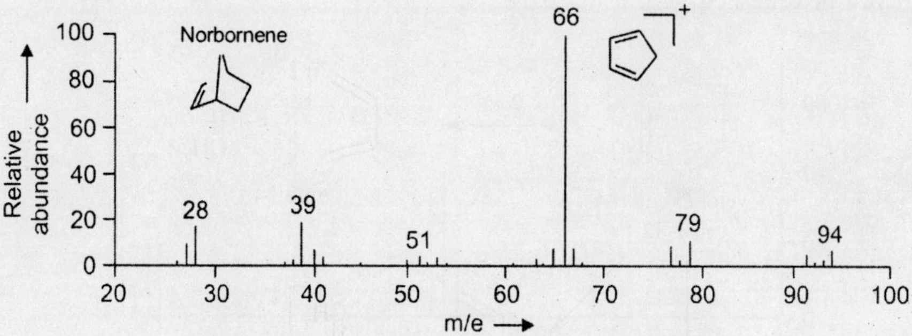

Fig. 6.11. Mass spectrum of Neobornene.

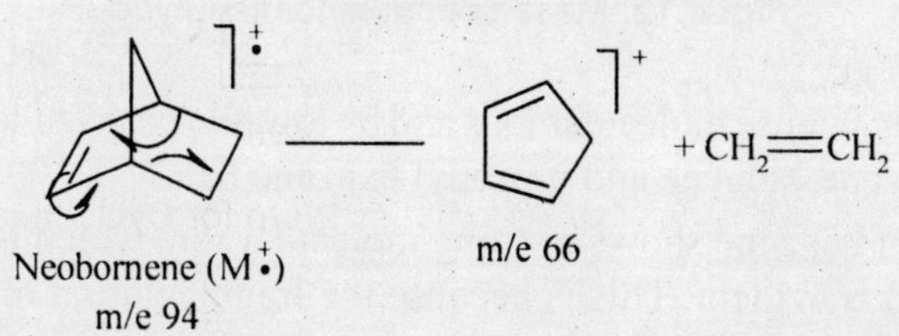

6.1.4.3 Alkynes

The mass spectra of alkynes are virtually identical to those of alkenes. The molecular ion peak is intense, and fragmentation parallels to the alkenes. Two differences are worth mentioning: terminal alkynes fragment to form propargyl ions (m/e 39), and can also lose the terminal hydrogen, yielding a strong M–1 peak. These two modes of fragmentation are outlined in Scheme 6.7 for 1–butyne, and the complete mass spectrum for 1–butyne is given in Fig. 6.12.

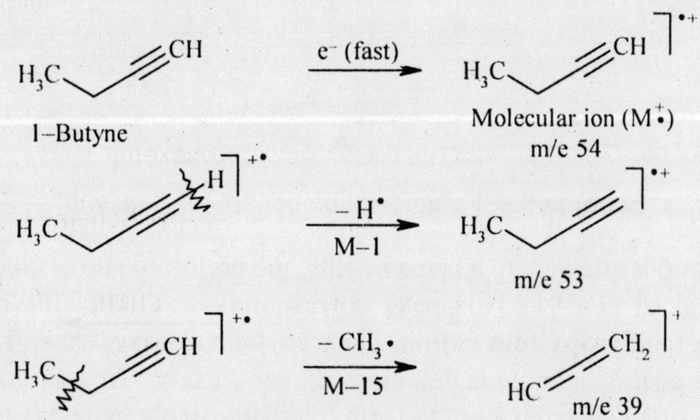

Scheme 6.7. Fragmentation pattern for 1-Butyne.

6.1.5 Aromatic Hydrocarbons

Unlike other hydrocarbons, the mass spectra of aromatic hydrocarbons are characterized by the

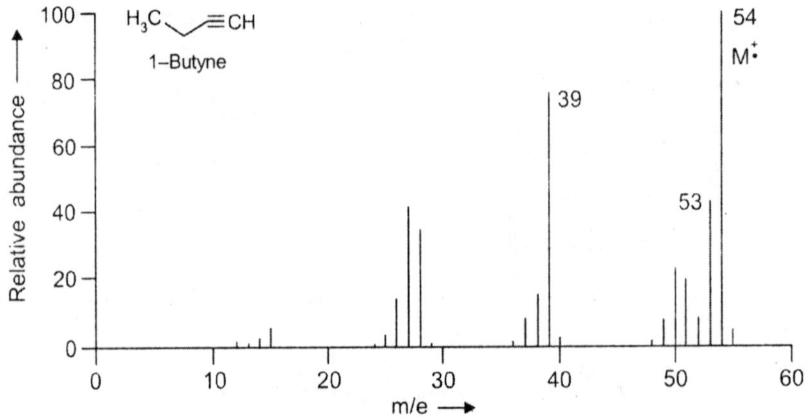

Fig. 6.12. Mass spectrum for 1-Butyne.

presence of comparatively intense molecular ions and by low m/e peaks of low intensity, as illustrated by the EI spectra of benzene, toluene and n-propyl benzene below.

The mass spectrum of benzene shows a strong molecular ion, which is the base peak, and little additional fragmentation is evident. This is because the fragmentation of a benzene ring is a high energy process and simple pathways for the formation of stable ions do not exist. However, some detectable peaks (Fig 6.13) are evident as shown in Scheme 6.8.

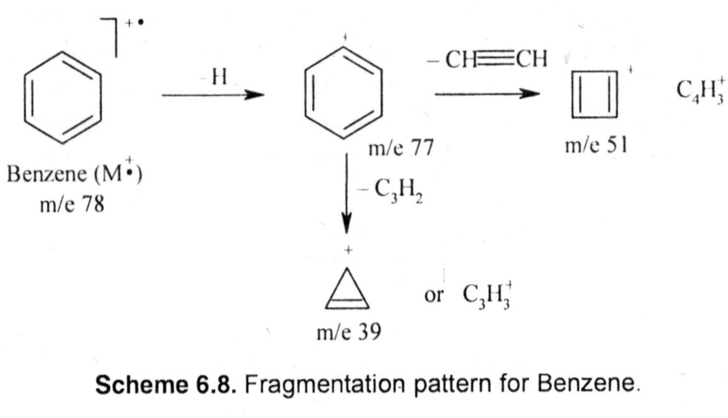

Scheme 6.8. Fragmentation pattern for Benzene.

When an alkyl group is attached to a benzene ring, the preferred site of cleavage is at the benzyl carbon to give a peak at *m/e* 91. This peak corresponds to $C_7H_7^+$, the benzyl cation, or its rearrangement product, the **tropylium cation**. The tropylium cation is exceptionally stable because it is aromatic and the positive charge is delocalized over all seven ring carbons. The base peak in toluene is due to loss of a hydrogen atom to form relatively stable benzyl cation which undergoes rearrangement to form the very stable tropylium cation.. The frequently observed peak at m/e 65 is due to the loss of neutral acetylene from the tropylium ion and the minor peaks below this arise from more complex fragmentation (Scheme 6.9).

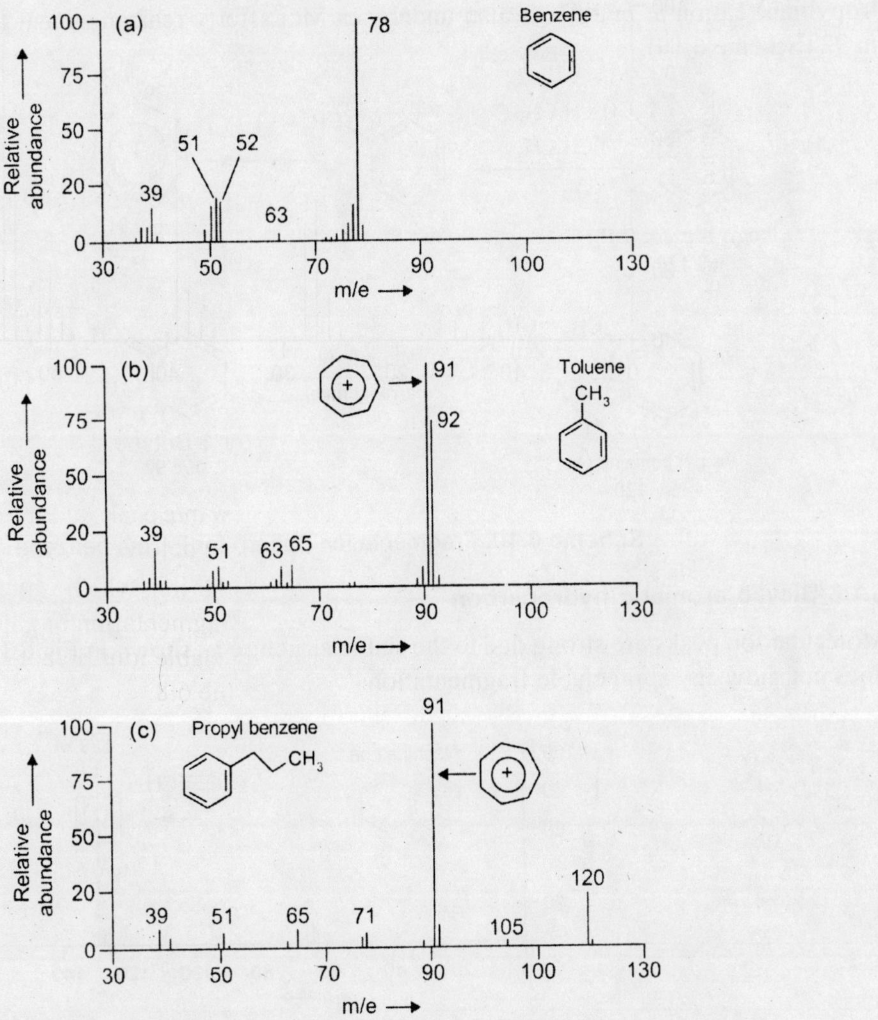

Fig. 6.13. Mass spectrum of (a) Benzene, (b) Toluene and (c) Propyl benzene.

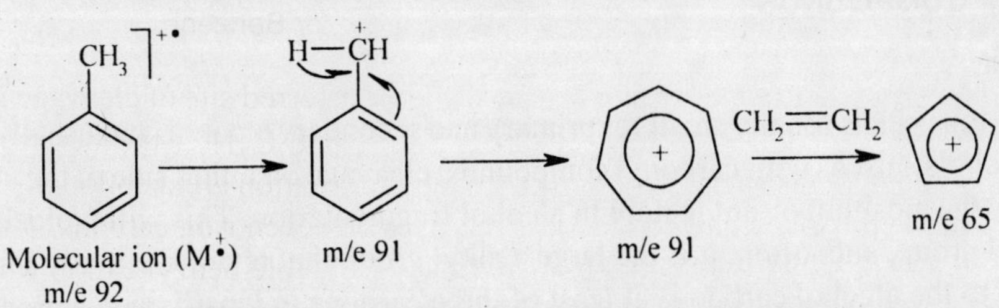

Scheme 6.9. Fragmentation pattern for Toluene.

The mass spectrum of propyl benzene is shown in Fig. 6.13. A decent molecular ion is evident at *m/e* 120, with the major cleavage being loss of an ethyl radical (M–29) to give the benzyl (or tropylium) cation at *m/e* 91. It also undergoes McLafferty rearrangement to exhibit the peak at m.92 (Scheme 6.10).

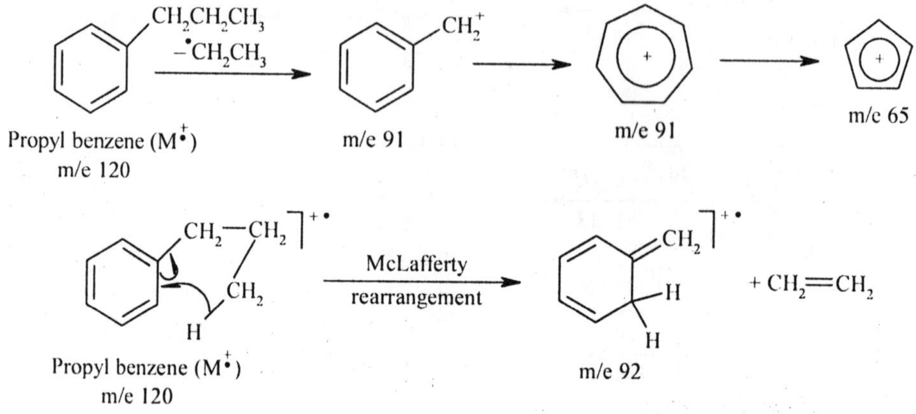

Scheme 6.10. Fragmentation pattern for Propyl benzene.

6.1.6 Bicylic aromatic hydrocarbon

Molecular ion peaks are strong due to the stable structure as shown in Fig 6.14 for naphthalene. It does not show any appreciable fragmentation.

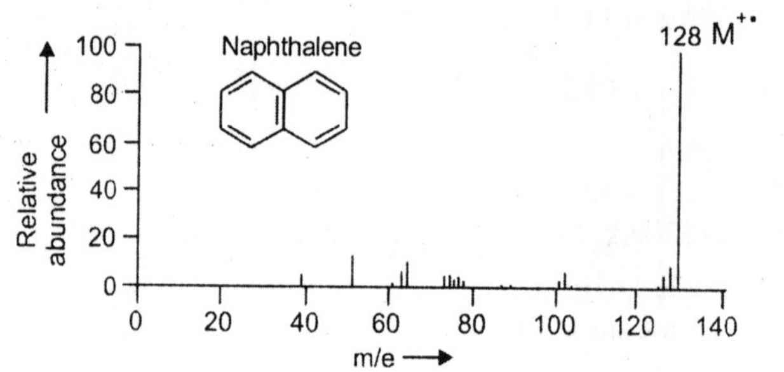

Fig. 6.14. Mass spectrum of Naphthalene.

6.2 HYDROXY COMPOUNDS

6.2.1 Alcohols

The Molecular ion peak is usually small for primary and secondary alcohol, and usually undetectable for tertiary alcohols. Just as with carbonyl compounds, cleavage on either side of the alcohol carbon (α-cleavage) is the most important feature in alcohol fragmentation. This will typically involve the loss of an alkyl group, and, often, it is the largest alkyl group that is preferentially lost. If the alkyl chain attached to the alcohol carbon is at least of three carbons in length, then a process similar to McLafferty rearrangements seen for carbonyl compounds can take place. Transfer of a γ-hydrogen to the alcohol oxygen leads to the loss of water from the molecule. This dehydration can be a very important indication for the presence of alcohol functionality. The mechanism for alcohol fragmentation is given in Scheme 6.11 for 2–pentanol.

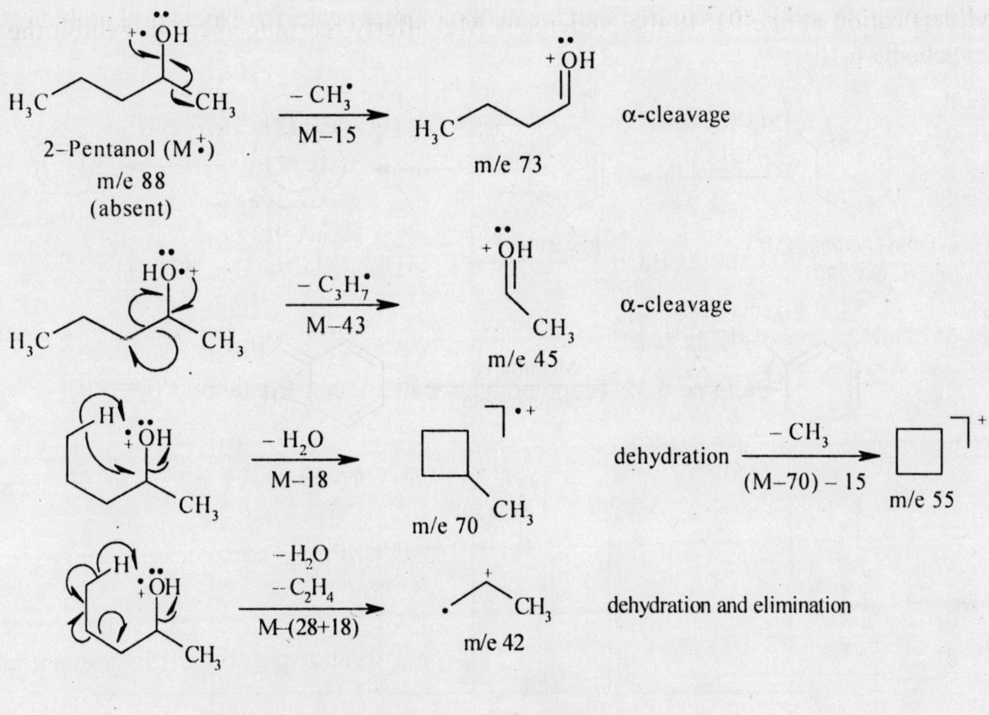

Scheme 6.11. Fragmentation pattern for 2-Pentanol.

The complete mass spectrum of 2-pentanol is given in Fig. 6.15, which illustrates most of these points.

t-Pentanol shows three significant fragment ions. Fragment due to α-cleavage (loss of an ethyl radical) forms the m/e 59 base peak. Loss of water from this gives a m/e = 41 fragment, and loss of ethene from m/e 59 gives a m/e 31 fragment (Scheme 6.13).

In mass spectrum, 1-Pentanol shows a peak at 70 (Fig 6.16). This is an [M-18] peak due to loss

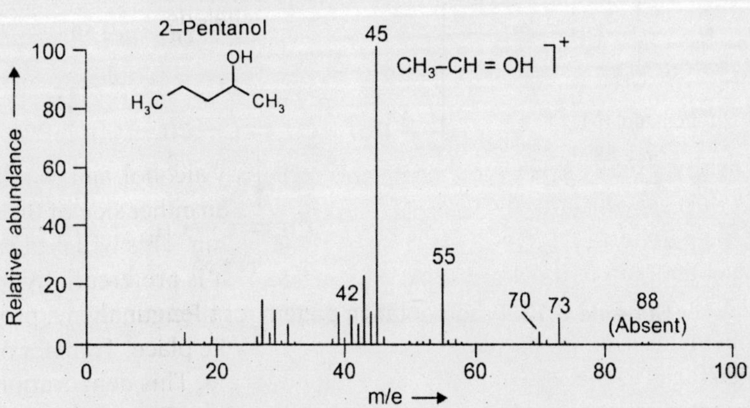

Fig. 6.15. Mass spectrum of 2-Pentanol.

of water molecule and is characteristic of an alcohol. Other peaks for 1-pentanol include at m/e 31 (Scheme 6.12).

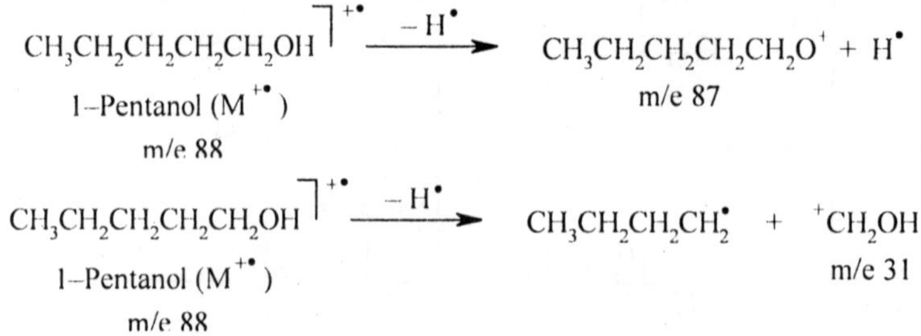

Scheme 6.12. Fragmentation pattern for 1-Pentanol.

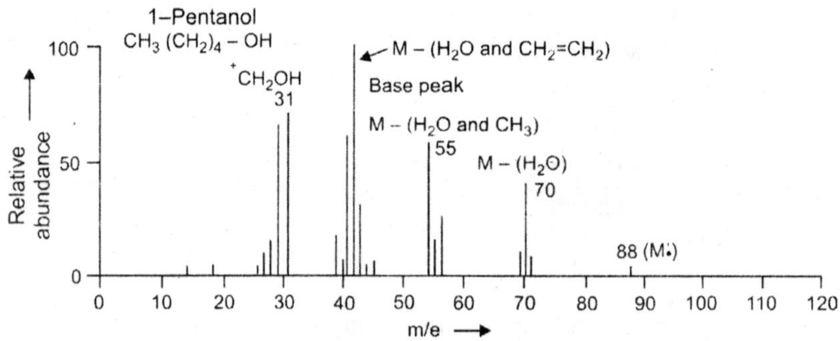

Fig. 6.16. Mass spectrum of 1-Pentanol

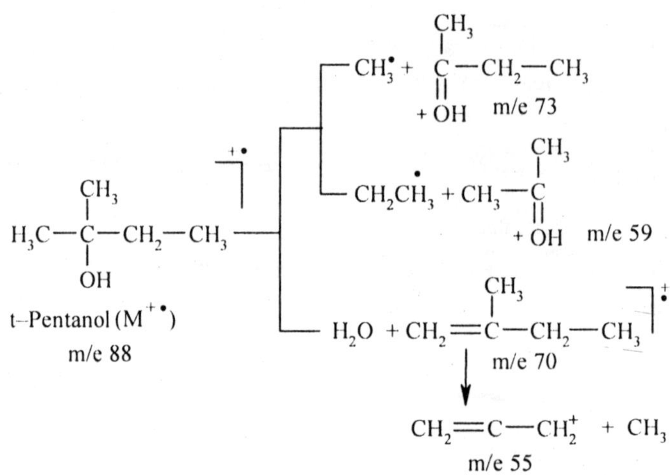

Scheme 6.13. Fragmentation pattern for t-Pentanol.

6.2.2 Cyclic alcohol

Cyclic alcohol (Fig. 6.17) undergoes fragmentation by at least three ways and these are exemplified with the spectrum of cyclohexanol. The first fragmentation is the α-cleavage and loss of hydrogen

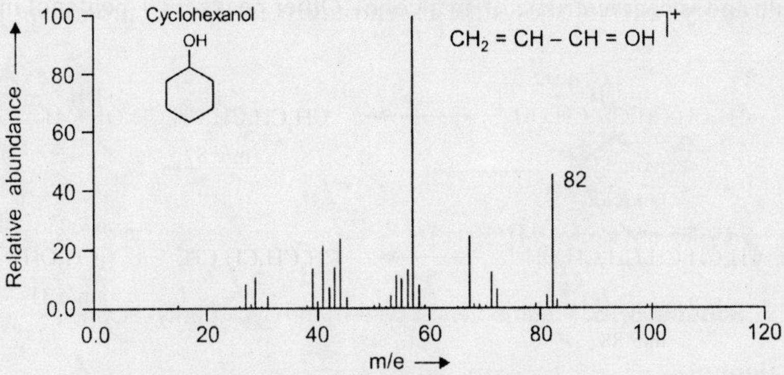

Fig. 6.17. Mass spectrum of cyclohexanol.

atom to give the M–1 peak. The second fragmentation path begins with initial alpha cleavage of a ring bond adjacent hydroxyl group bearing carbon atom followed by 1,5 hydrogen migration. This moves the radical site back to a resonance stabilized position adjacent to oxonium ion. A second α-cleavage results in loss of propyl radical and formation of a protonated acrolein ion with m/e 57. This fragmentation pathway is identical one that operates with cyclohexanone (Scheme 6.14). The third pathway is dehydration via abstraction of hydrogen atom from three or four carbon atoms away to produce bicyclic radical cations with m/e 82.

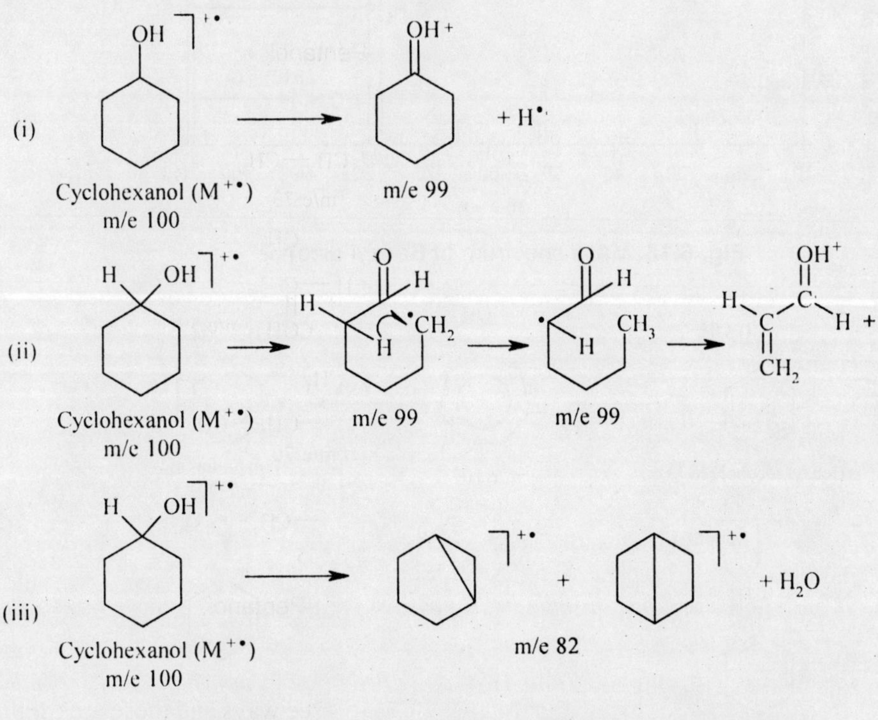

Scheme 6.14. Fragmentation pattern for Cyclohexanol.

Similarly, cyclopentyl alcohol shows the H-rearrangement for the prominent peak at m/e 57 (Scheme 6.15).

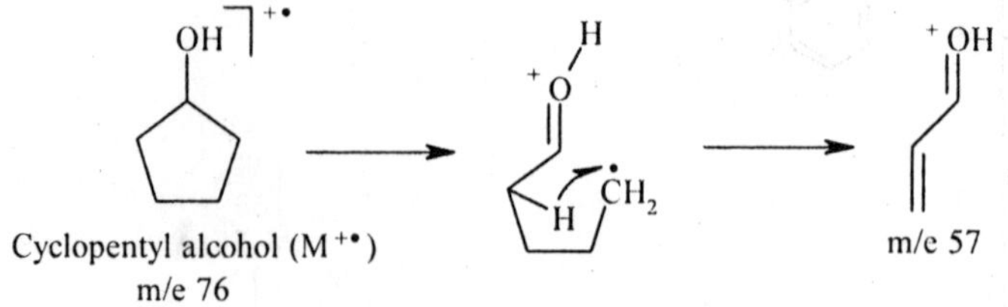

Scheme 6.15. Fragmentation pattern for Cyclopentyl alcohol.

6.2.3 Aromatic alcohol

The mass spectrum of benzyl alcohol (Fig. 6.18) shows the **molecular ion** at m/e 108. Fragmentation via loss of 17 (–OH) gives a common fragment seen for alkyl benzenes at m/e 91. Loss of 31 (–CH_2OH) from the molecular ion gives 77 corresponding to the phenyl cation (Scheme 6.16).

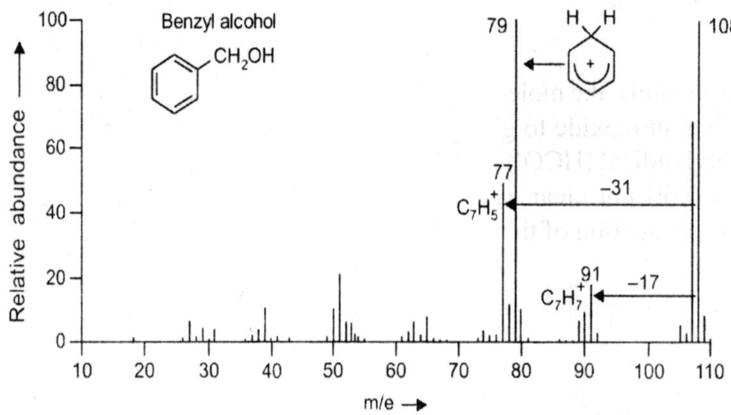

Fig. 6.18. Mass spectrum of Benzyl alcohol.

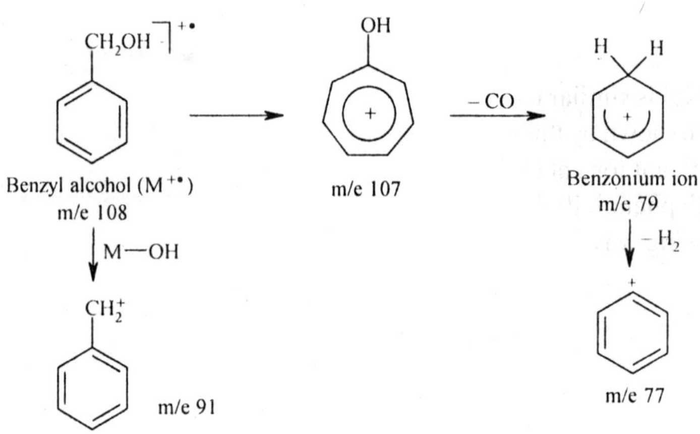

Scheme 6.16. Fragmentation pattern for Benzyl alcohol.

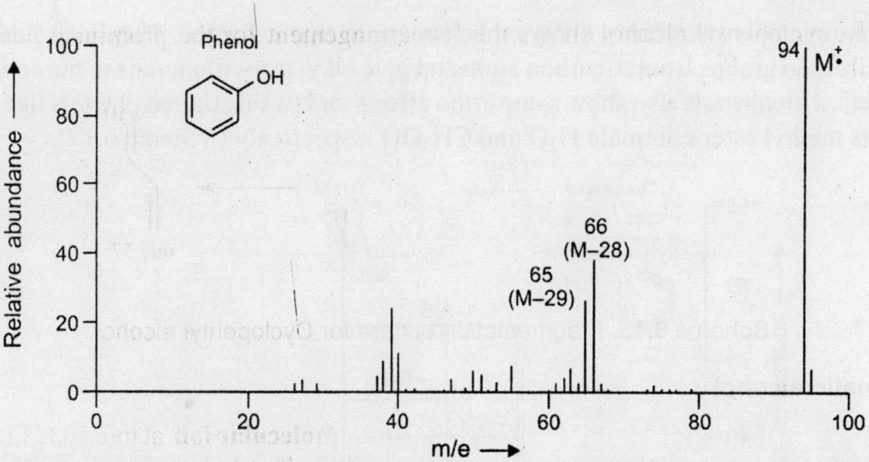

Fig. 6.19. Mass spectrum of phenol.

6.2.4 Phenol

Unlike for aliphatic alcohols, the molecular ion peak for phenols are quite intense. Phenols can lose the elements of carbon monoxide to give abundant fragment ions at M–28, and can also lose the elements of the formyl radical (HCO•) to give abundant fragment ions at M–29. The mechanism of this fragmentation is still not clear. However, Fig. 6.19 contains the mass spectrum of phenol, which highlights the production of the fragment ions.

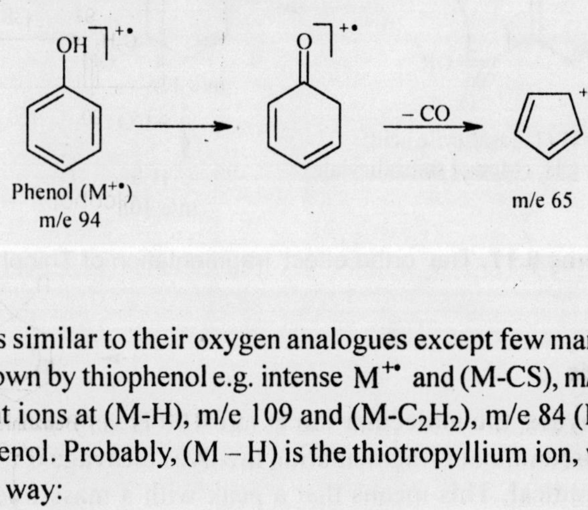

6.2.5 Thiols

The behaviour of thiol is similar to their oxygen analogues except few marked differences. The two expected features are shown by thiophenol e.g. intense $M^{+\bullet}$ and (M-CS), m/e 66 (Fig. 6.20). However there are also significant ions at (M-H), m/e 109 and (M-C_2H_2), m/e 84 (M-SH), m/e 77; these has no resemblance with phenol. Probably, (M – H) is the thiotropyllium ion, which can lose CS to give m/e 65 in the following way:

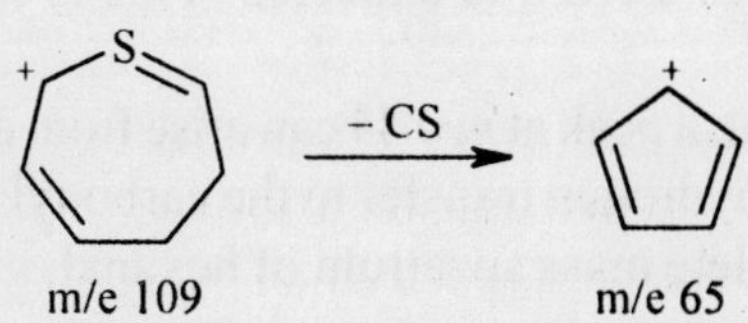

Alkyl thiophenols also shows different behaviour to that expected. They lose side chain much more readily than groups from α-carbon atom and give alkyl tropyllium ions in the series of m/e 91, 105, 119, etc. Thiophenols also show same ortho effects and so substituted phenols like thiosalicylic acid and its methyl ester eliminate H_2O and CH_3OH respectively (Scheme 6.17).

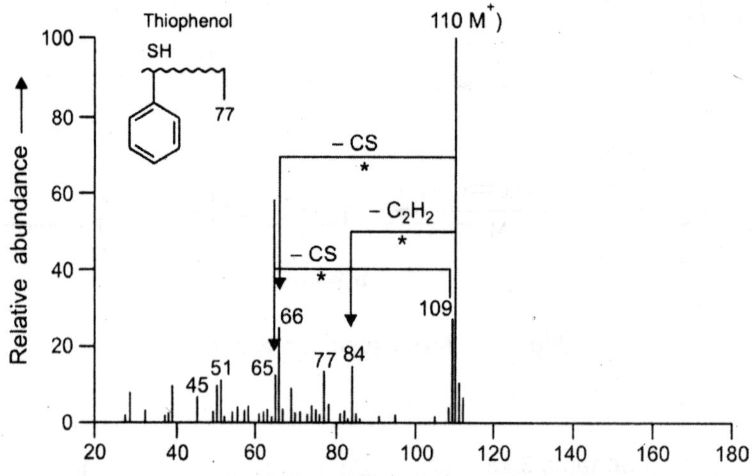

Fig. 6.20. Mass spectrum of Thiophenol.

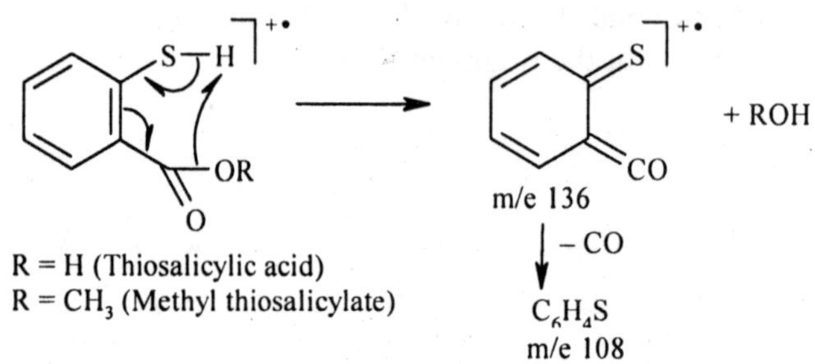

Scheme 6.17. The 'ortho effect' fragmentation of Thiophenol.

6.3 ALDEHYDE

6.3.1 Aliphatic aldehyde

In simple aliphatic aldehydes, the molecular ion at m/e 100 is very weak but detectable, as is the M–1 ion at m/e 99. The predominant fragmentation involves cleavage α to the carbonyl group with loss of the larger alkyl radical. This means that a peak with a mass-to-charge ratio (*m/e*) of 29, corresponding to the formation of CHO^+, is expected. This is illustrated for n-hexanal below in Scheme 6.18.

If a gamma hydrogen is present, a peak at *m/e* 44 can arise from a process known as the McLafferty rearrangement. This involves γ- hydrogen transfer to the carbonyl oxygen atom with the subsequent formation of $C_2H_5O^+$. The complete mass spectrum of hexanal, given in Fig. 6.21, illustrates these points.

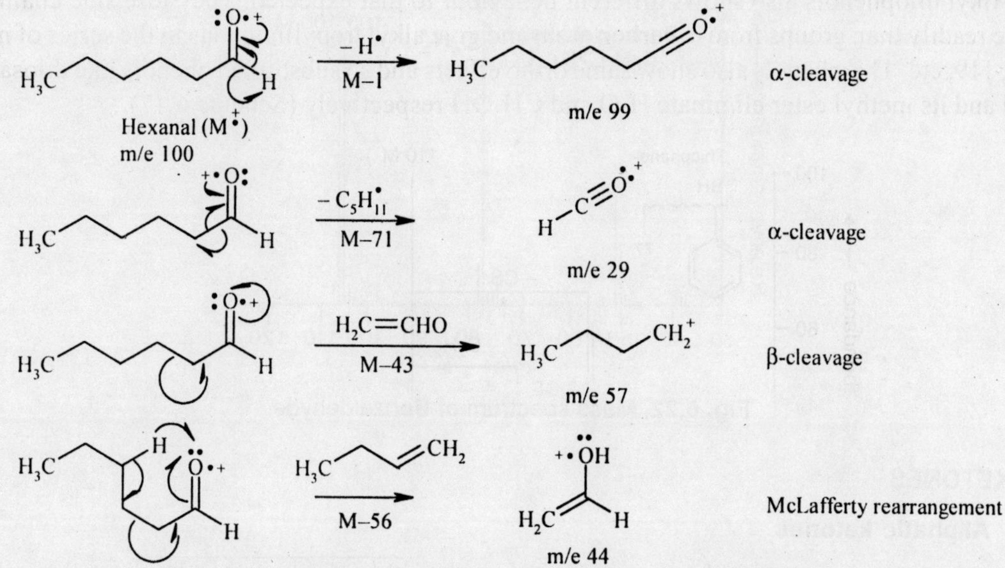

Scheme 6.18. Fragmentation pattern for Hexanal.

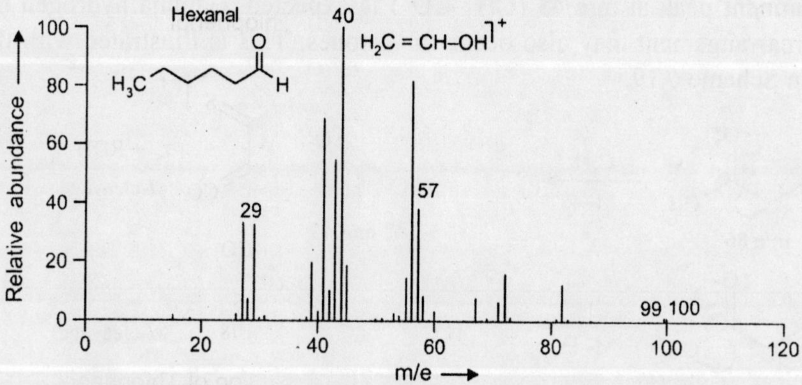

Fig. 6.21. Mass spectrum of Hexanal.

6.3.2 Aromatic aldehydes

Aromatic aldehydes, such as benzaldehyde Fig. 6.22, typically display intense molecular ions and M–1 peaks. In the mass spectrum of benzaldehyde, the oxocarbocation formed by loss of a hydrogen atom, expels CO to give the phenyl cation, $C_6H_5^+$ at *m/e* 77.

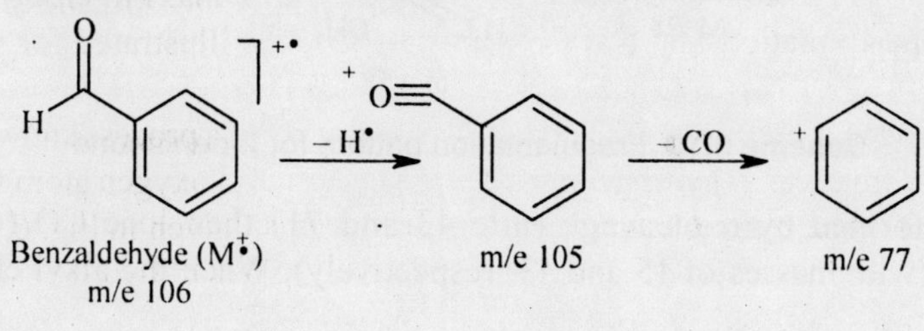

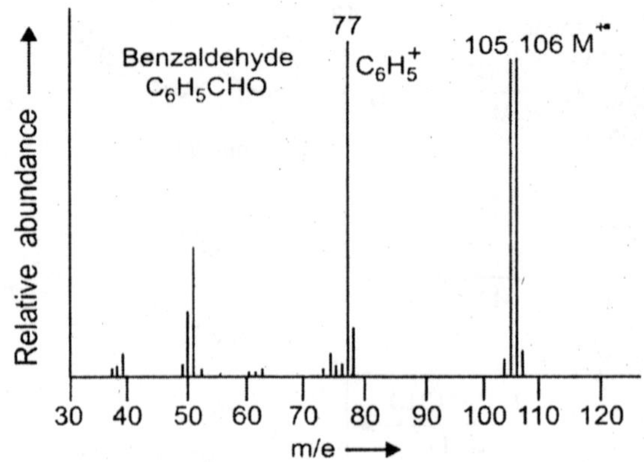

Fig. 6.22. Mass spectrum of Benzaldehyde.

6.4 KETONES

6.4.1 Aliphatic ketones

α-cleavage is also common for ketones and may occur at either of the two bonds next to the carbonyl group. In general, loss of the larger alkyl fragment is preferred. Thus, for methyl ketones (CH_3–CO–R) a prominent peak at m/e 43 (CH_3–CO^+) is expected. Gamma hydrogen transfer due to MacLafferty rearrangement may also occur for ketones. This is illustrated with the example of 2-pentanone in Scheme 6.19.

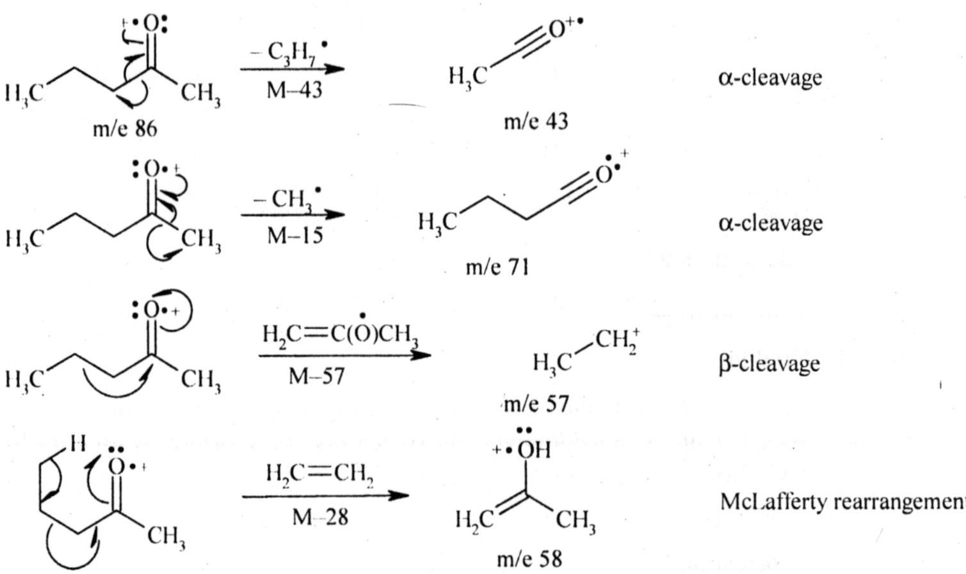

Scheme 6.19. Fragmentation pattern for 2-pentanone.

The two ions formed by α-cleavage (m/e 43 and 71) then lose CO (decarbonylate) to give carbocations (with masses of 15 and 43, respectively). When the alkyl chains are long, the

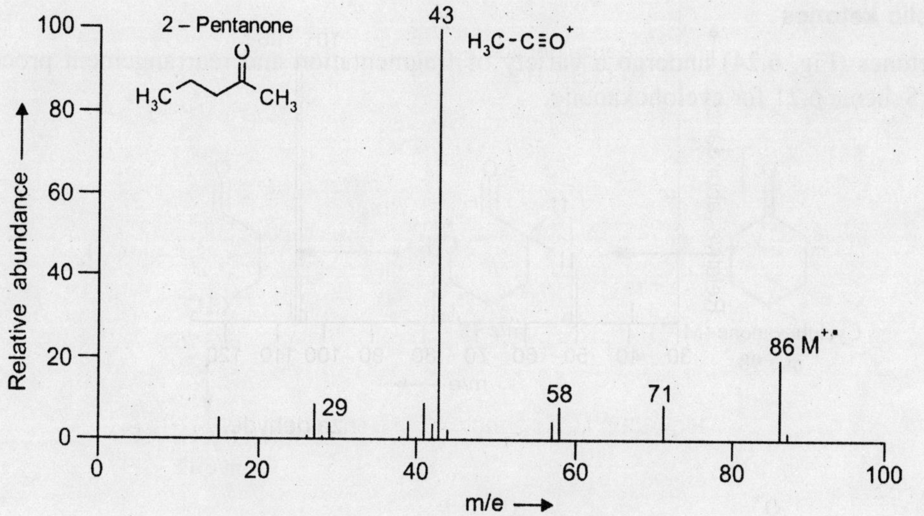

Fig. 6.23. Mass spectrum of 2-Pentanone.

resulting alkene will fragment by losses of alkenes and other neutrals (e.g., H_2), in accord with EE ion rule.

If there is a chain of three or more carbons atoms in each chain of the ketone, then a second McLafferty rearrangement is possible. This is illustrated below for octan-4-one in Scheme 6.20.

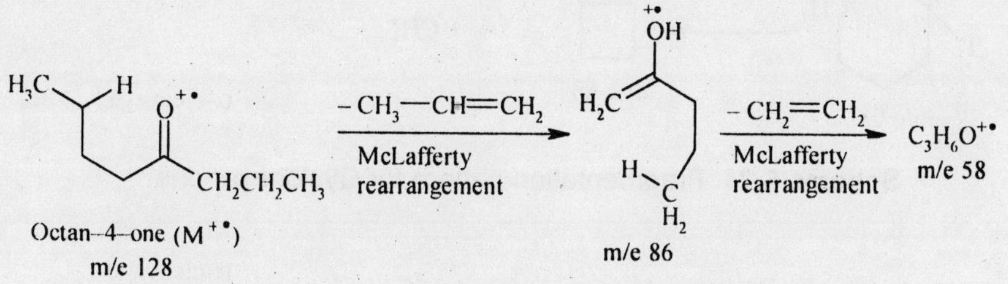

Scheme 6.20. Fragmentation pattern for Octan–4–one.

The mass spectrum of unsaturated ketone, 2-propenyl ethanoate (allyl acetate) shows a small molecular ion peak, and a pair of peaks at m/e 57 and 58.

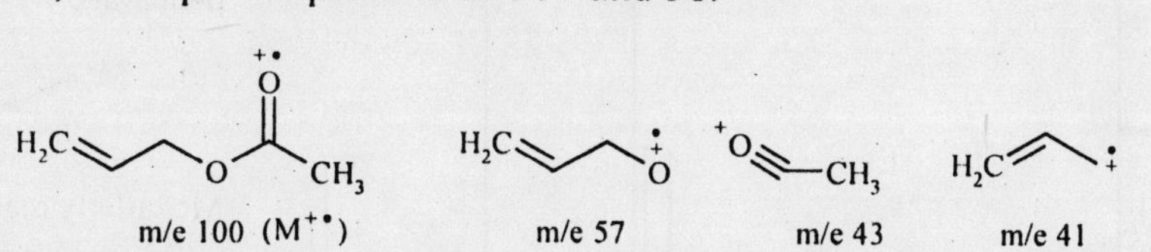

m/e 100 ($M^{+\bullet}$) m/e 57 m/e 43 m/e 41

The peak at m/e 57 corresponds to loss of m/e 43, which is the base peak and corresponds to the acylium ion ($CH_3C\equiv O^+$). The m/e 57 fragment corresponds to C_3H_5O, suggesting the original compound was an allyl (–O–CH_2CH = CH) or methylvinyl (–O–CH–$CHCH_3$) ester. Either of these would generate the peak observed at m/e 41. The peak at m/e 58 corresponds to the protonated m/e 57 cation radical.

6.4.2 Cyclic ketones

Cyclic ketones (Fig. 6.24) undergo a variety of fragmentation and rearrangement processes as shown in Scheme 6.21 for cyclohexanone.

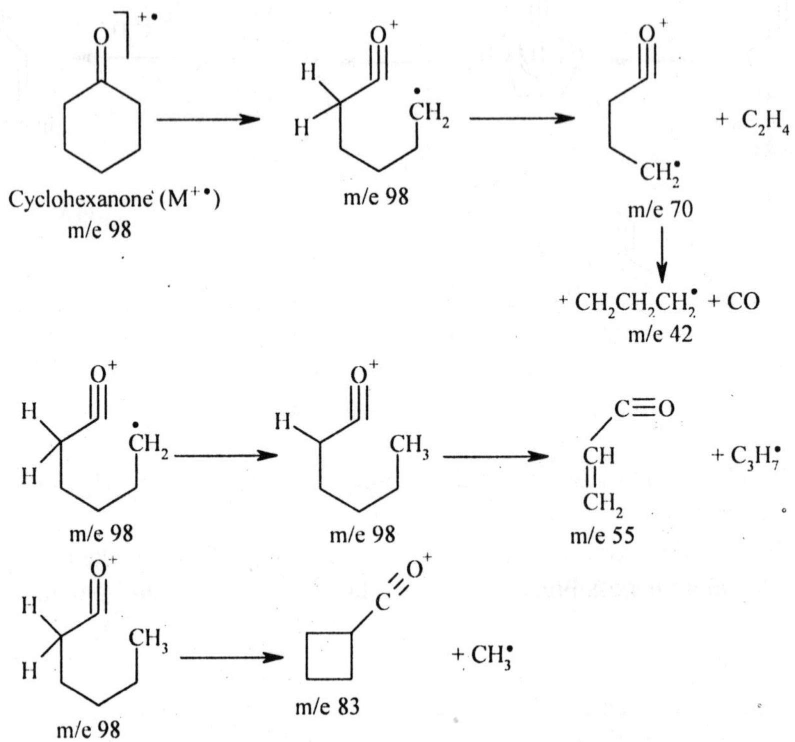

Scheme 6.21. Fragmentation pattern for Cyclohexanone.

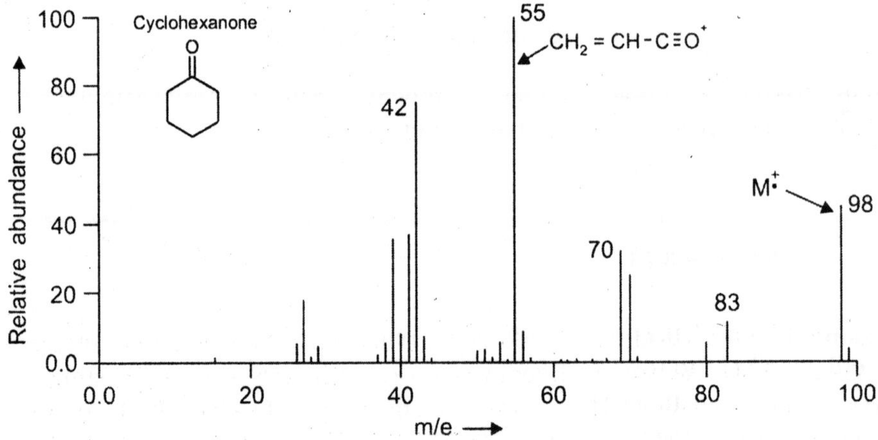

Fig. 6.24. Mass spectrum of Cyclohexanone.

Similarly, cyclopentanone reveals the presence of α-cleavage and other fragmentation pathways as per Scheme 6.22.

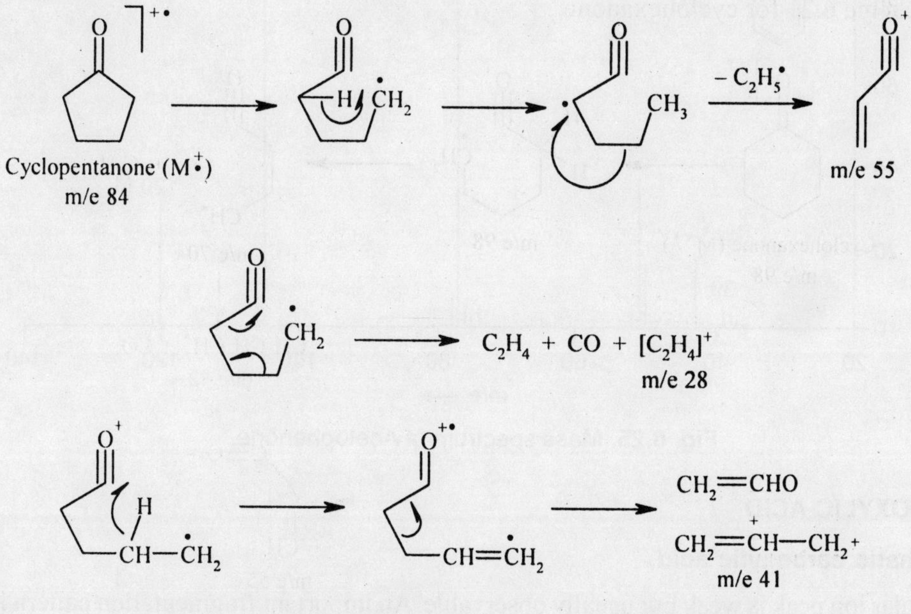

Scheme 6.22. Fragmentation pattern for Cyclopentanone

6.4.3 Aromatic ketones

For aromatic ketones, α-cleavage usually involves cleavage of the alkyl group leaving behind an acylium ion. This is subsequently followed by a loss of carbon monoxide from the molecule as indicated in Scheme 6.23 for Acetophenone. If the aromatic ketone has a 3 carbon alkyl chain (or longer), then McLafferty rearrangements (as described above for 2-pentanone) are possible.

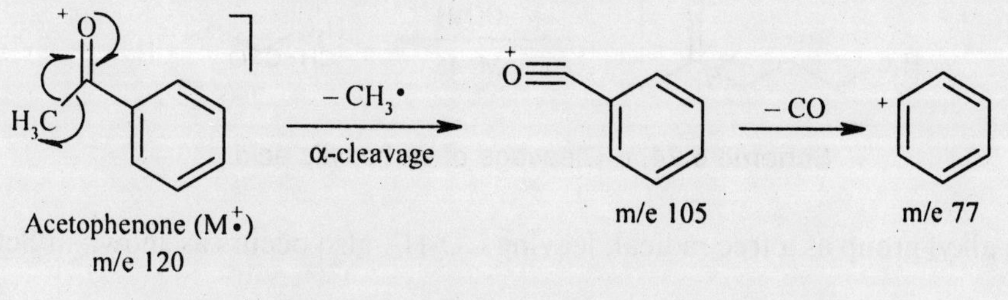

Scheme 6.23. Fragmentation pattern for Acetophenone.

The phenyl cation (m/e 77, the product of decarbonylation) subsequently loses acetylene, C_2H_2, or an allene diradical, C_3H_2, to form fragment ions with m/e 51 and 39, respectively. This is very characteristic of the phenyl cation and the overall process is a "signature" for the benzoyl group, which is common in organic chemistry. The complete mass spectrum of acetophenone is given in Fig. 6.25, which illustrates these points.

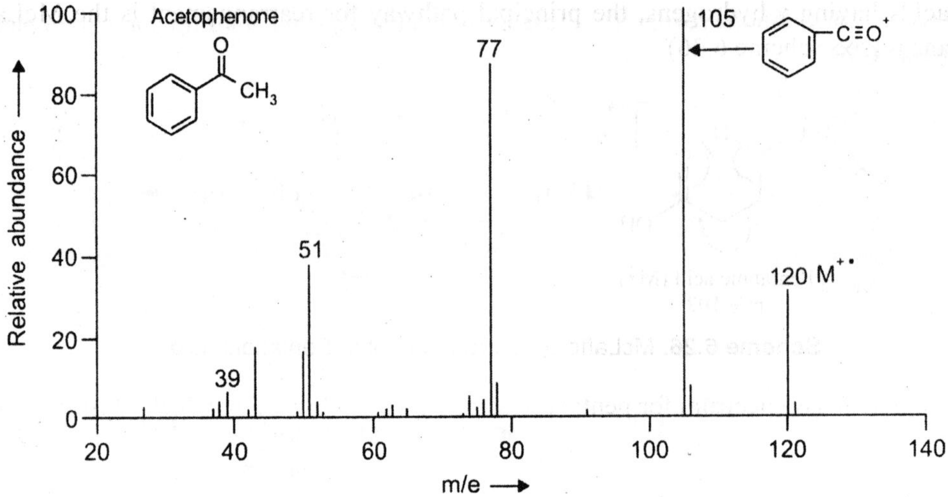

Fig. 6.25. Mass spectrum of Acetophenone.

6.5 CARBOXYLIC ACID

6.5.1 Aliphatic carboxylic acid

The molecular ion peak is weak but usually observable. An important fragmentation pattern involves α-cleavage (breaking either bond to the carbonyl carbon) as shown in Scheme 6.24.

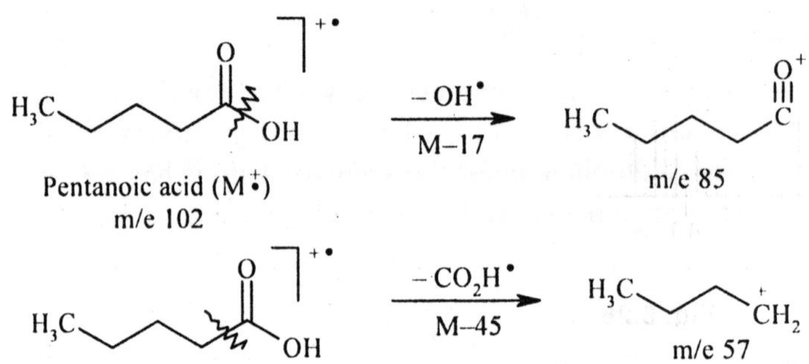

Scheme 6.24. α-Cleavage of carboxylic acid.

Loss of the alkyl group as a free radical, leaving CO_2H^+, also occurs as shown in Scheme 6.25.

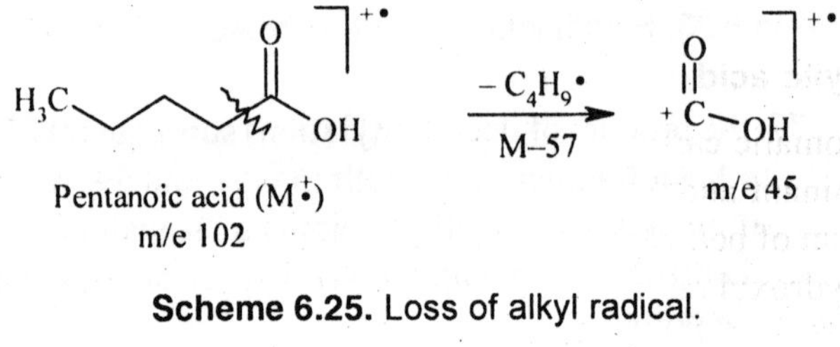

Scheme 6.25. Loss of alkyl radical.

With acids having γ hydrogens, the principal pathway for rearrangement is the McLafferty rearrangement (see Scheme 6.26).

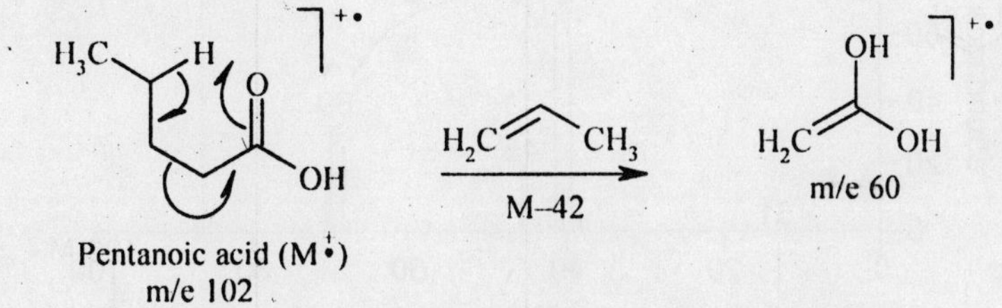

Scheme 6.26. McLafferty rearrangement in Pentanoic acid.

The complete mass spectrum for pentanoic acid is given in Fig. 6.26, which illustrates most of these points.

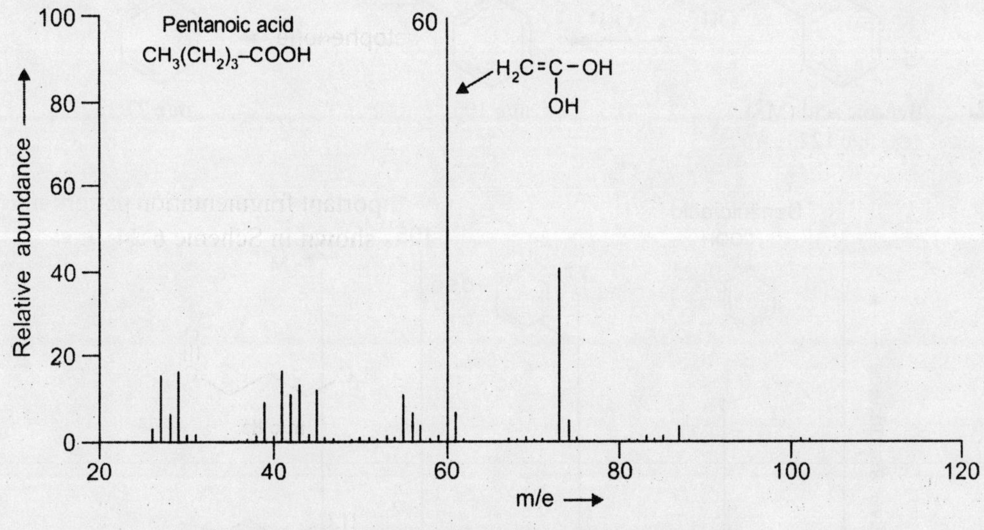

Fig. 6.26. Mass spectrum for Pentanoic acid.

6.5.2 Unsaturated carboxylic acids

The unsaturated carboxylic acids e.g. methyl acrylic acid (Fig. 6.27) also show M–OH (m/e 69), M–COOH (m/e 41) ion in the spectrum. The unsaturated acids show intense molecular ion peak.

6.5.3 Aromatic carboxylic acid

The fragmentation in aromatic carboxylic acids is similar to that observed in simple esters, with "cleavage being predominant and McLafferty rearrangements being observed with longer side-chains. The mass spectrum of benzoic acid (Fig. 6.28) shows a strong molecular ion, a peak at m/e 105, due to loss of the hydroxyl radical, and loss of CO to give the phenyl cation at *me* 77.

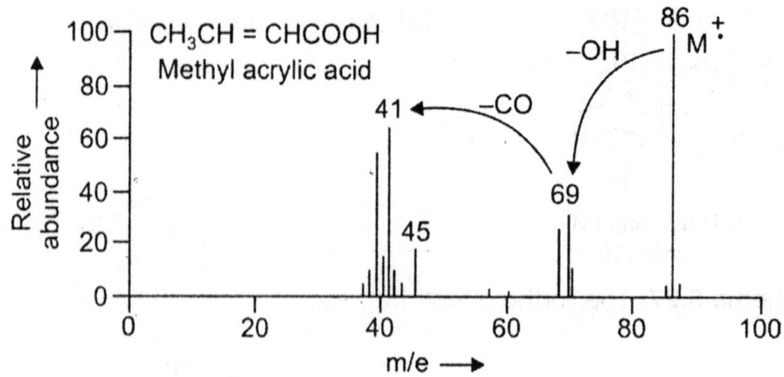

Fig. 6.27. Mass spectrum of Methyl acrylic acid.

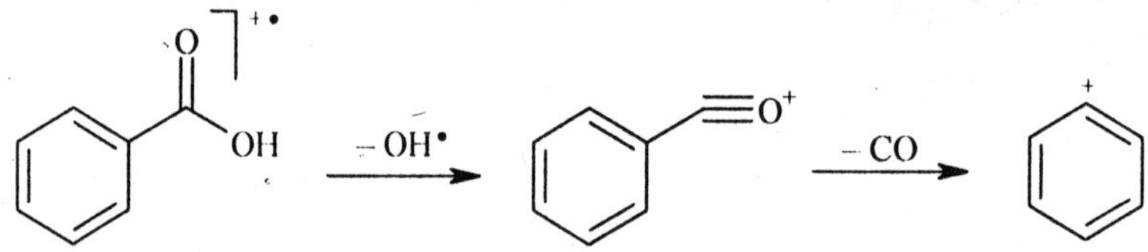

Benzoic acid ($M^{+\bullet}$) m/e 122 | m/e 105 | m/e 77

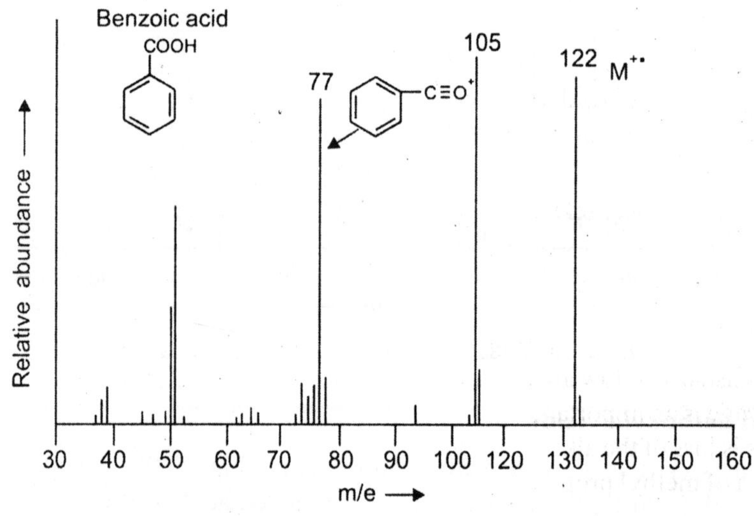

Fig. 6.28. Mass spectrum of Benzoic acid.

The benzoic acids substituted with alkyl, amino, or hydroxy substituents at the *ortho* position readily dehydrate via proton transfer from the *ortho* substituent to the hydroxyl group (ortho effect). Water is lost, resulting in a major M–18 ion in the mass spectrum. Scheme 6.27 outlines this process for *o*-toluic acid.

The mass spectrum of *o*-toluic acid (Fig. 6.29) indicates the facile nature of this dehydration event (the signal for the product ion is the base peak).

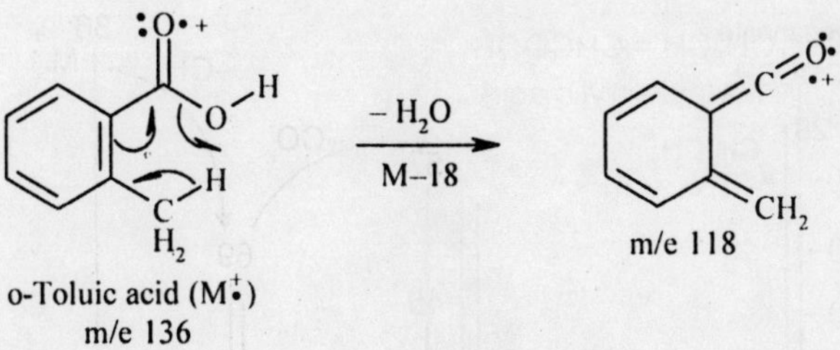

Scheme 6.27. The "ortho effect" fragmentation of *o*-Toluic acid.

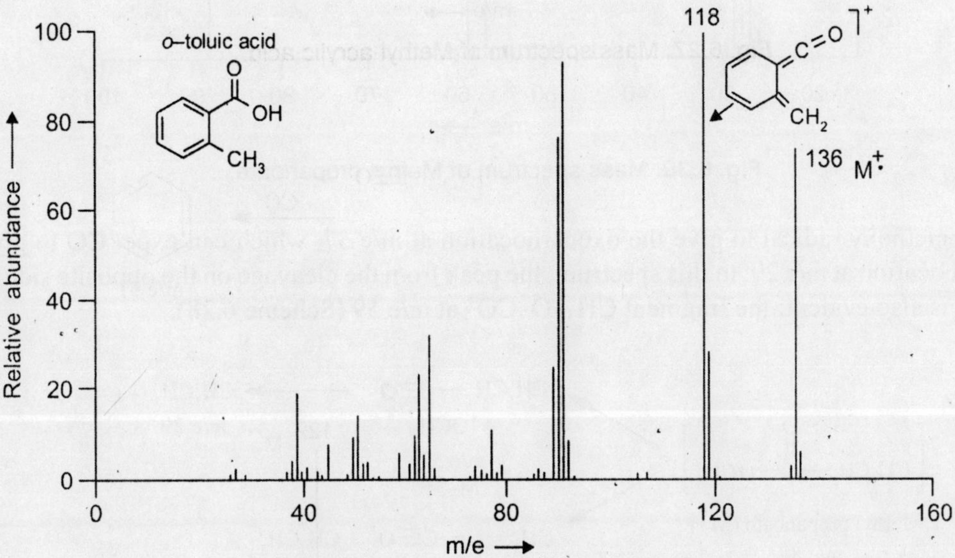

Fig. 6.29. Mass spectrum of *o*-Toluic acid.

6.6. ESTER

6.6.1 Aliphatic esters

The molecular ion is usually of low abundance but generally observable for esters. As in all carbonyl compounds, α-cleavage is an important fragmentation process The most important cleavage reaction of carboxylate esters is loss of the alkoxy group (summarize in Table 6.1) to form the oxocarbocation. In the mass spectrum of methyl propanoate (Fig. 6.30), the molecular ion at m/e 88 fragments with

Table 6.1. Alkoxy Radicals formed from the most common esters.

Ester	*Alkoxy Radical Formed*	*Ion to Observe*
Methyl	$CH_3O\bullet$	M–31
Ethyl	$CH_3CH_2O\bullet$	M–45
Propyl (and isopropyl)	$CH_3CH_2CH_2O\bullet$	M–59
Phenyl	$C_6H_5O\bullet$ (PhO•)	M–93
Benzyl	$C_6H_5CH_2O\bullet$ (BzO•)	M–105

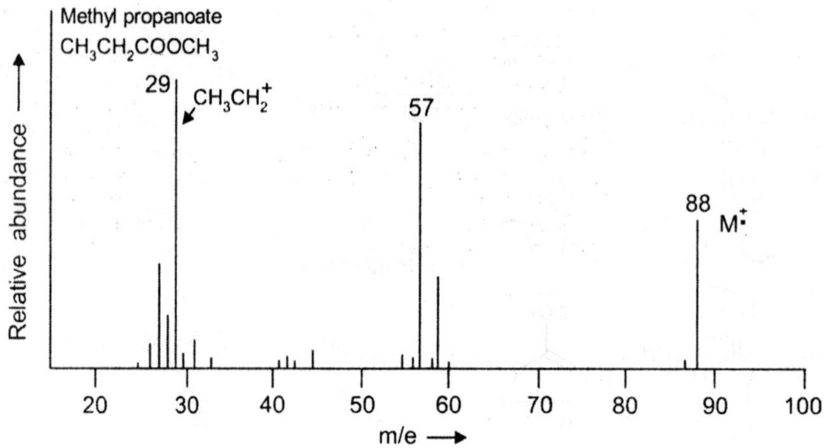

Fig. 6.30. Mass spectrum of Methyl propanoate.

loss of a methoxy radical to give the oxocarbocation at m/e 57, which can expel CO to give the ethyl carbocation at m/e 29. In this spectrum, the peak from the cleavage on the opposite side of the carbonyl is also evident; the fragment CH_3–O–CO^+ at m/e 59 (Scheme 6.28).

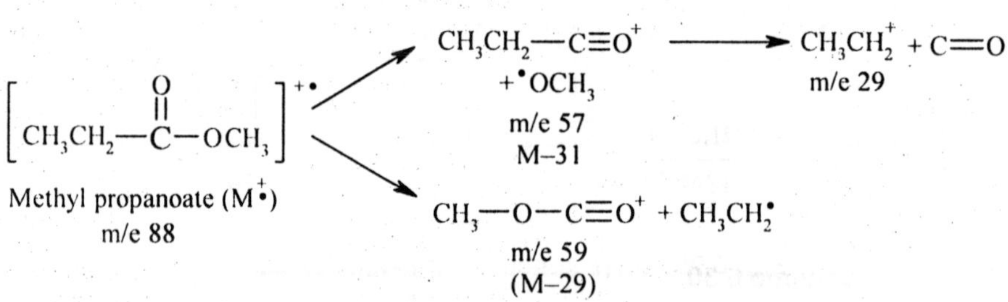

Scheme 6.28. Fragmentation pattern for Methyl propanoate.

Methyl esters with alkyl side-chains readily undergo McLafferty rearrangement reactions producing cation radicals with m/e 74 (Scheme 6.29).

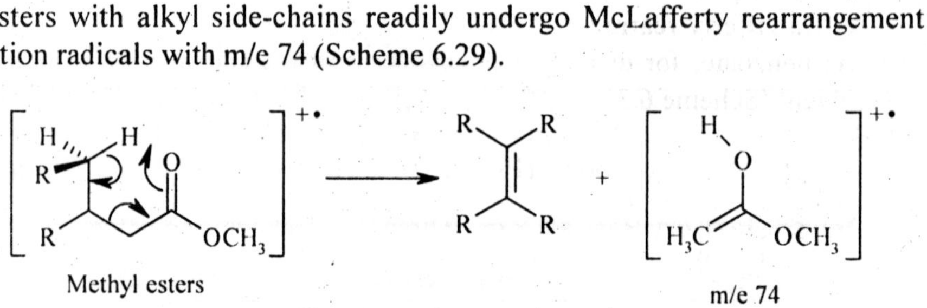

Scheme 6.29. McLafferty rearrangement in methyl esters.

Since methyl esters are very common and their formation is used in the derivatization of fatty acids for GC/MS, the example below is presented to indicate the most common fragmentation patterns observed for a simple methyl ester, methyl butyrate. Loss of the alkoxy group is the most important of these fragmentations as shown in Scheme 6.30.

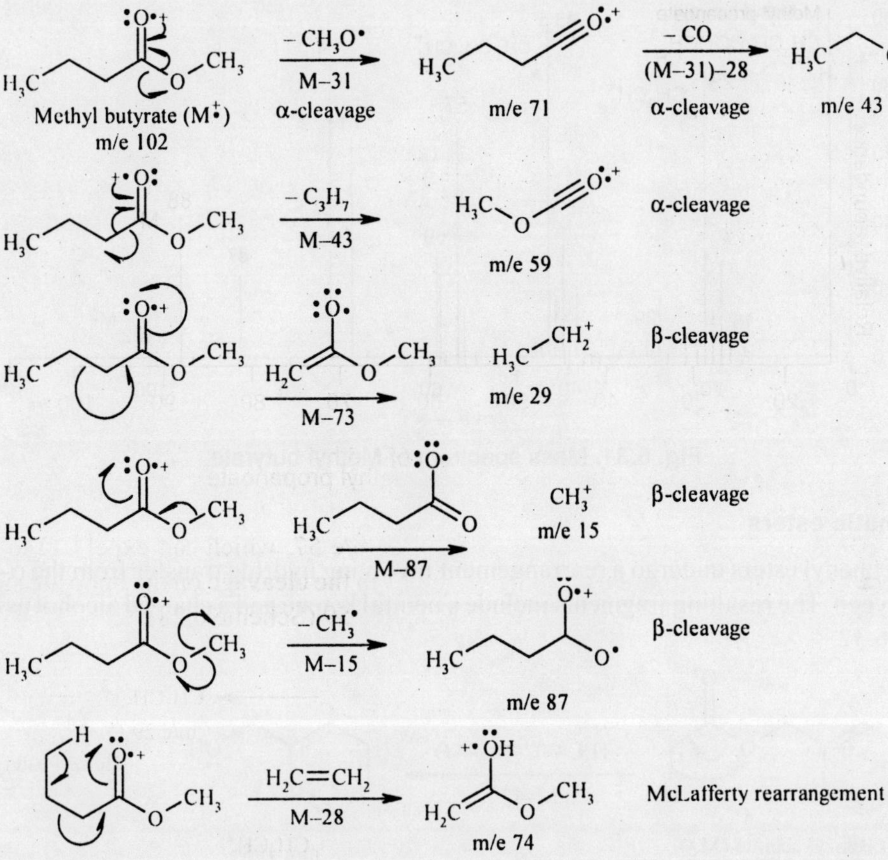

Scheme 6.30. Fragmentation pattern for Methyl butyrate.

The complete mass spectrum of methyl butyrate is given in Fig. 6.31, which illustrates most of these points. Ethyl, and particularly larger alkyl esters, do a double rearrangement - sometimes called a "double McLafferty rearrangement" - to make a protonated acid $RCOOH_2^+$. The mass spectrum of butyl benzoate, for example, gives the abundant ion of *m/e* 123 arising from this double rearrangement (Scheme 6.31).

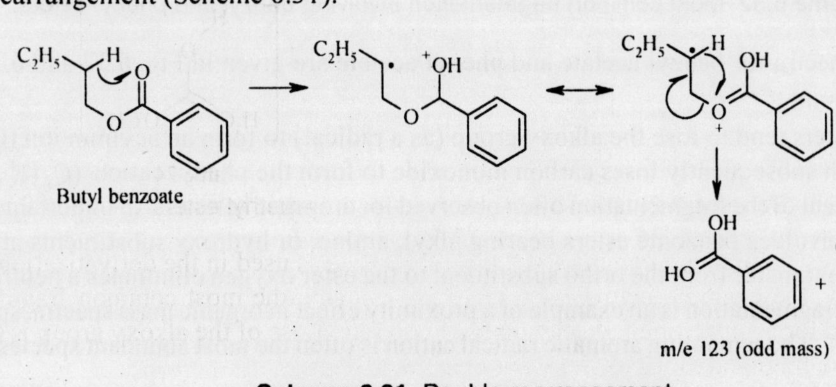

Scheme 6.31. Double rearrangement.

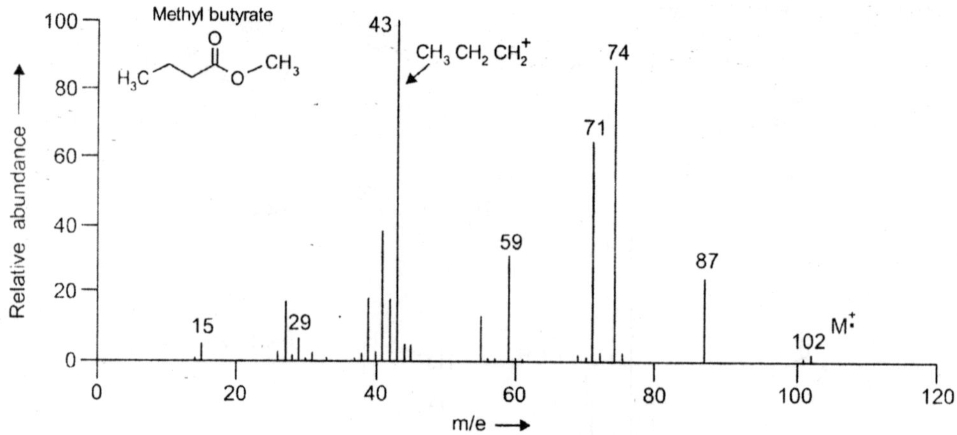

Fig. 6.31. Mass spectrum of Methyl butyrate.

6.6.2 Aromatic esters

Benzyl and phenyl esters undergo a rearrangement involving hydride transfer from the α-carbon to the ester oxygen. The resulting fragments include a neutral ketene and a charged alcohol as described in Scheme 6.32.

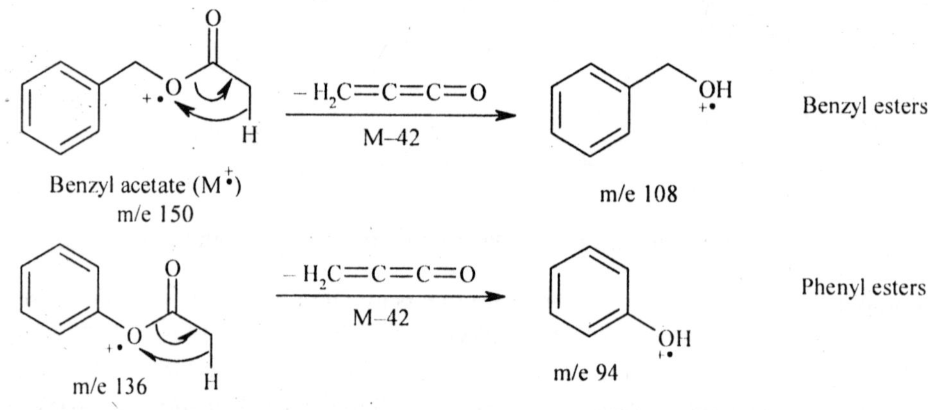

Scheme 6.32. Most common fragmentation involving benzyl and phenyl esters.

The mass spectra for benzyl acetate and phenyl acetate are given in Fig. 6.32 and 6.33, which illustrates the point.

Benzoate esters tend to lose the alkoxy group (as a radical) to form an acylium ion ($C_6H_5CO^+$, m/e 105), which subsequently loses carbon monoxide to form the phenyl cation ($C_6H_5^+$, m/e 77). This is reminiscent of the fragmentation often observed for aromatic ketones. An important exception to this pattern involves benzoate esters bearing alkyl, amino, or hydroxy substituents at the ortho position. Proton transfer from the ortho substituent to the ester oxygen eliminates a neutral alcohol fragment. This fragmentation is an example of a proximity effect in organic mass spectra, specifically an "ortho effect". The remaining aromatic radical cation is often the most abundant species detected.

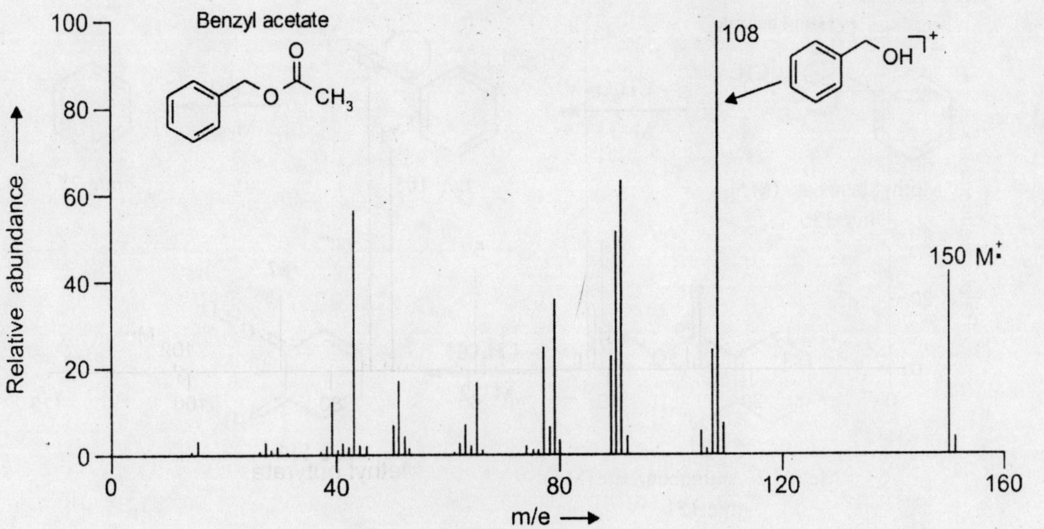

Fig. 6.32. Mass spectrum of Benzyl acetate.

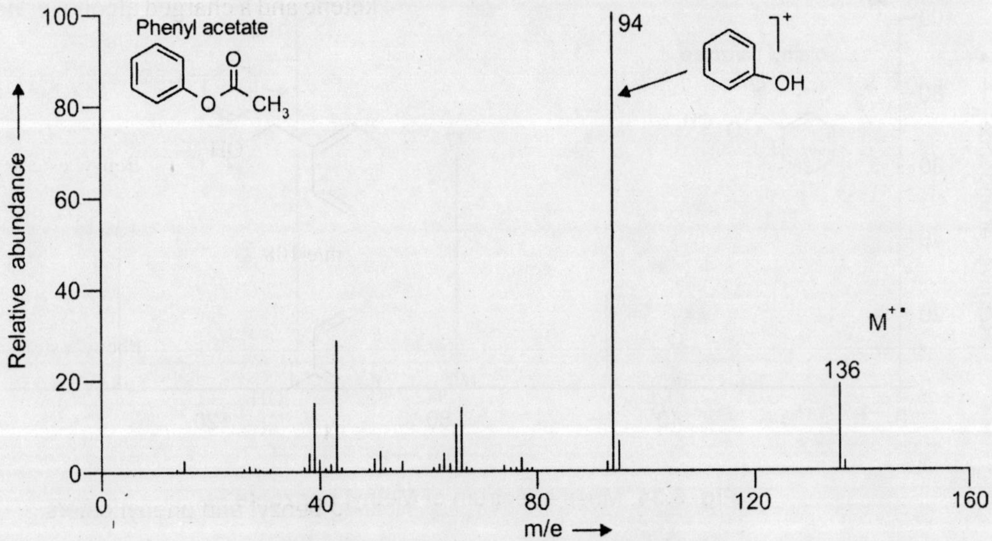

Fig. 6.33. Mass spectrum of Phenyl acetate.

Illustrations of these two common pathways are given in Scheme 6.33. The mass spectra for both methyl benzoate and methyl 2-aminobenzoate, given in Fig. 6.34 and 6.35, show that the ortho substituted benzoate ester undergoes a facile loss of methanol resulting in an abundant M - 32 (m/e 119) ion in the mass spectrum. Ortho effects offer one way of distinguishing *ortho* from *meta* and *para* isomers by mass spectrometry. When this process cannot occur, the mass spectra of *ortho*, *meta*, and *para* isomers are usually very similar and nearly indistinguishable (e.g., *o*-, *m*-, and *p*-ethyl toluene have nearly identical spectra).

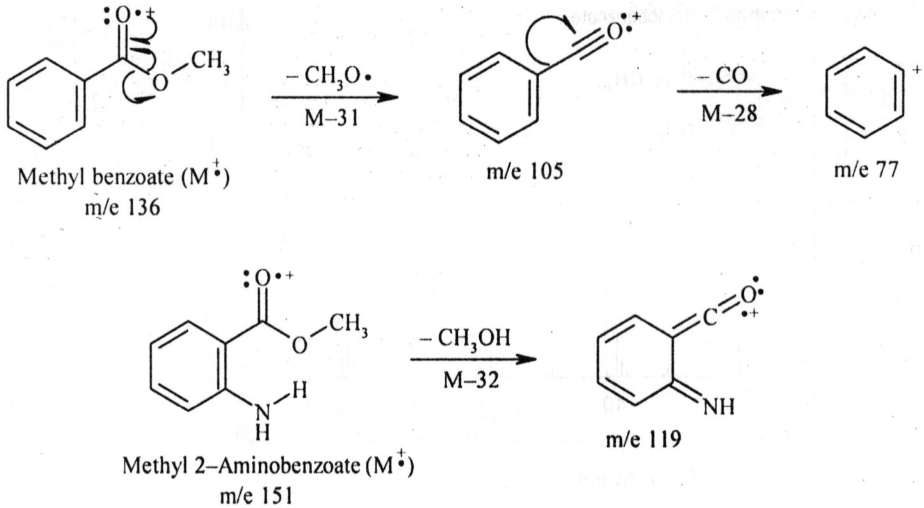

Scheme 6.33. Most common fragmentation involving benzoate and *ortho* substituted benzoate esters.

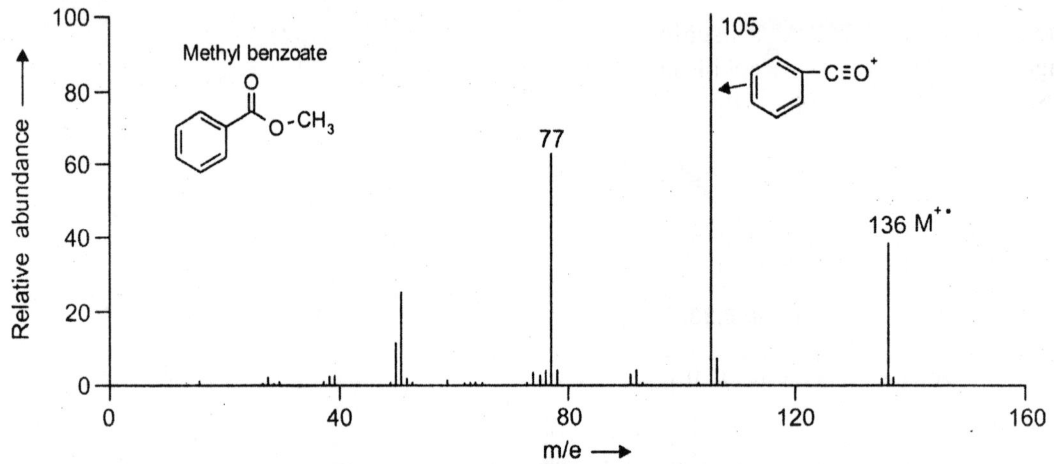

Fig. 6.34. Mass spectrum of Methyl benzoate.

6.7 LACTONES

The cleavage adjacent to the oxygen atom is a characteristic fragmentation pattern of γ and δ lactone spectrum. The peaks at m/e 42,70 and 71 are typical of δ-lactone spectrum.

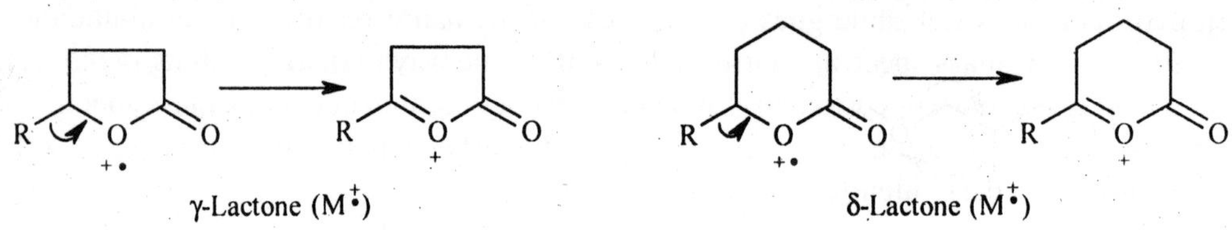

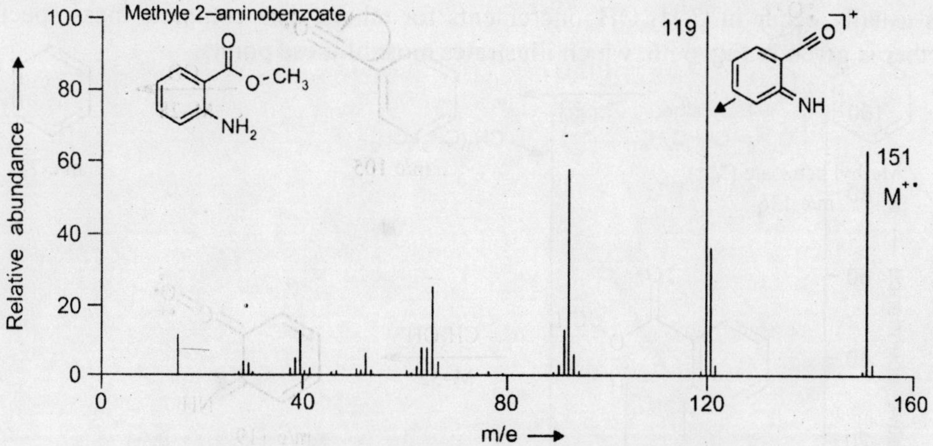

Fig. 6.35. Mass spectrum of Methyl 2-aminobenzoate.

6.8 ETHERS

6.8.1 Aliphatic ethers

The molecular ion peak is usually weak, however, larger than for alcohols. An important fragmentation process for alcohols involves the cleavage of the C–C bond to the α-carbon as shown in Scheme 6.34.

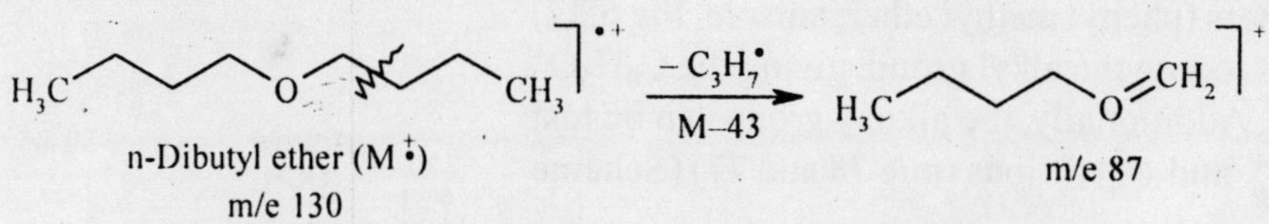

Scheme 6.33. Cleavage of the C-C bond to the α-carbon.

A second common mode of fragmentation involves cleavage of the C-O bond (see scheme 6.35).

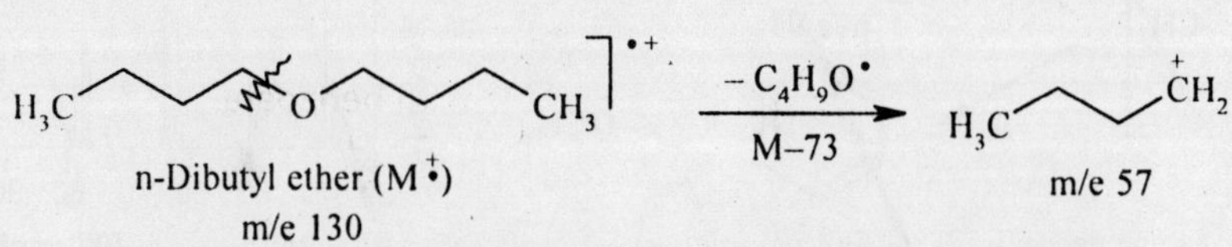

Scheme 6.35. Cleavage of the C-O bond in an ether.

Hydride transfer from a β-carbon is an important rearrangement process in ethers as shown in Scheme 6.36.

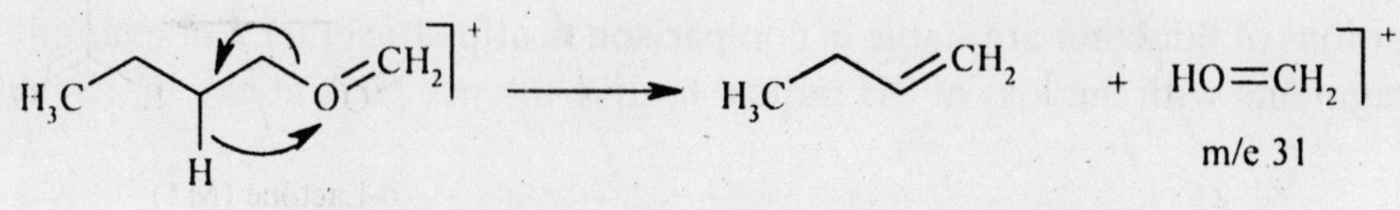

Scheme 6.36. Rearrangement in an ether.

Peaks usually occur in $C_nH_{2n}OH^+$ increments for ethers. The complete mass spectrum for n-butyl ether is given in Fig. 6.36, which illustrates most of these points.

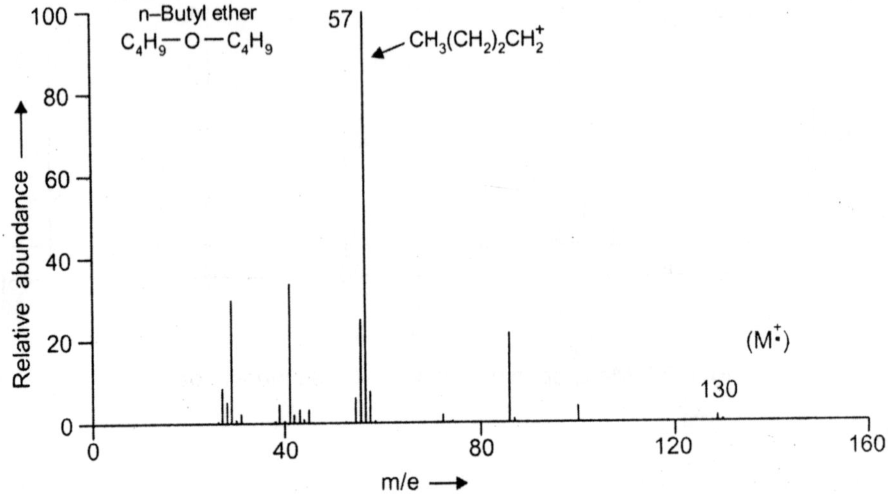

Fig. 6.36. Mass spectrum for n-Butyl ether.

6.8.2 Aromatic ethers

Aromatic ethers (phenyl methyl ether; anisole, Fig 6.37) can fragment to lose the alkyl group, giving the $C_6H_5O^+$ ion (m/e 93). Additionally, the alkoxy group can be lost to give $C_6H_6^+$ and $C_6H_5^+$ ions (m/e 78 and 77) (Scheme 6.37).

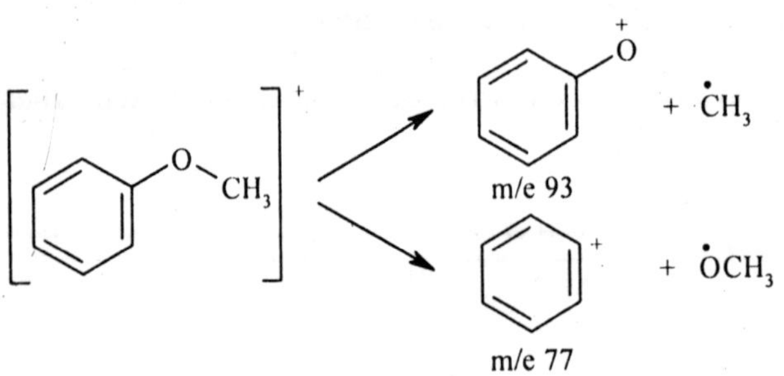

Scheme 6.37. Fragmentation pattern for Anisole.

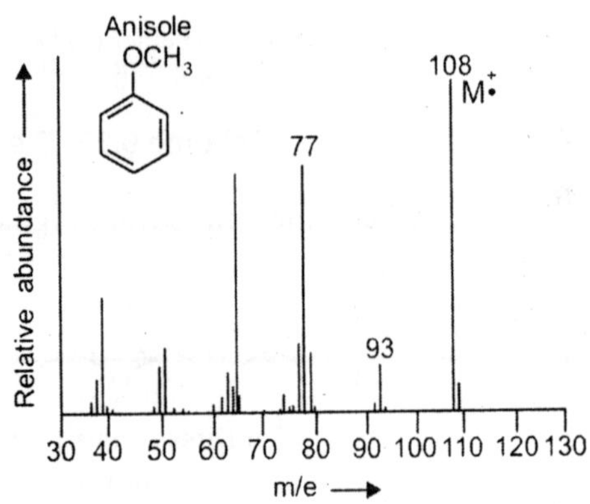

Fig. 6.37. Mass spectrum of Anisole.

6.8.3 Thio ether

The molecular ions of thioether are stable in comparison to aliphatic ether. For example, thioanisole (Fig. 6.38) fragments with the loss of SH radical to give intense peak at m/e 91 (Scheme 6.38).

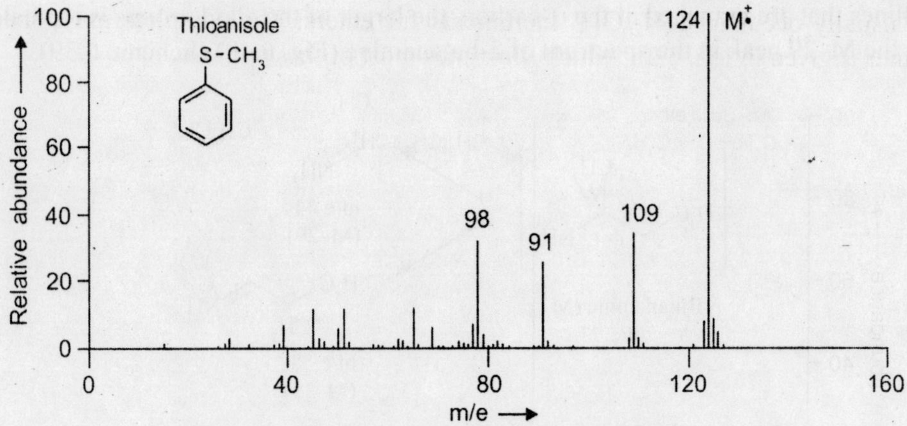

Fig. 6.38. Mass spectrum of Thioanisole.

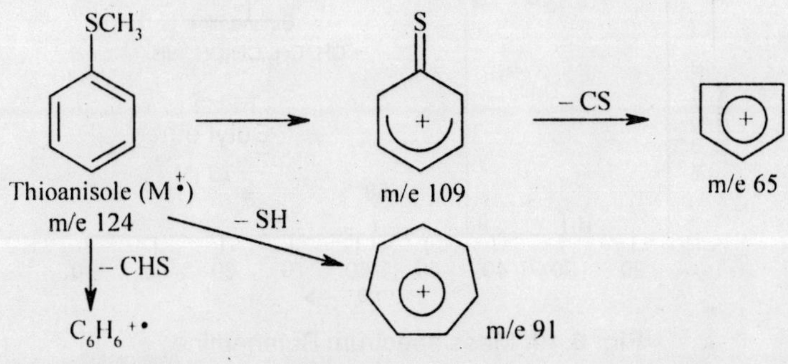

Scheme 6.38. Fragmentation pattern for Thioanisole.

6.9 AMINES

6.9.1 Aliphatic amines

The molecular ion peak is weak or absent. When observable, is a good indication of the presence of an amine (nitrogen rule). The most intense peak in the mass spectrum of most simple aliphatic amines results from α-cleavage to give the ammonium cation. For primary amines, this results in an intense peak at m/e 30, as seen in the mass spectrum of propylamine (Fig. 6.39).

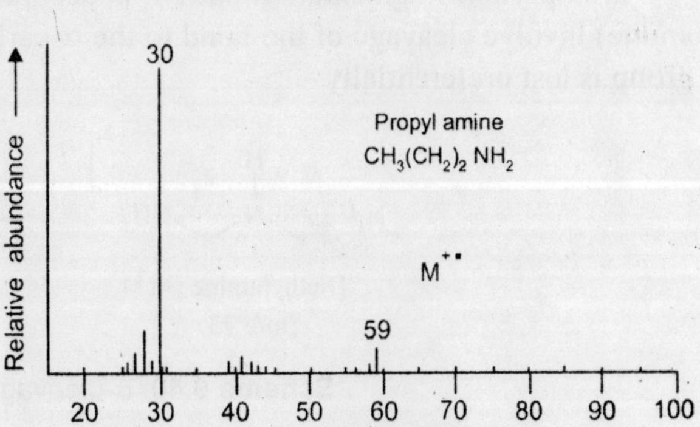

Fig. 6.39. Mass spectrum of Propyl amine.

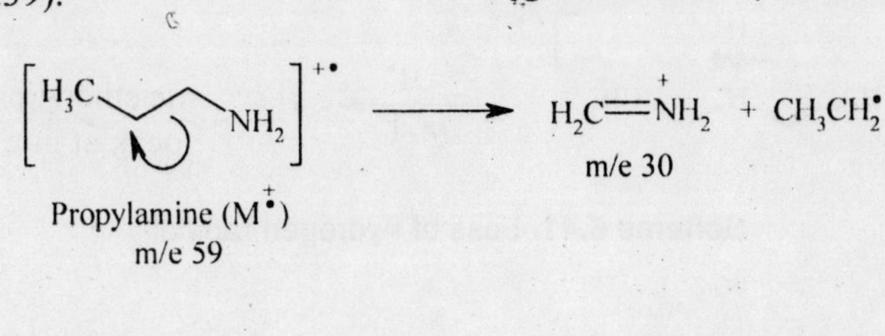

For amines that are branched at the α-carbon, the larger of the alkyl groups is typically lost, as shown by the M–29 peak in the spectrum of 2-butanamine (Fig. 6.40) (Scheme 6.39).

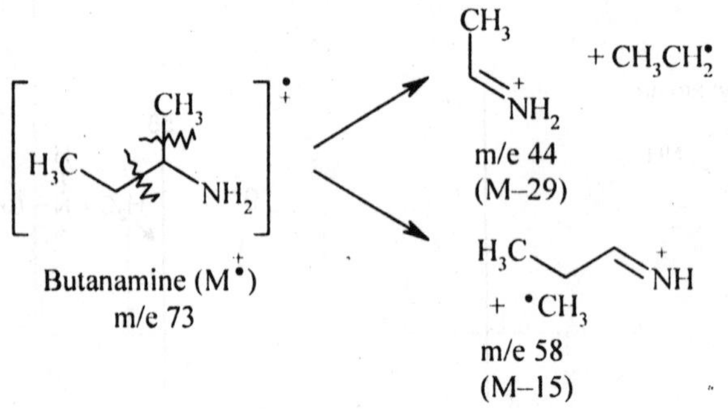

Scheme 6.39. Mass fragmentation pattern for Butanamine.

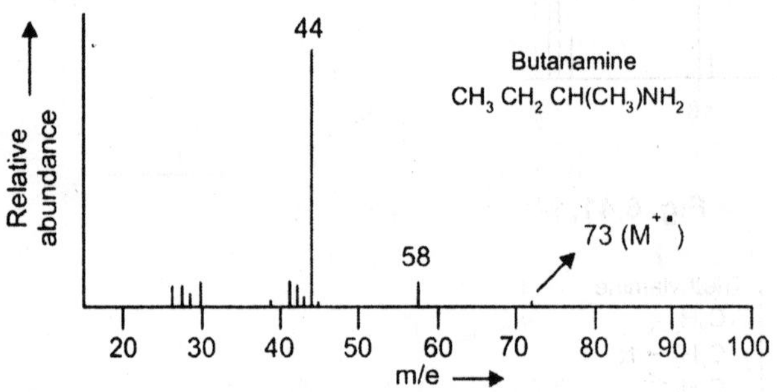

Fig. 6.40. Mass spectrum Butanamine.

An important fragmentation pattern in secondary (diethyl amine) and tertiary amine (triethyl amine) involve cleavage of the bond to the α-carbon as shown in Scheme 6.40. The largest alkyl group is lost preferentially.

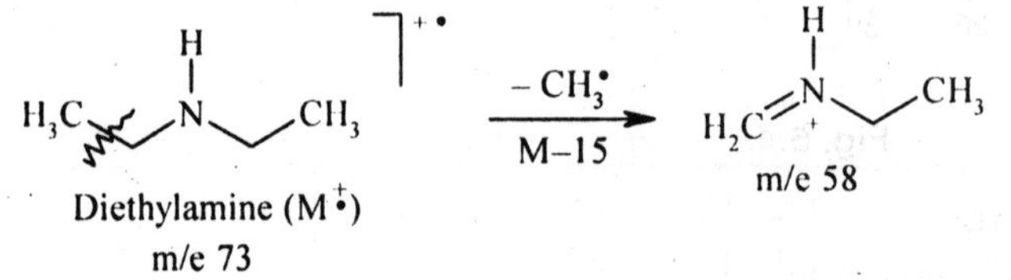

Scheme 6.40. α-cleavage in Secondary amine.

Loss of hydrogen radical, is quite common in amines as shown in Scheme 6.41.

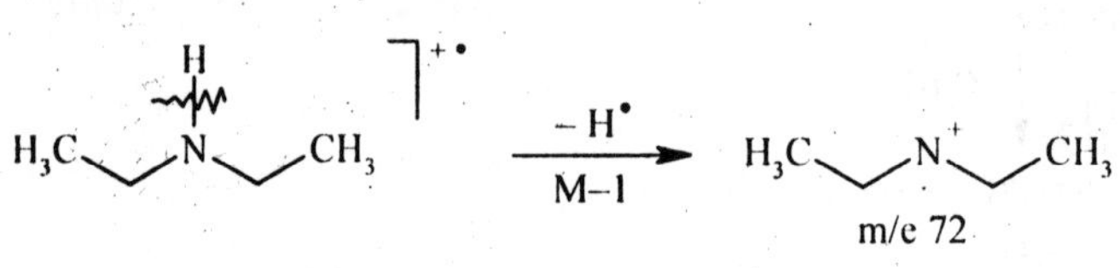

Scheme 6.41. Loss of hydrogen radical.

The complete mass spectrum for diethyl amine and triethyl amine is given in Fig. 6.41 and 6.42, which illustrates most of these points. The secondary and tertiary amines also show rearrangement as per Scheme 6.42.

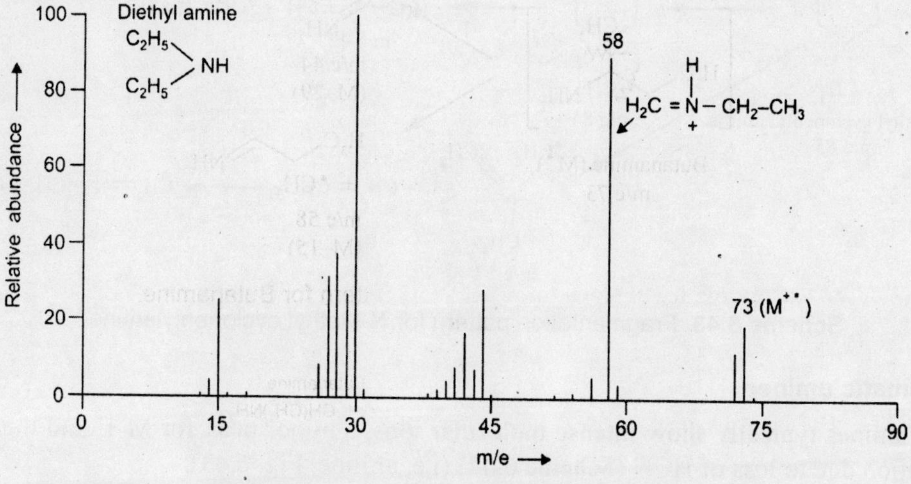

Fig. 6.41. Mass spectrum for Diethyl amine.

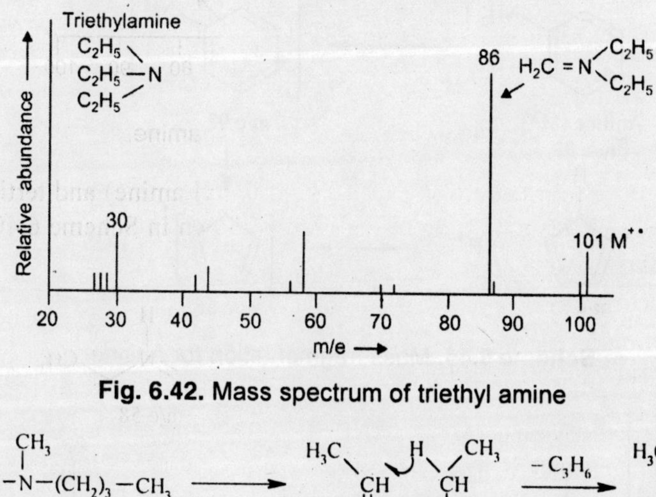

Fig. 6.42. Mass spectrum of triethyl amine

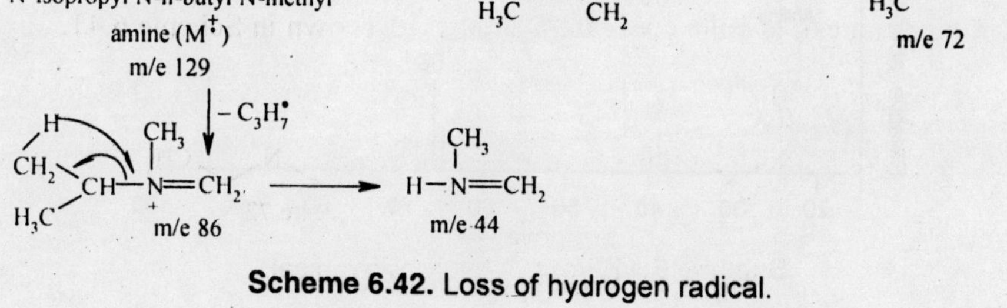

Scheme 6.42. Loss of hydrogen radical.

Cyclic aliphatic amines produce molecular ion peaks. Their principal modes of fragmentation are as follows:

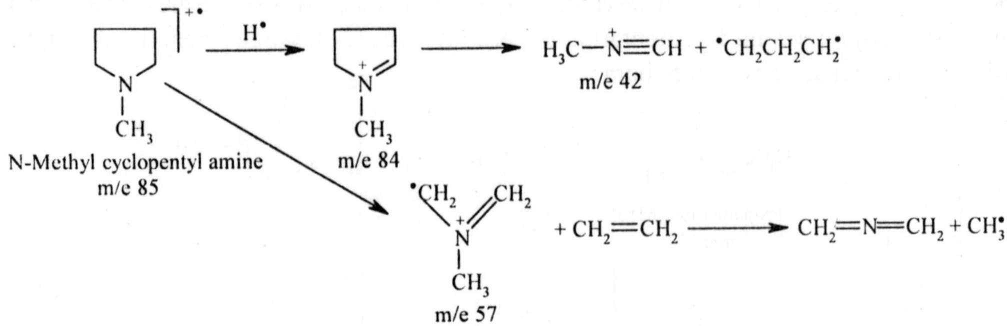

Scheme 6.43. Fragmentation pattern for N-Methyl cyclopentylamine.

6.9.2 Aromatic amines

Aromatic amines typically show intense molecular ions, a minor peak for M-1, and then further fragmentation due to loss of HCN (Scheme 6.44) (i.e. aniline, Fig. 6.43).

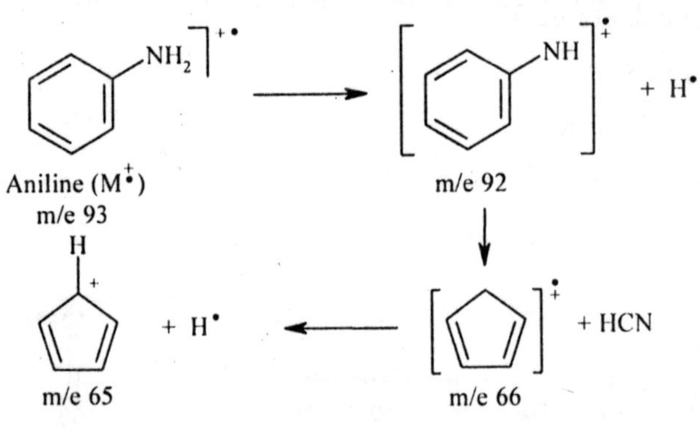

Scheme 6.44. Mass fragmentation for Aniline.

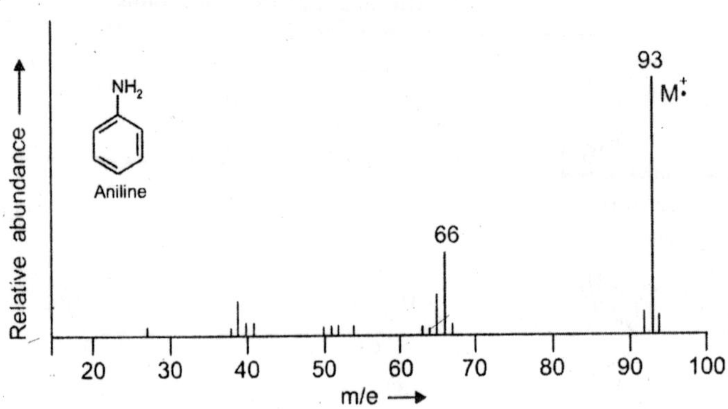

Fig. 6.43. Mass spectrum of Aniline.

6.10 AMIDE

6.10.1 Aliphatic amides

The molecular ion peak is usually observable, and is a good indication of the presence of an amide (nitrogen rule). An important fragmentation pattern involves α-cleavage (breaking either bond to the carbonyl carbon) as shown in Scheme 6.45.

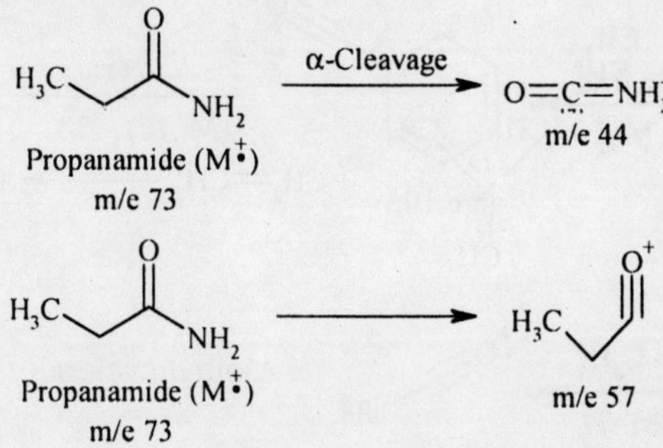

Scheme 6.45. Mass fragmentation for Propanamide.

The mass spectrum of simple primary amides typically shows a moderate molecular ion and an intense peak at m/e 44 due to loss of an alkyl radical (propanamide, Fig. 6.44). It also exhibits loss of amino group to give peak at m/e 57.

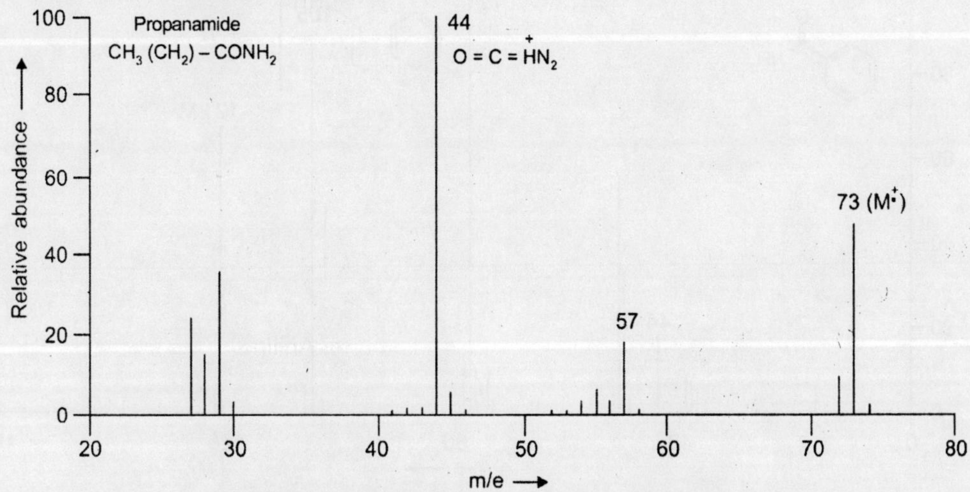

Fig. 6.44. Mass spectrum for Propanamide.

McLafferty rearrangement can take place for amides possessing long chain alkyl portion (see Scheme 6.46).

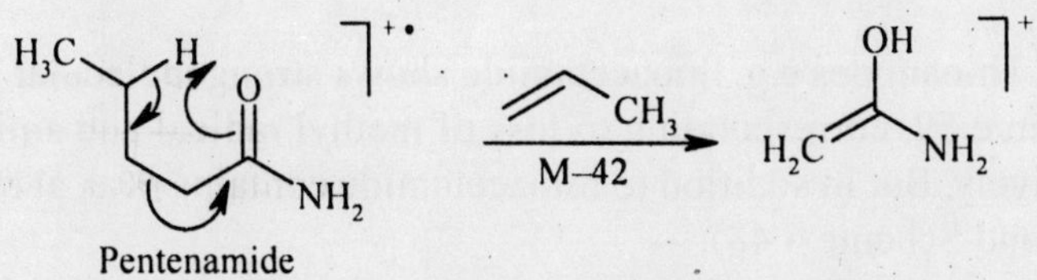

Scheme. 6.46. McLafferty rearrangement of an amide.

6.10.2 Aromatic amides

The aromatic amides show intense molecular ion peak. Like aliphatic amides, all show important fragmentation pattern involves α-cleavage (breaking either bond to the carbonyl carbon) as shown in Scheme 6.47 with the example of Benzamide (Fig. 6.45).

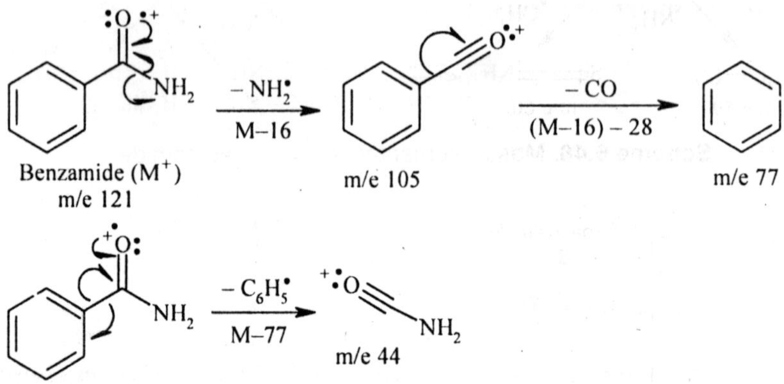

Scheme 6.47. Fragmentation pattern for Benzamide.

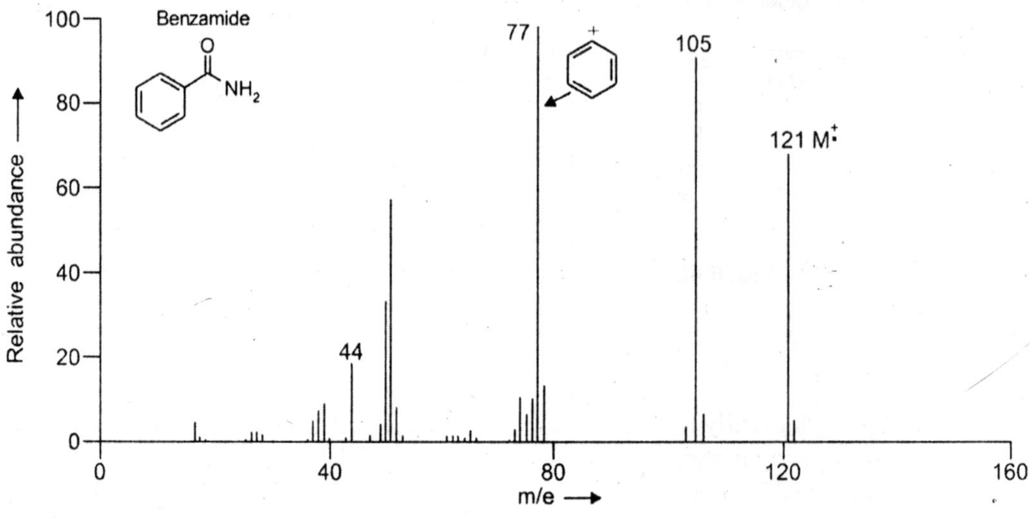

Fig. 6.45. Mass spectrum of Benzamide.

6.10.3 Thioamides

The mass spectrum of Thioamides e.g. thioacetamide shows strong molecular ion peak. It exhibits the peak at m/60 and m/e 59, corresponding to loss of methyl radical and amino radical from the molecular ion respectively. But in addition to thioacetamide contains peak at m/e 42 due to loss an M–'SH ion (Fig 6.46 and Scheme 6.48).

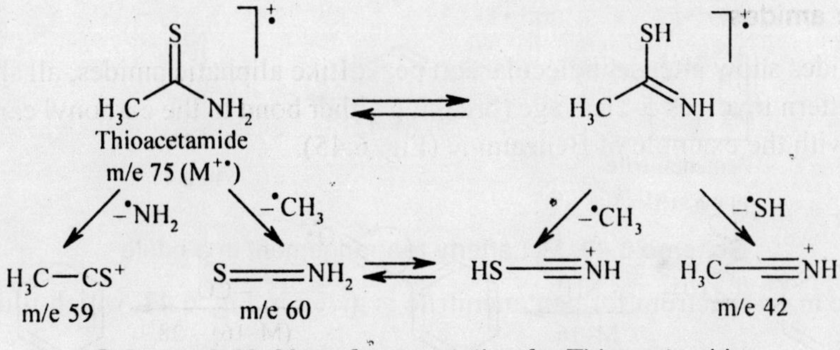

Scheme 6.48. Mass fragmentation for Thioacetamide.

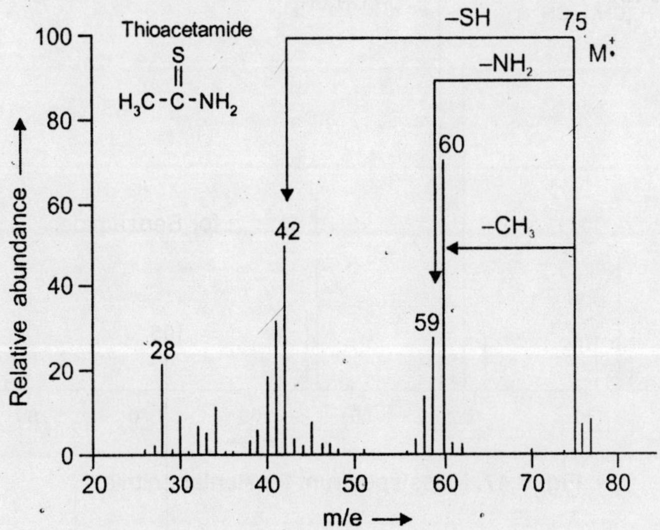

Fig. 6.46. Mass spectrum of Thioacetamide.

6.11 NITRILES

6.11.1 Aliphatic nitriles

The molecular ion peak is usually too weak to be observed. However, the loss of hydrogen radical will almost always produce an observable peak. For nitriles then, the M–1 peak is usually more prominent than the M^+ peak (see Scheme 6.49).

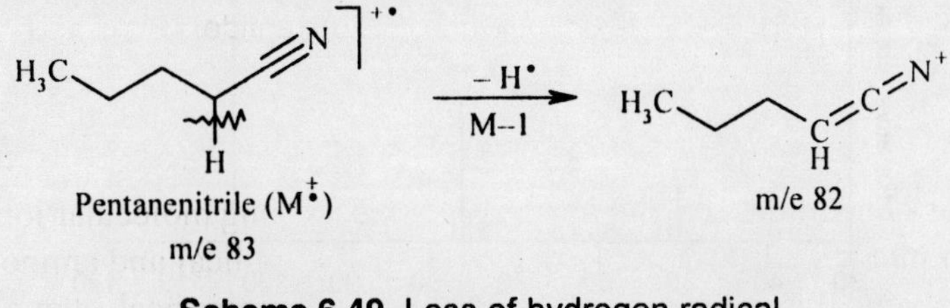

Scheme 6.49. Loss of hydrogen radical.

McLafferty rearrangement can take place for nitriles (see Scheme 6.50).

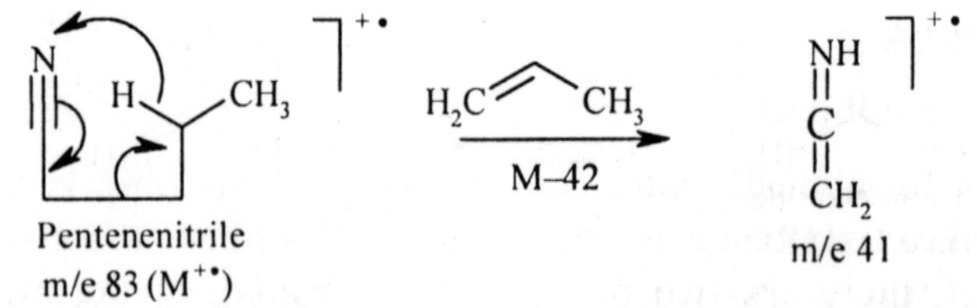

Scheme 6.49. McLafferty rearrangement in a nitrile.

The complete mass spectrum for pentanenitrile is given in Fig. 6.47, which illustrates most of these points.

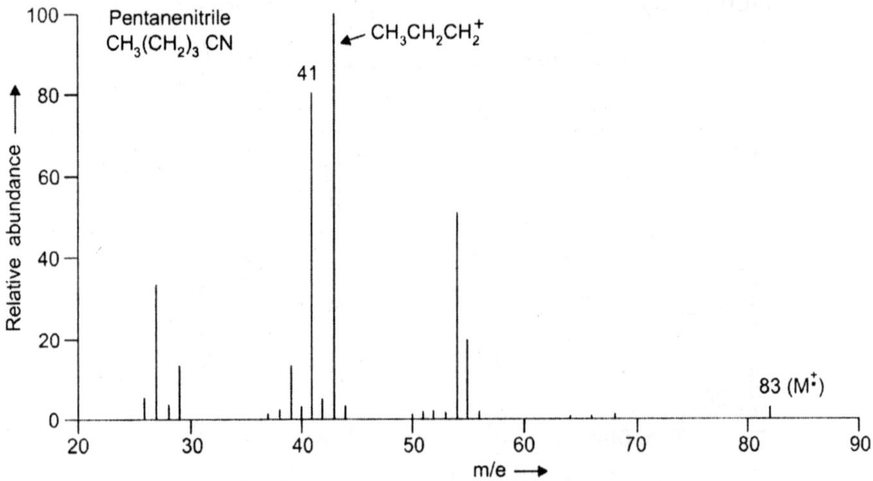

Fig. 6.47. Mass spectrum for Pentanenitrile.

6.11.2 Aromatic nitriles

Aromatic nitriles show strong molecular ions (benzonitrile, Fig. 6.48) and peaks for the loss of cyanide and the elements of HCN (m/e 77 and 76, respectively).

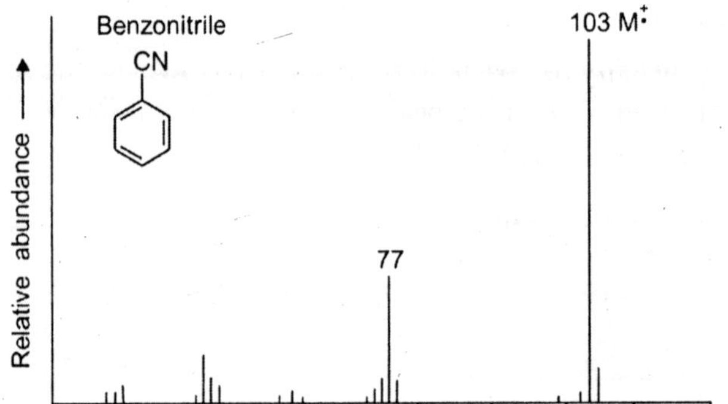

Fig. 6.48. Mass Spectrum of Benzonitrile.

6.12 NITRO COMPOUNDS

6.12.1 Aliphatic nitro compounds

The molecular ion peak for aliphatic nitro compounds is seldom observed. The mass spectrum observed for aliphatic nitro compounds is usually due to the fragmentation of the alkyl portion of the molecule. However, there are two peaks quite indicative of the nitro group: one peak corresponding to the NO^+ ion (m/e 30), and another corresponding to the NO_2^+ ion (m/e 46). The complete mass spectrum for 1-nitropropane is given in Fig. 6.49, which illustrates these points.

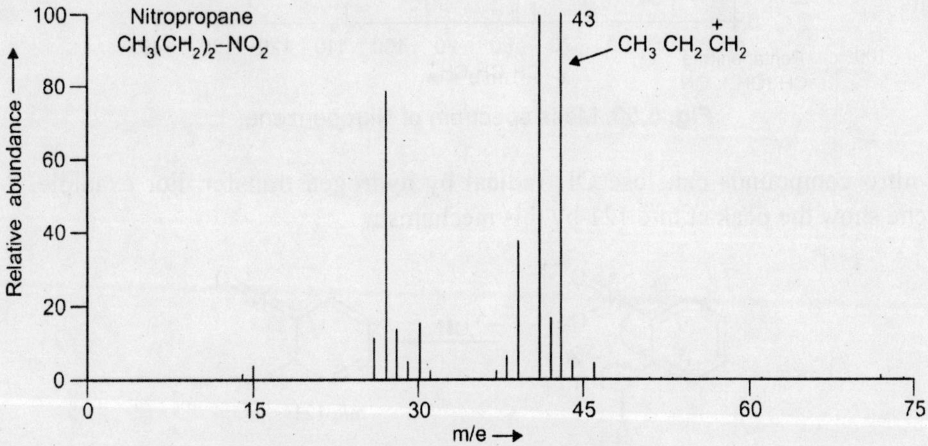

Fig. 6.49. Mass Spectrum of Nitropropane.

6.12.2 Aromatic nitro compounds

Aromatic nitro compounds have good molecular ion peak and lose nitro radical to show the peak of Ar^+. Many $ArNO_2$ compounds like nitrobenzene show a signal of $(M–O)^+$ which is quite distinctive (Scheme 6.51).

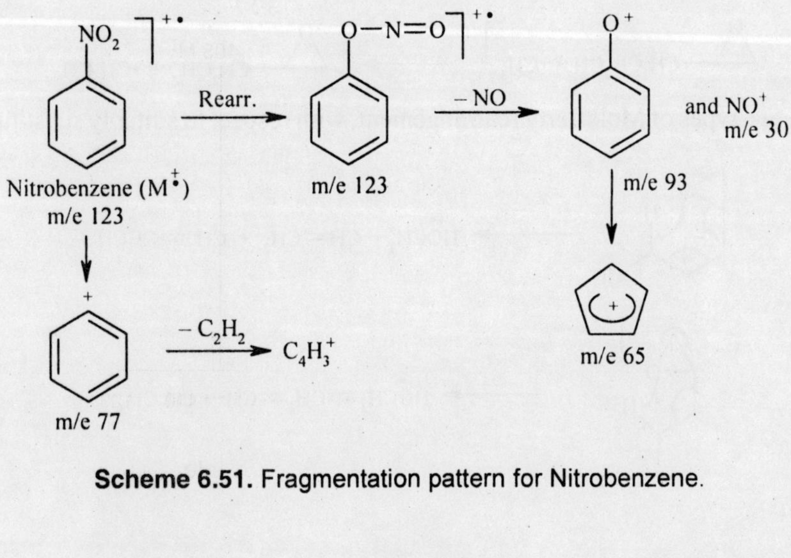

Scheme 6.51. Fragmentation pattern for Nitrobenzene.

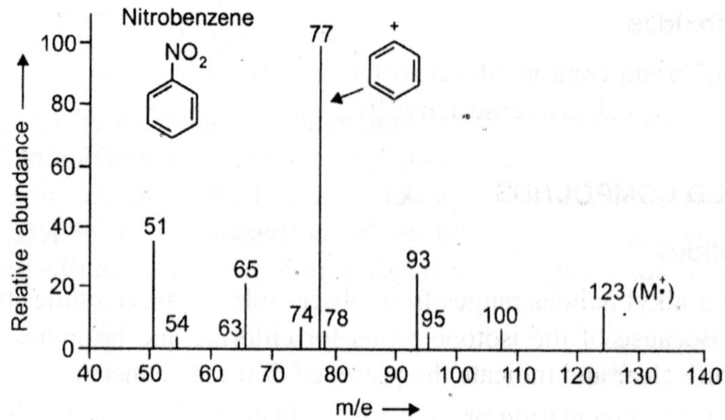

Fig. 6.50. Mass spectrum of Nitrobenzene.

Ortho nitro compounds can lose OH radical by hydrogen transfer. For example, 2-Amino nitrobenzene show the peak at m/e 121 by this mechanism.

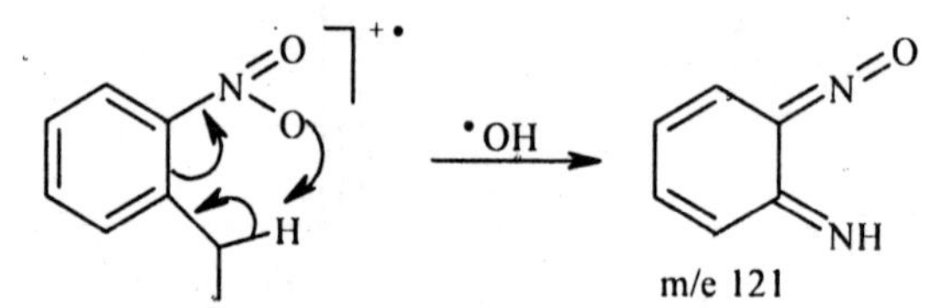

2-Amino nitrobenzene ($M^{+\bullet}$)
m/e 138

6.13 EPOXIDES

6.13.1 Aliphatic epoxides

The molecular ion peak is weak. The molecular ion undergoes γ fission with respect to the epoxide ring giving an intense peak.,

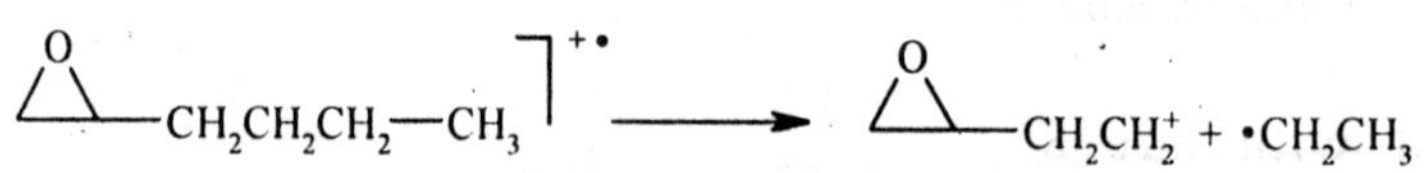

There can be two types of Mclafferty rearrangement, with respect to suitably substituted epoxides.

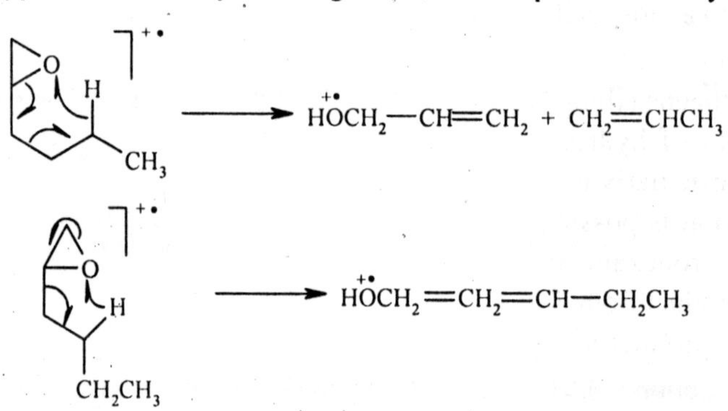

6.13.2 Aromatic epoxides

There is an intense M-1 peak. Transannular cleavage gives the tropyllium ion, which is intense at m/e 91.

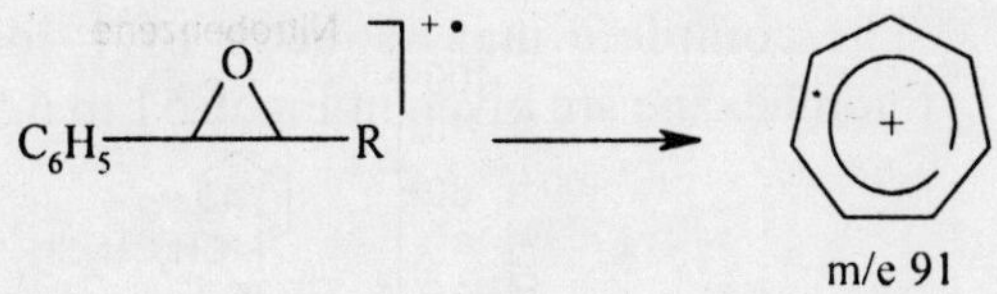

6.14 HALOGENATED COMPOUNDS

6.14.1 Aliphatic halides

The molecular ion for alkyl halides ranges from observable for alkyl iodides to barely detectable for alkyl fluorides. Because of the isotope ratios for chlorine and bromine, the M^+ and $M + 2$ observed ions are quite clear and indicate the presence of these elements.

The most important fragmentation process for the heavier alkyl halides (bromine and iodine) involves simply losing the halogen to form an alkyl carbocation (*ipso*-cleavage). For this reason, the mass spectra for these halogenated compounds are dominated by the fragmentation of an alkyl ion and, thus, mimic the mass spectra of simple alkanes. Competing with this loss (for sufficiently long chain primary halides) is a δ cleavage (e.g., the loss of an ethyl group in the fragmentation of 1-bromohexane (to give ions of m/e 135/137) and 1–chlorohexane (to give ions of m/e 91/93)) - (see Scheme 6.52 and Scheme 6.53). The product ions are 5-membered ring halonium ions.

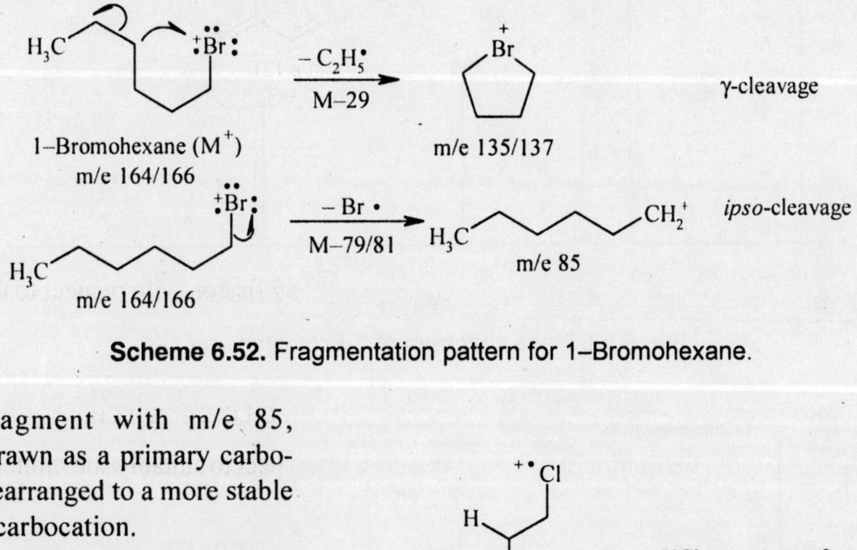

Scheme 6.52. Fragmentation pattern for 1–Bromohexane.

The fragment with m/e 85, although drawn as a primary carbocation, is rearranged to a more stable secondary carbocation.

For the lighter halogens (fluorine and chlorine) the loss of hydrogen halide is important particularly when a 1,3 or 1,4–elimination is possible. In the cases of 1–chlorohexane and 1–fluorohexane, the product from loss of HCl (or HF) is the product ion of m/e 84.

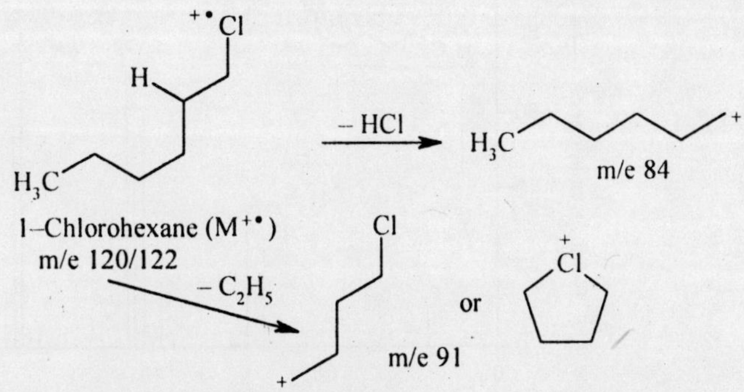

Scheme 6.53. Fragmentation pattern for 1-Chlorohexane.

The complete mass spectra of 1–iodohexane, 1–bromohexane, 1–chlorohexane, and 1–fluorohexane are given in Fig. 6.51 to 6.54, respectively.

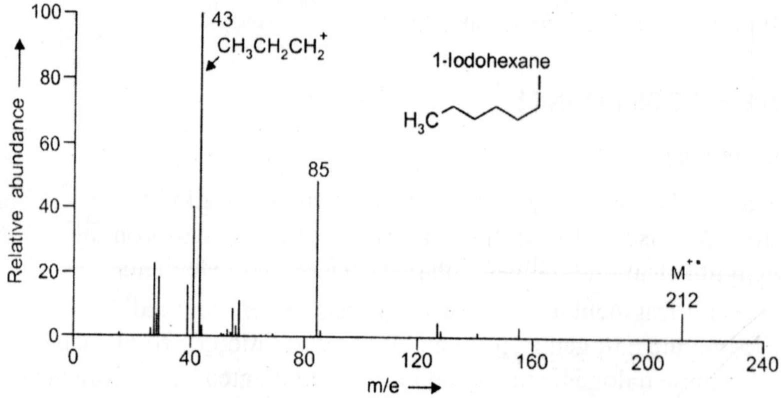

Fig. 6.51. Mass spectrum of 1-Iodohexane.

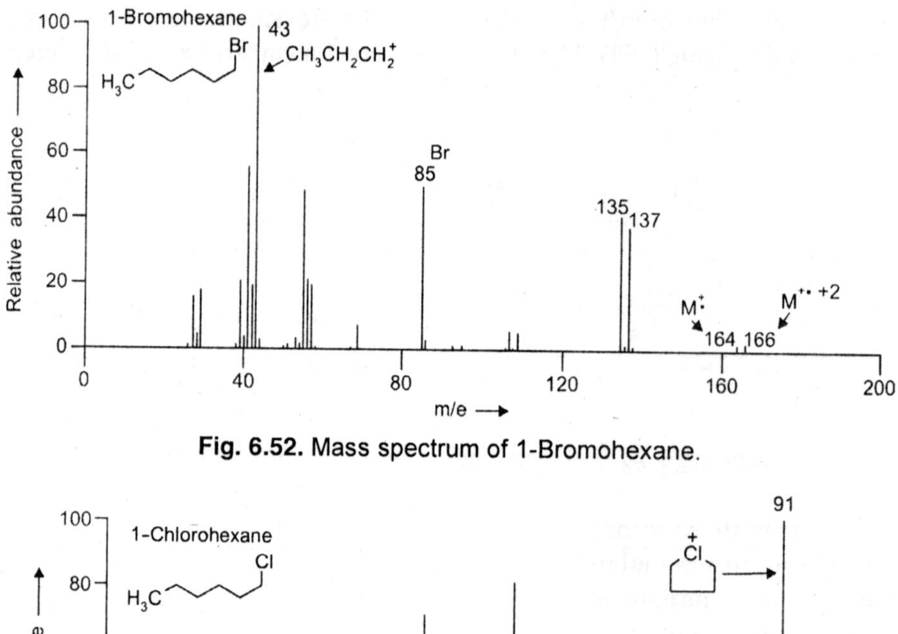

Fig. 6.52. Mass spectrum of 1-Bromohexane.

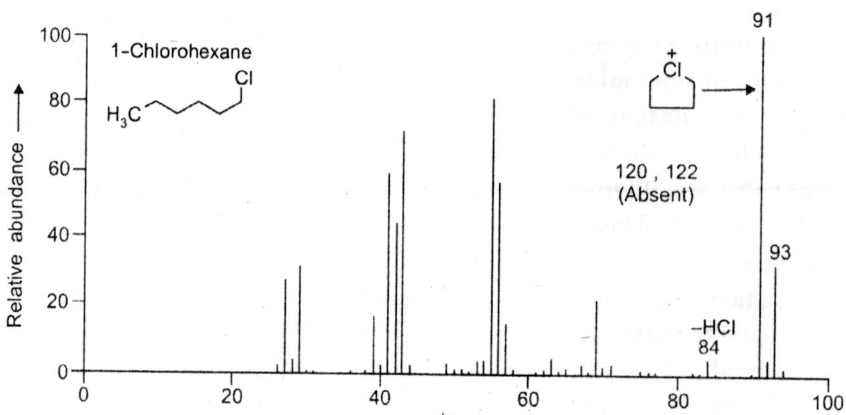

Fig. 6.53. Mass spectrum of 1-Chlorohexane.

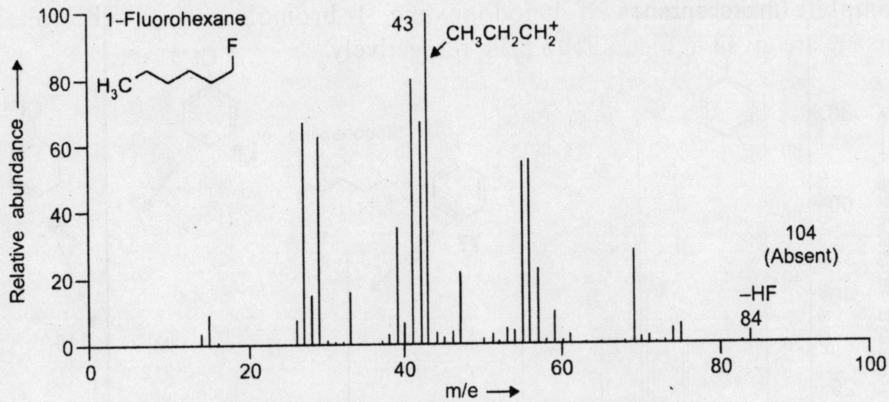

Fig. 6.54. Mass spectrum of 1-Fluorohexane

6.14.2 Aromatic halides

The molecular ion peak is strong in aryl halides. M-halide ion in intense in all compounds containing halogen atom directly attached to the ring. For example, mechanism of fragmentation of halobenzene is given in Scheme 6.54. For reference, mass spectrum (Fig. 6.55) of chlorobenzene is given here.

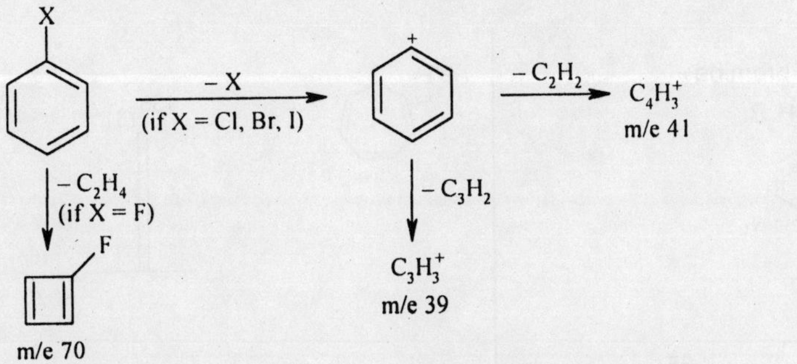

Scheme 6.54. Fragmentation pattern for Aromatic halides.

Benzyl halide ions shows strong molecular ion peak and also lose halide ion to form benzyl cation which changes to form more stable tropyllium ion. For example, the spectrum of Benzyl bromide shows two small peaks of equal intensity in the molecular ion region, strongly suggesting that the molecule contains bromine (equal concentrations of the ^{79}Br and ^{81}Br isotopes). The base peak represents loss of this bromine to give the peak at m/e 91, which is highly suggestive of a benzyl fragment, which rearranges to form the tropylium cation (Scheme 6.55).

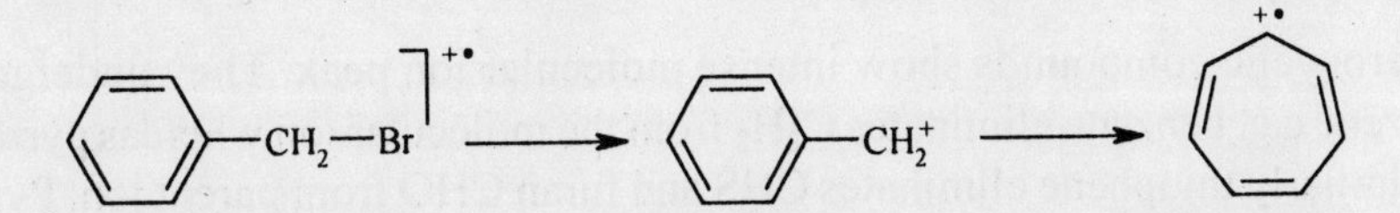

Scheme 6.55. Mass Fragmentation pattern for Benzyl Bromide

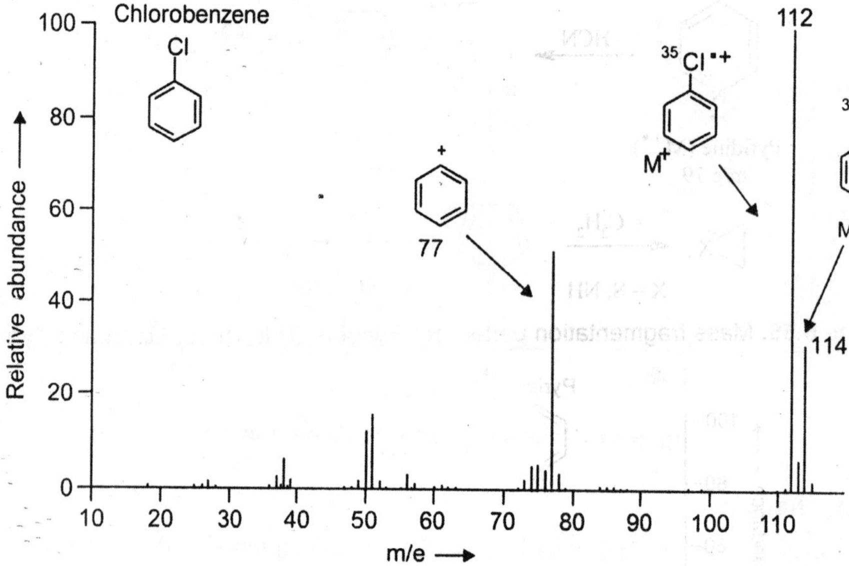

Fig. 6.55. Mass spectrum of Chlorobenzene.

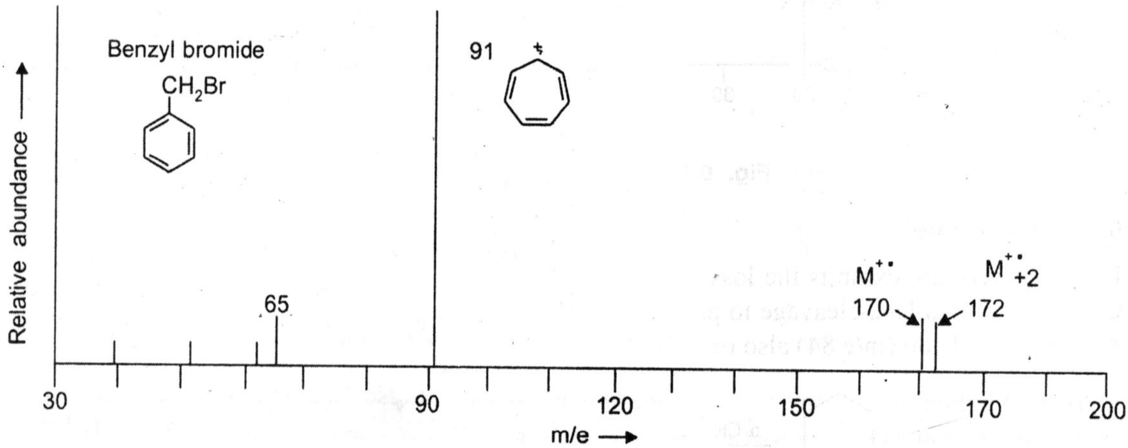

Fig. 6.56. Mass spectrum of Benzyl bromide.

6.15 HETEROCYCLIC COMPOUNDS

6.15.1 Pyridine, Pyrrole, Furan, Thiophene

Aromatic heterocyclic compounds show intense molecular ion peak. They undergo fragmentation similar to benzene e.g. benzene eliminates C_2H_2 from the molecular ion whereas pyrrole and pyridine loose HCN. Similarly thiophene eliminates CHS and furan CHO from parent ion. Pyrrole, thiophene and furan also elim inate $C_3H_3^{\cdot}$ from their molecular ion to give HC≡S and HC≡O ions respectively (Scheme 6.56).

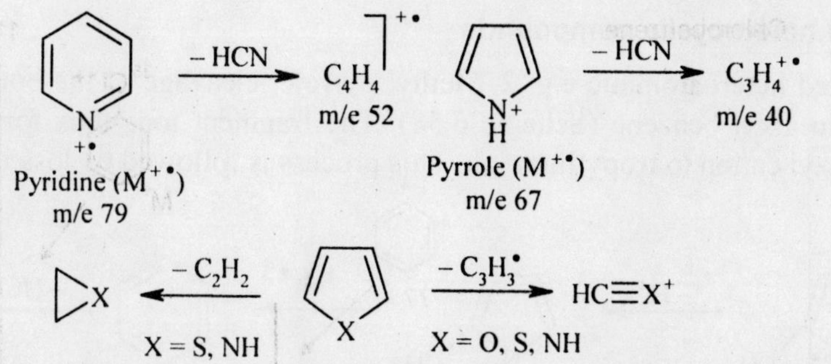

Scheme 6.56. Mass fragmentation pattern for Pyridine, Thiophene, Furan and Pyrrole.

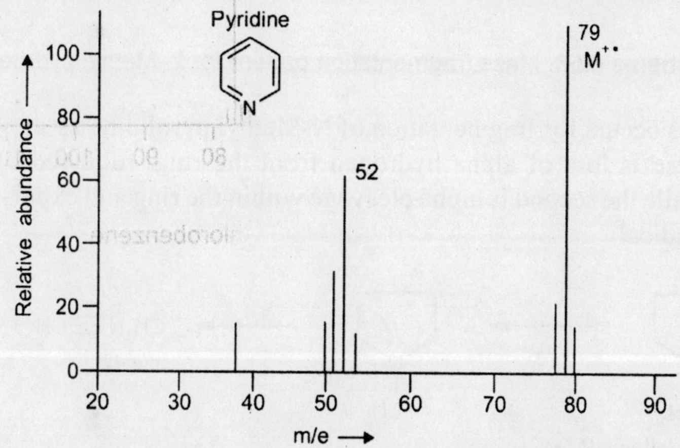

Fig. 6.57. Mass spectrum of Pyridine.

6.15.2 Piperidine

Ionized piperidine exhibits the loss of $^•CH_3$ and $^•C_2H_5$ due to hydrogen transfer reaction and of C_2H_5 due to double α-cleavage to produce ions at m/e 70,56 and 57 respectively (Scheme 6.57). Abundant M–1 ion (m/e 84) also result due to loss of alpha H.

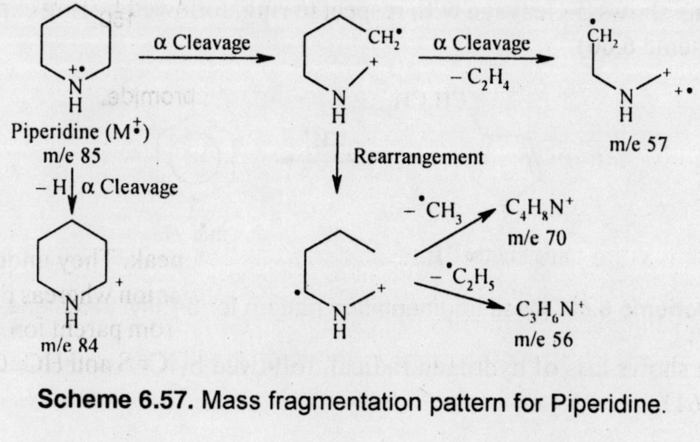

Scheme 6.57. Mass fragmentation pattern for Piperidine.

6.15.3 Alkylated heterocyclic compounds

In alkyl substituted heteroaromatic e.g. 2–Methyl pyrrole, cleavage of the bond β to the ring is favored similar to alkyl benzene (Scheme 6.58). The fragment ions thus formed undergo ring expansion as benzyl cation to tropyllium ion. This process is followed by loss if HCN in nitrogen heterocycles.

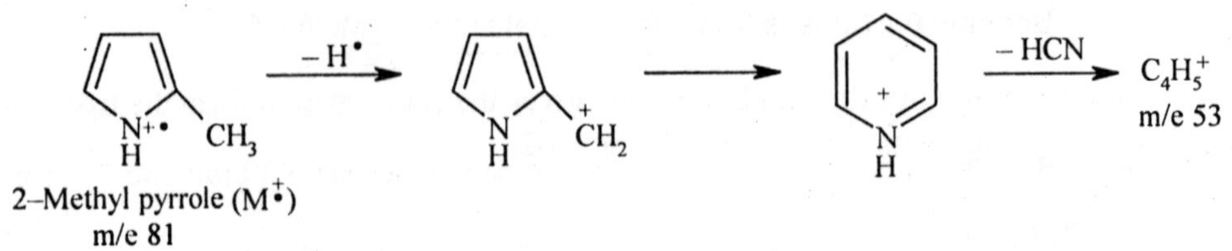

Scheme 6.58. Mass fragmentation pattern for 2–Methyl pyrrole.

Two main process occurs for fragmentation of N-Methyl pyrolidine as shown in Scheme 6.59. The first one of these is loss of alpha hydrogen from the ring, followed by the formation of CH_3–N^+= CH ion while the second is alpha cleavage within the ring and expulsion of the alkene to form ^+N=CH_2CH_2 radical.

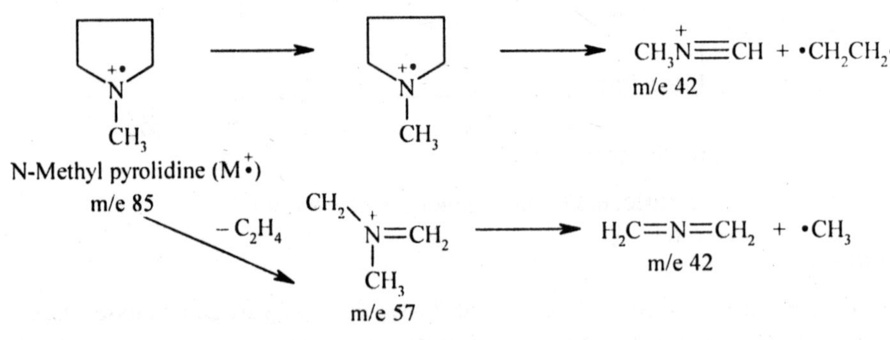

Scheme 6.59. Mass fragmentation pattern for N-Methyl pyrolidine.

3-Ethyl thiophene shows β-cleavage with respect to ring, followed by ring expansion to give the peak at m/e 97 (Scheme 6.60).

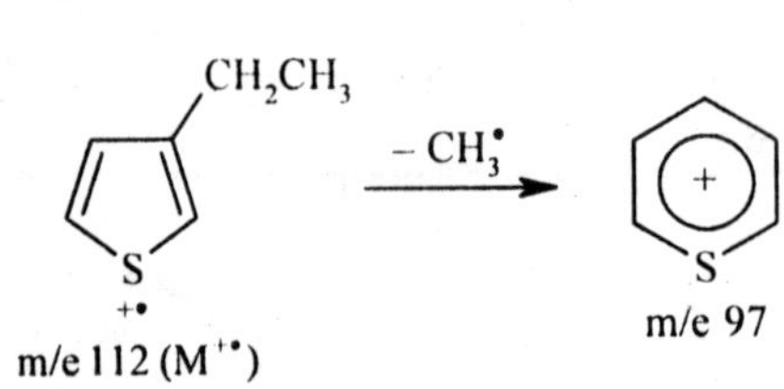

Scheme 6.60. Mass fragmentation pattern for 3-Ethyl thiophene.

2-Methyl Furan shows loss of hydrogen radical, followed by CO molecule to give the peak at m/e 53 (Scheme 6.61).

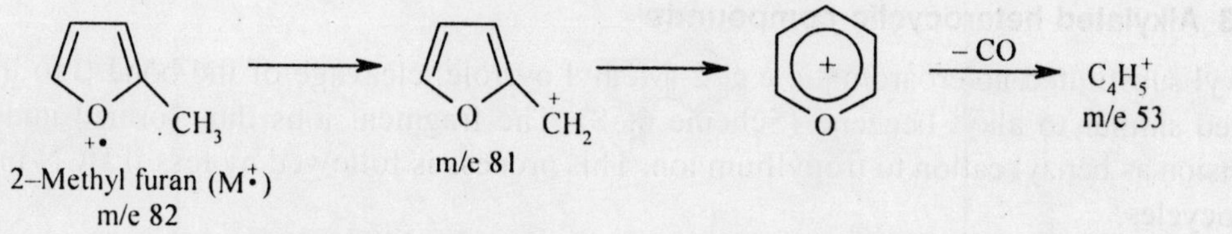

Scheme 6.61. Mass fragmentation pattern for 2-Methyl furan.

The substituted 3–Ethyl pyridine on β cleavage gives the cation which form the tropyllium ion, m/e 106. This shows fragmentation as per Scheme 6.62.

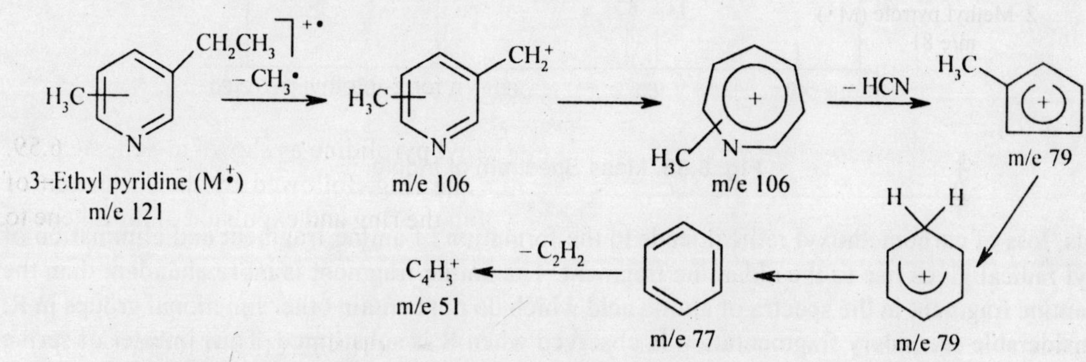

Scheme 6.62. Mass fragmentation pattern for Substituted 3-Ethyl pyridine.

6.15.4 Benzfused heterocyclic compounds

Indole. Indole shows intense molecular ion peak at m/e 117 (Fig. 6.58). It fragments by the loss of hydrogen cyanide (Scheme 6.63). Alkyl substituted indoles decompose by α cleavage and undergo ring expansion reactions.

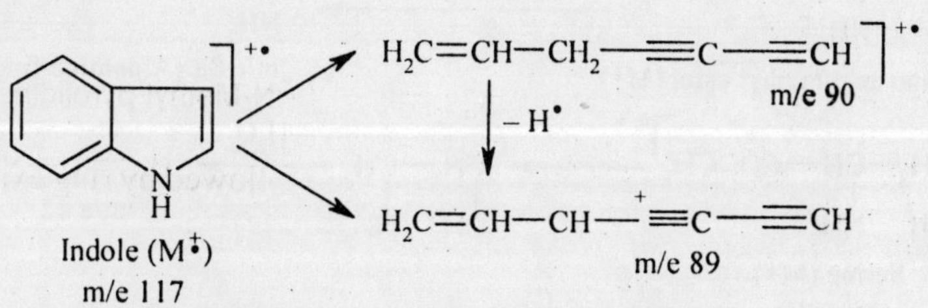

Scheme 6.63. Mass fragmentation pattern for Indole.

6.16 NATURAL PRODUCTS

6.16.1 Amino acid

The amino acids are non volatile in nature and so they are derivatized for mass analysis. Some of these derivatives include ethyl ester, N-acetyl, N-trimethylsilyl, etc. The mass spectra of esters furnish more clear structural information than those of all other derivatives. The major fragmentation mode of an α-amino acid is α-cleavage (cleavage of carbon-carbon bond next to amino group).

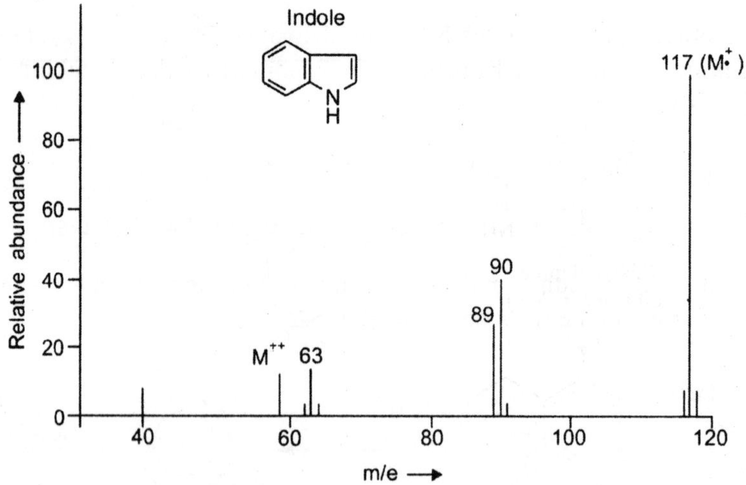

Fig. 6.58. Mass Spectrum of Indole.

Thus, loss of carbomethoxyl radical leads to the formation of amine fragment and elimination of alkyl radical gives rise to the aldamine fragment. The amine fragment is more abundant than the aldamine fragment in the spectra of amino acid which do not contain other functional groups in R. Considerable secondary fragmentation is observed when R is substituted. Thus in ester of serine and threonine the presence of the hydroxyl group triggers both the elimination of water and McLafferty rearrangement (Scheme 6.64).

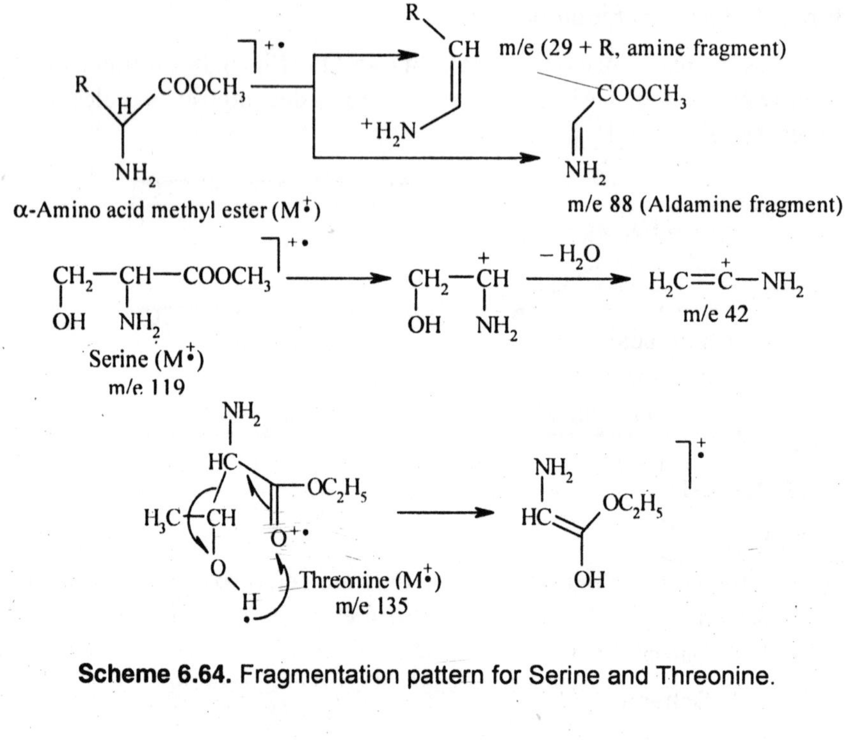

Scheme 6.64. Fragmentation pattern for Serine and Threonine.

Phenyl alanine ethyl ester undergoes benzylic cleavage. The charge is retained by either of fragment. The aldamine fragments (Scheme 6.65) are in abundance due to stability if benzyl radical.

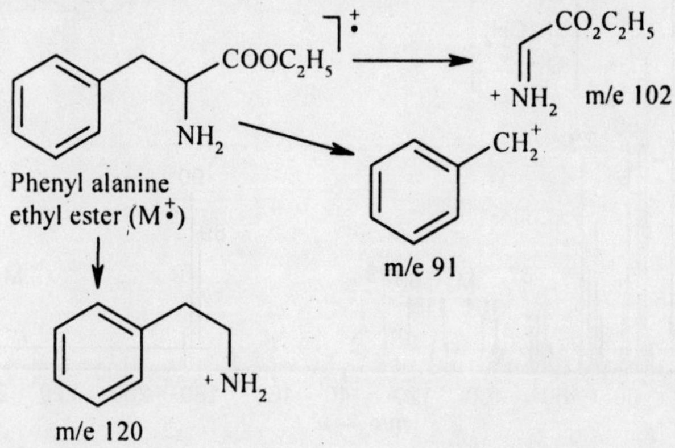

Scheme 6.65. Fragmentation pattern for Phenyl alanine ethyl ester.

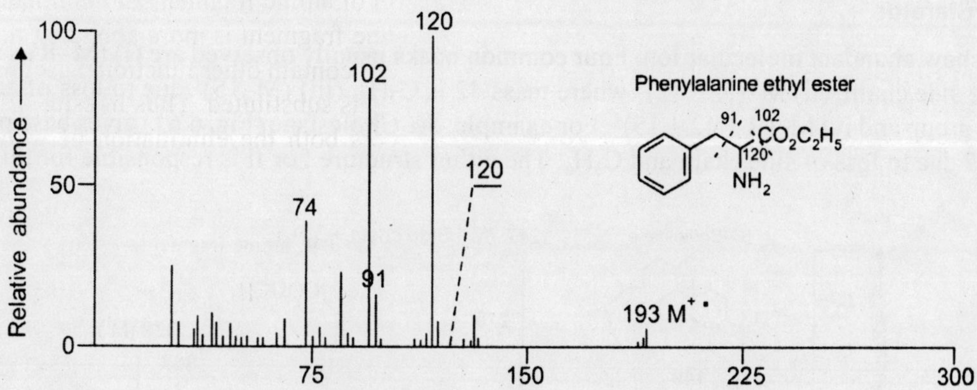

Fig. 6.59. Mass spectrum of Phenyl alanine ethyl ester.

6.16.2 Fatty acids

Mass fragmentation of fatty acid includes characteristic peak at m/e 60 due to transfer of gamma hydrogen as shown in mass spectrum of stearic acid (Fig. 6.60).

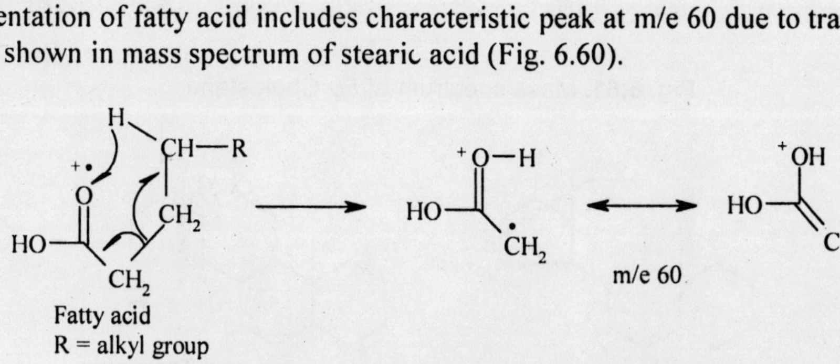

Scheme 6.66. Fragmentation pattern for Fatty acid.

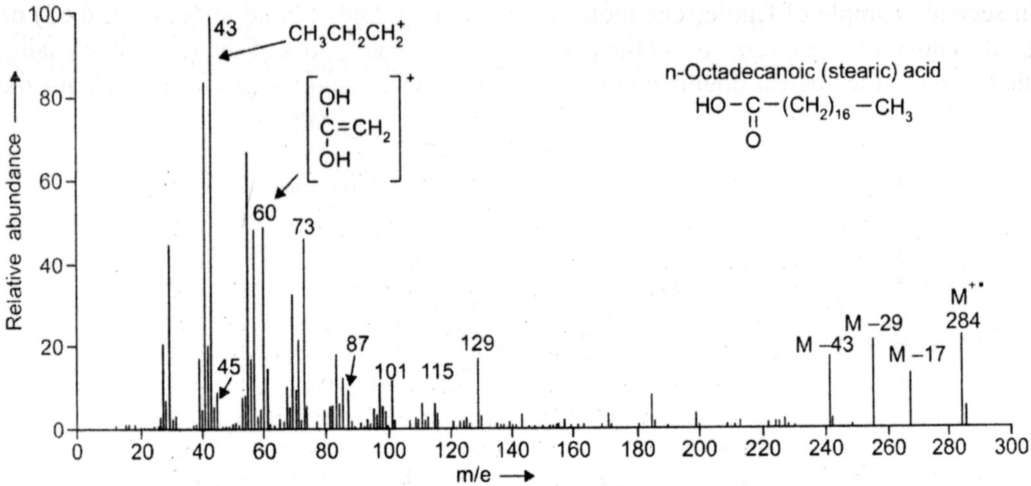

Fig. 6.60. Mass spectrum of Stearic acid.

6.16.3 Steroids

These show abundant molecular ion. Four common peaks usually observed are (i) $(M–R)^+$, where R is the side chain, (ii) $M–(R + 42)^+$ where mass 42 is C_3H_6, (iii) $(M–15)^+$ due to loss of angular methyl group and iv) $M–(R + 42 + 15)^+$. For example, 5α-Cholestane (Fig. 6.61) gives base peak at m/e 217 due to loss of side chain and C_3H_6. The either structure I or II is responsible for this base peak.

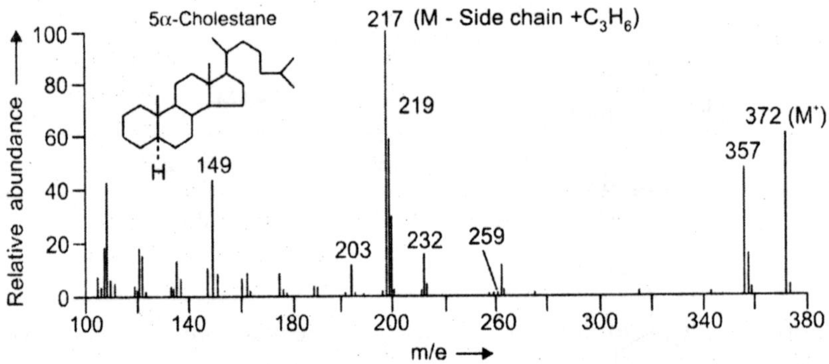

Fig. 6.61. Mass spectrum of 5α-Cholestane

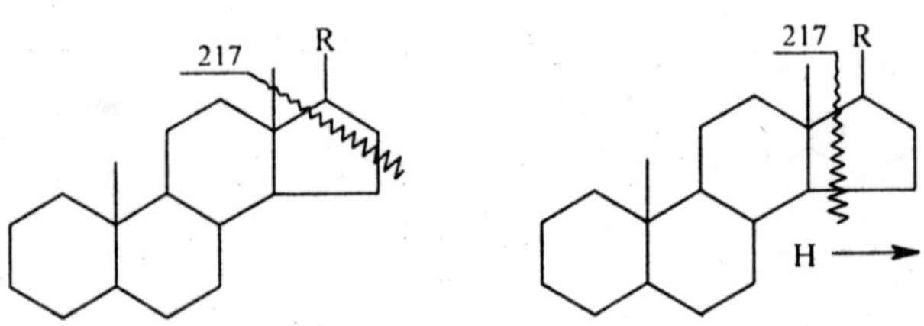

I

II

In second example of Cholestene molecule containing double bond at 5th (Fig. 6.62) or 7th (Fig. 6.63) position, spectrum shows the peak at m/e 257 due to loss of the C–17 side chain with allylic fission of the nuclear double bonds leading to species e and f respectively (Scheme 6.67).

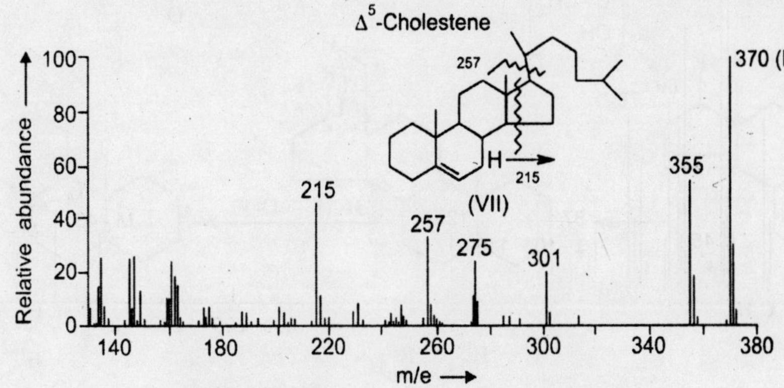

Fig. 6.62. Mass spectrum of Δ^5-Cholestene.

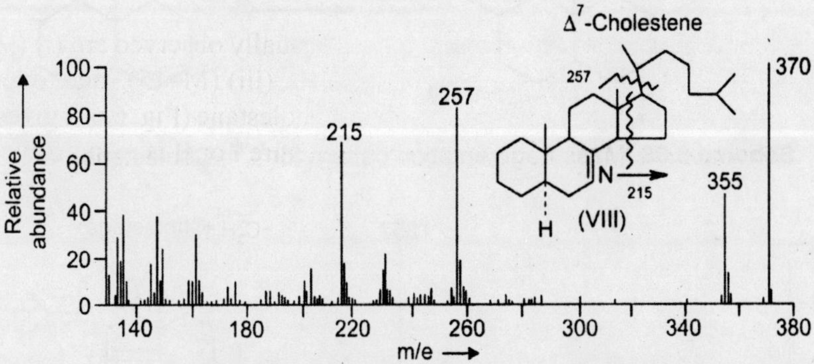

Fig. 6.63. Mass spectrum of Δ^7-Cholestene.

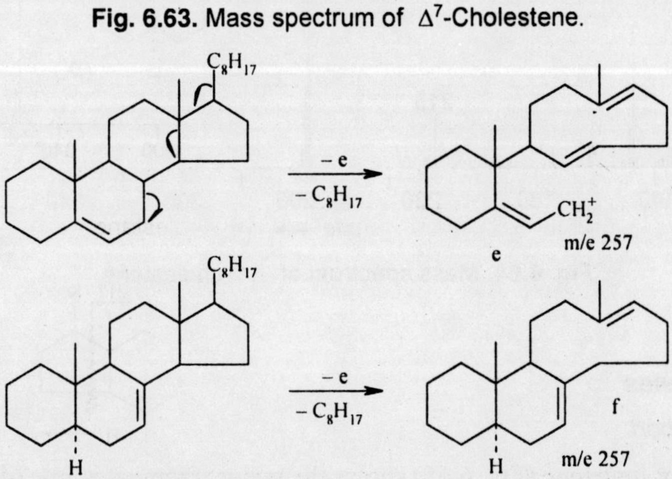

Scheme 6.67. Mass fragmentation pattern for Δ^5–Cholestene and Δ^7–Cholestene.

Such a supposition is clearly not feasible in Δ^{14}–cholestene (IX) and yet this is the substance where such side chain loss occurs to the greatest extent, virtually overshadowing all of the other fragment peaks and especially the molecular ion peak (Fig. 6.64). In this, peak at m/e 215 is very weak (Scheme 6.68).

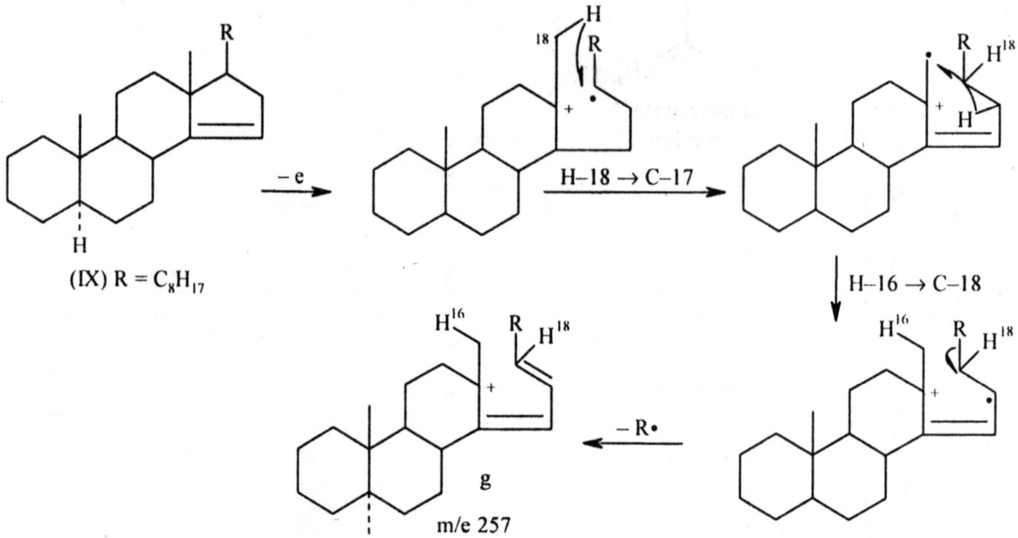

Scheme 6.68. Mass fragmentation pattern for Δ^{14}–Cholestene.

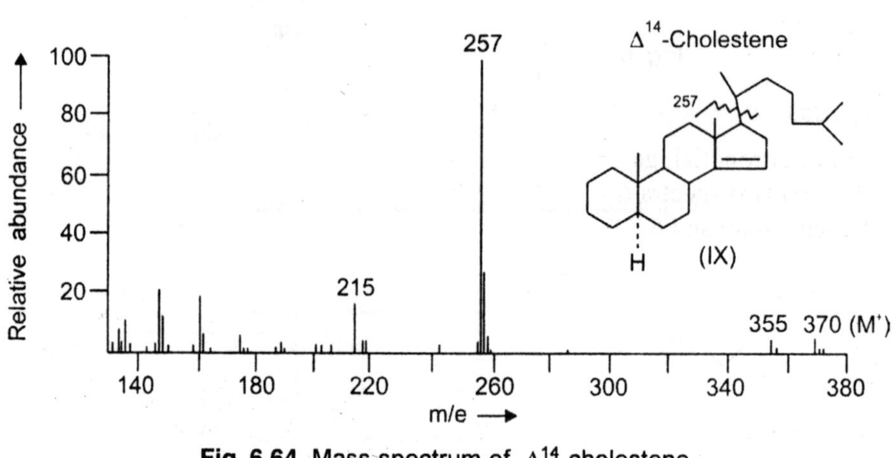

Fig. 6.64. Mass spectrum of Δ^{14}-cholestene.

6.16.4 Terpenes

6.16.4.1 Monoterpenes

6.16.4.1.1 Hydrocarbon

The mass spectrum of limonene (Fig. 6.65) shows the major fragment at m/e 68 by a reverse Diels Alder reaction.

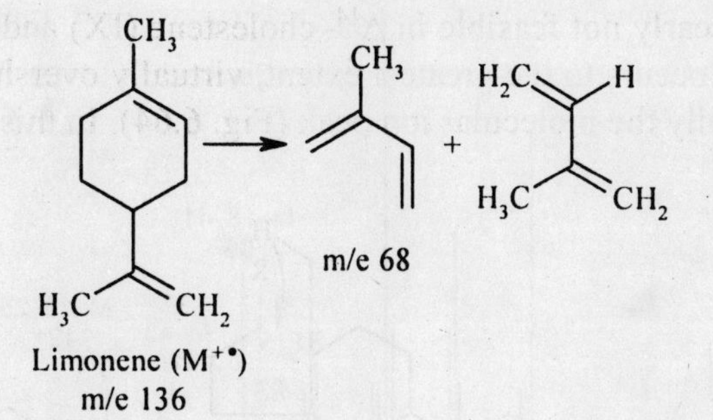

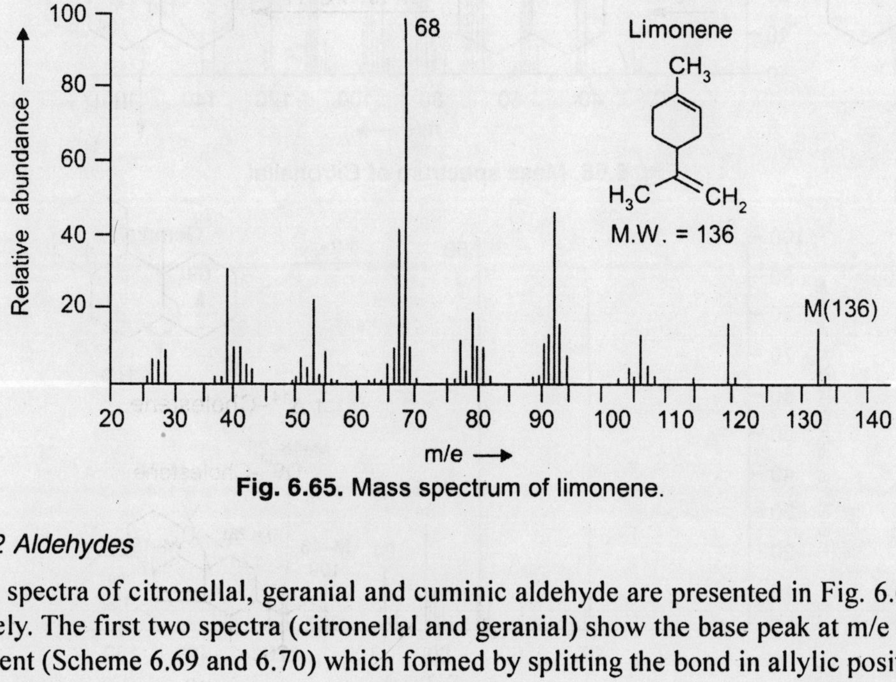

Fig. 6.65. Mass spectrum of limonene.

6.16.4.1.2 Aldehydes

The mass spectra of citronellal, geranial and cuminic aldehyde are presented in Fig. 6.66 to 6.68 respectively. The first two spectra (citronellal and geranial) show the base peak at m/e 69, due to the fragment (Scheme 6.69 and 6.70) which formed by splitting the bond in allylic position to the double bond.

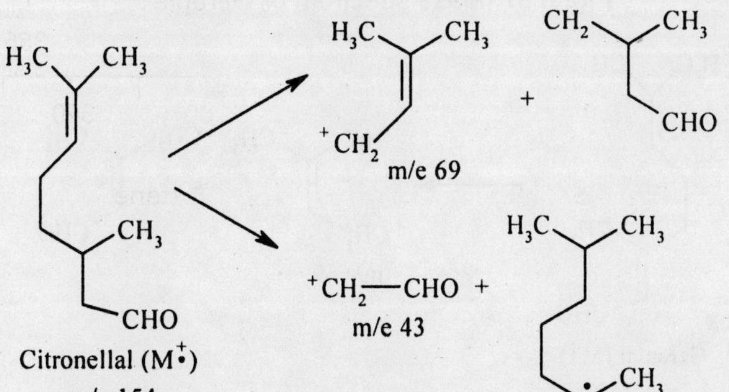

Scheme 6.69. Fragmentation pattern for Citronellal.

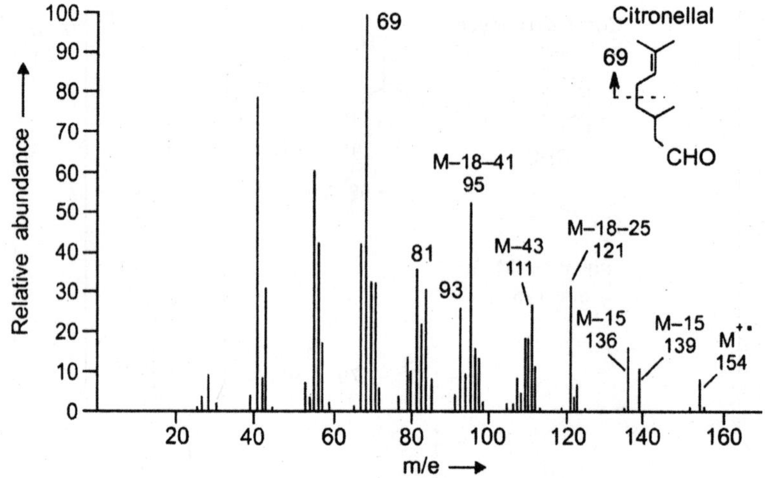

Fig. 6.66. Mass spectrum of Citronellal.

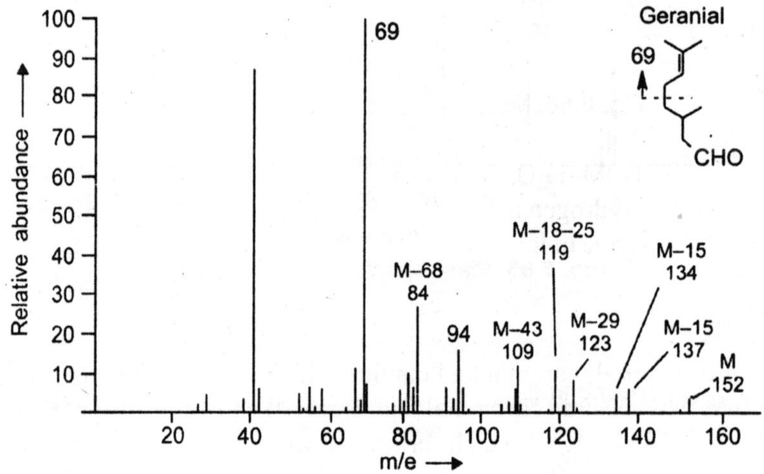

Fig. 6.67. Mass spectrum of Geranial.

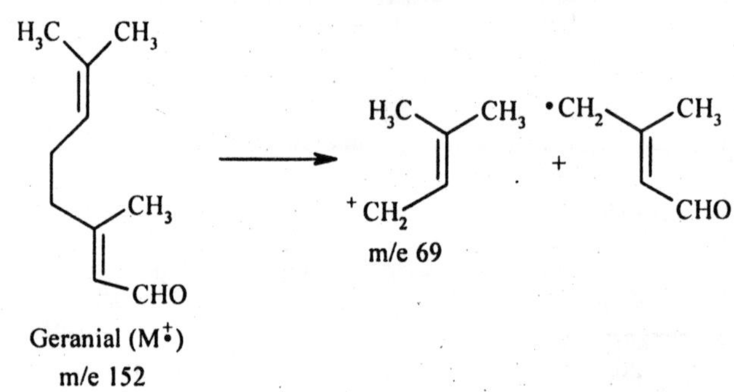

Scheme 6.70. Fragmentation pattern for Geranial.

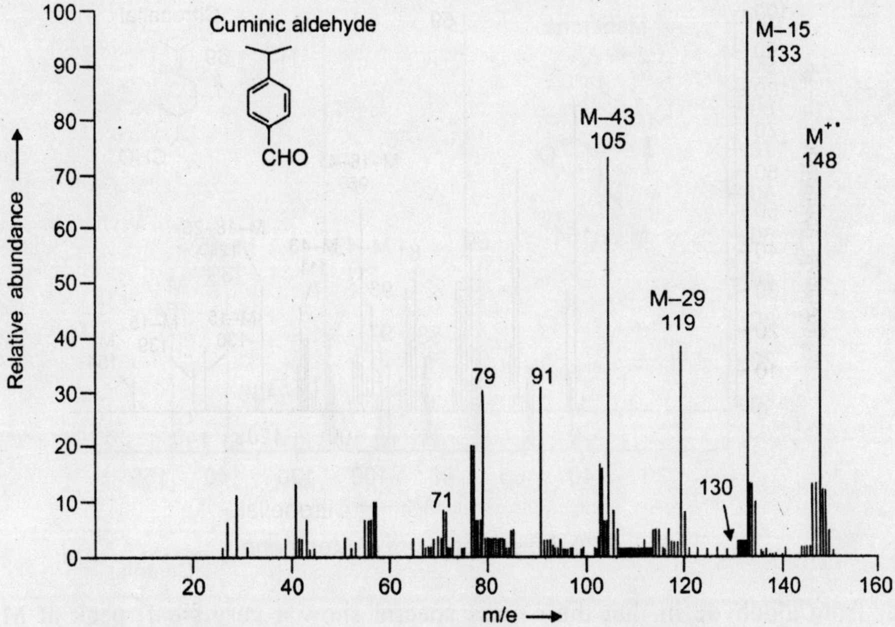

Fig. 6.68. Mass spectrum of Cuminic aldehyde.

The other peaks M–CH_3, M–H_2O, etc. are visible in the spectra. In case of cuminic aldehyde, there seems to be no extra hydrogen atom available for comparative loss of water for M–18 peak. The base peak at m/e 133 is due to loss of methyl group. The peak at m/e 105 (M–43) is due to loss of isopropyl group.

6.16.4.1.3 Ketones

The mass spectra of piperitone and menthone are presented in Fig 6.69 and 6.70) respectively.

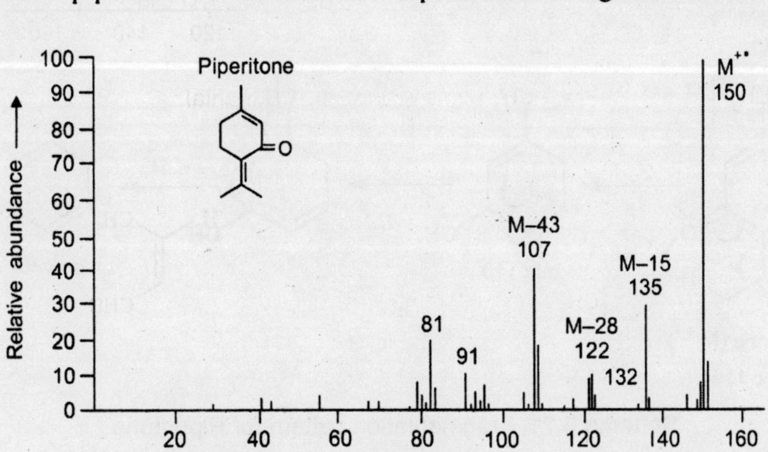

Fig. 6.69. Mass spectrum of Piperitone.

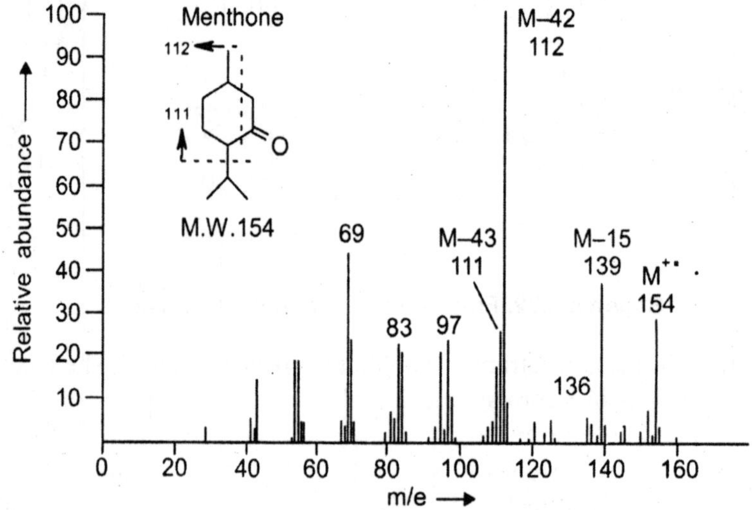

Fig. 6.70. Mass spectrum of Menthone.

They differ from aldehyde in that their mass spectra show a very small peak at M = M-18, corresponding to loss of one water molecule from the parent molecule. The piperitone shows the base peak at m/e 82 due to allylic cleavage (Scheme 6.71).

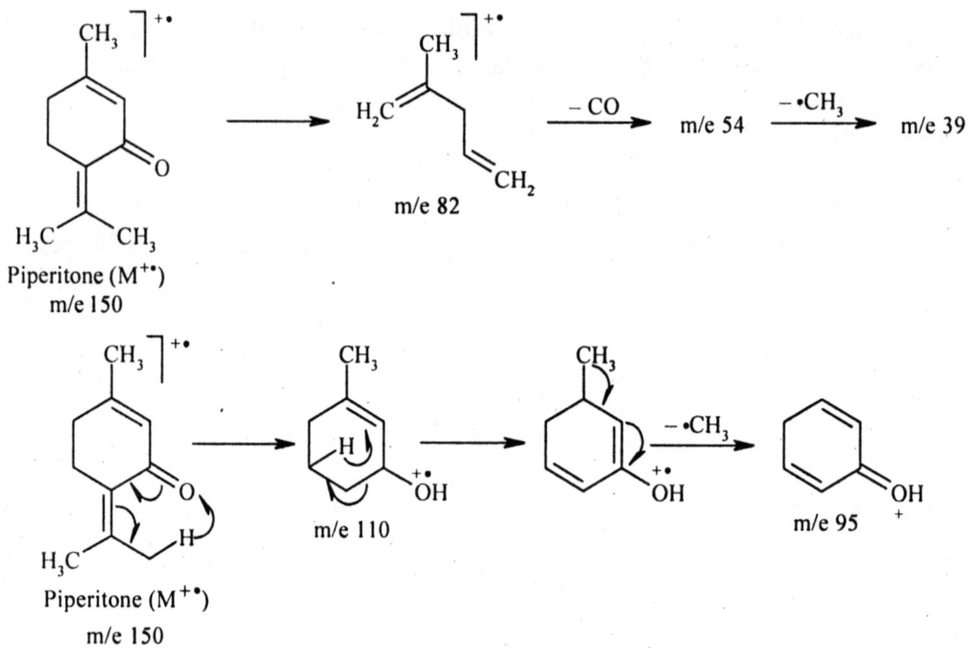

Scheme 6.71. Fragmentation pattern for Piperitone.

Menthone shows the base peak at m/e 112 due to release of stable fragment, $CH_3-CH=CH_2$ as shown in Scheme 6.72.

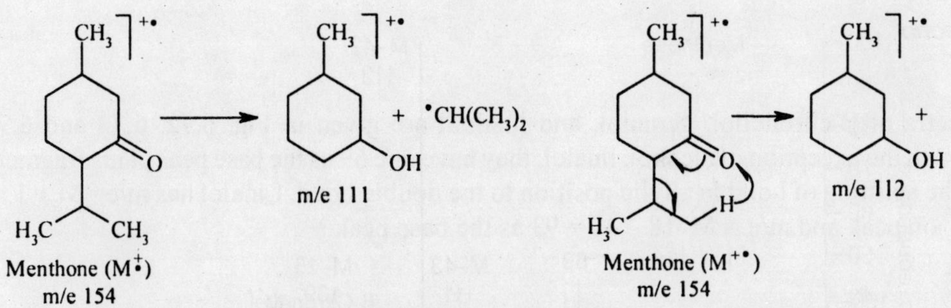

Scheme 6.72. Fragmentation pattern for Menthone.

Bicyclic ketones. The mass spectrum of camphor is given in Fig 6.71.The spectrum of camphor revealed one diffuse peak at 76.8 corresponding to the breakdown reaction of $152^+ \rightarrow 108^+ \rightarrow {}^+44$ (Scheme 6.73). The mass spectra of the monoterpene ketone show the presence generally have peaks at m/e = M–42 or M–44, while the spectra of the hydrocarbons and the alcohols generally have peaks at m/e 43, corresponding to loss of isopropyl group, or at m/e values derived from this fragment. It is therefore likely that loss of 42 or 44 units from ketones does not correspond to a loss of an isopropyl group but rather to an oxygen containing fragment (Scheme 6.73).

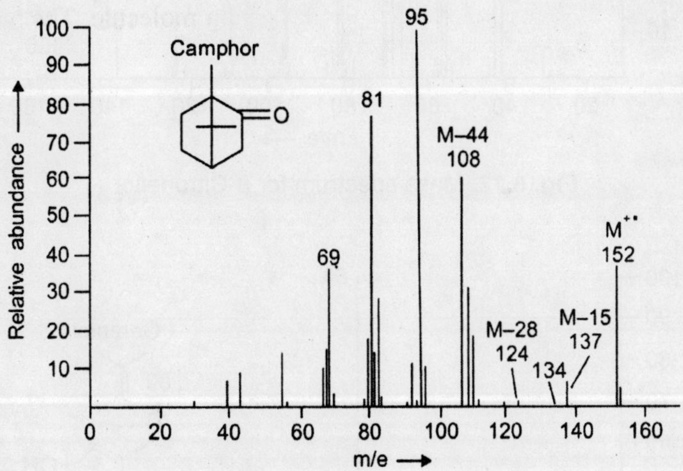

Fig. 6.71. Mass spectrum of camphor.

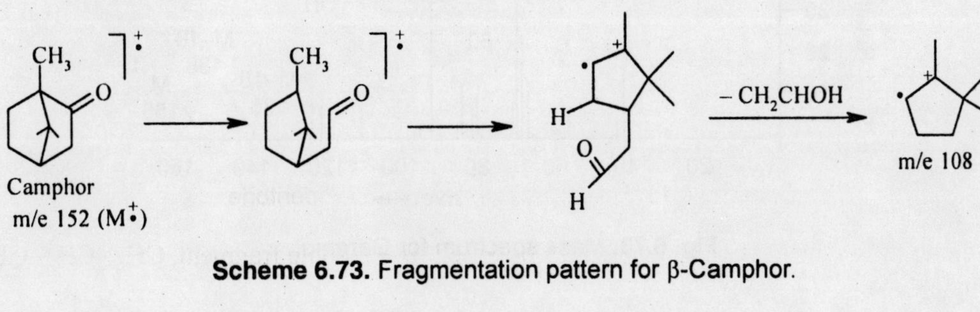

Scheme 6.73. Fragmentation pattern for β-Camphor.

6.16.4.1.4 Alcohol

(a) Acyclic

The mass spectra of β-citronellol, geraniol, and linalool are given in Fig. 6.72, 6.73 and 6.74 respectively. With the exception of alcohol, linalol, they have m/e 69 as the base peak. This fragment is formed by the splitting of bond in allylic position to the double bond. Linalol has m/e= M + 1 as the molecular ion peak and m/e = M–18 – 43 = 93 as the base peak.

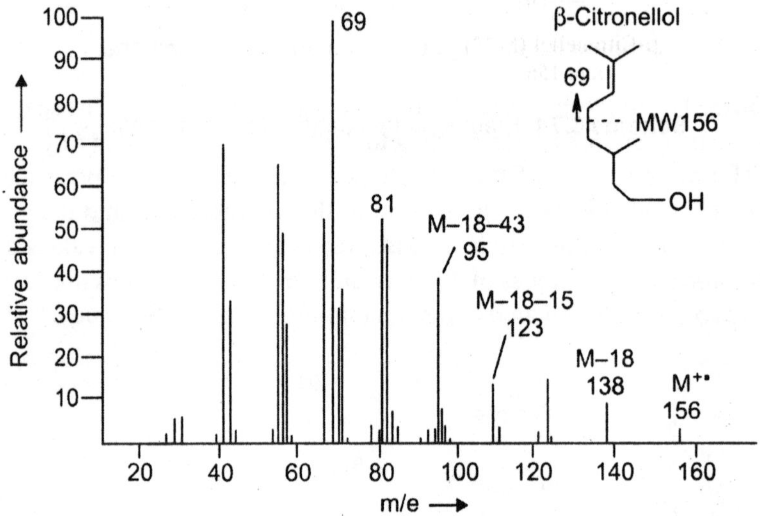

Fig. 6.72. Mass spectrum for β-Citronellol.

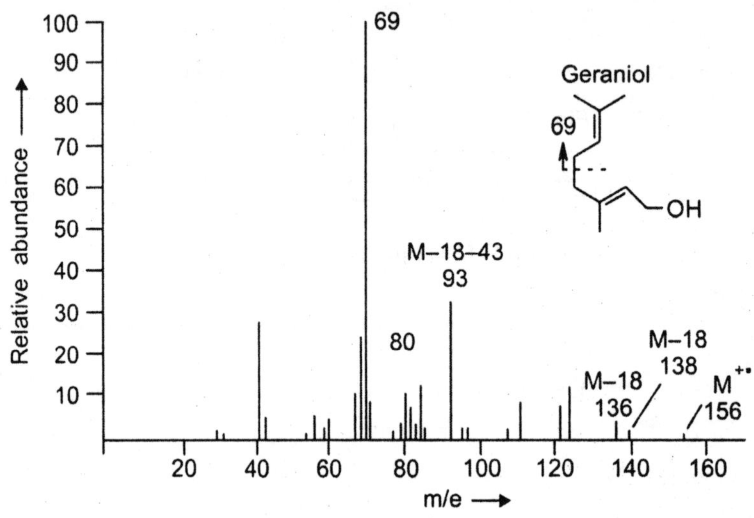

Fig. 6.73. Mass spectrum for Geraniol.

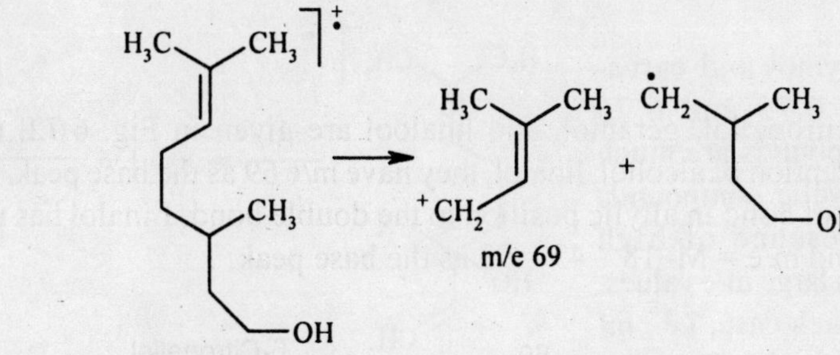

β-Citronellol ($M^{+\bullet}$)
m/e 156

Scheme 6.74. Fragmentation pattern for β-Citronellol.

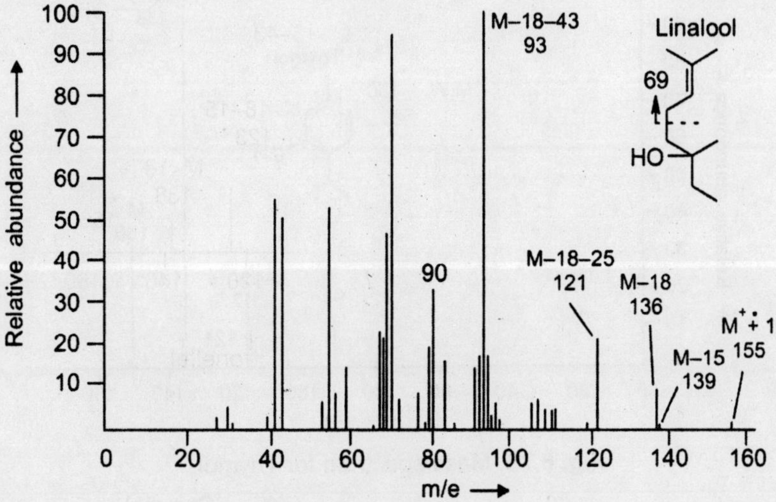

Fig. 6.74. Mass spectrum for Linalol.

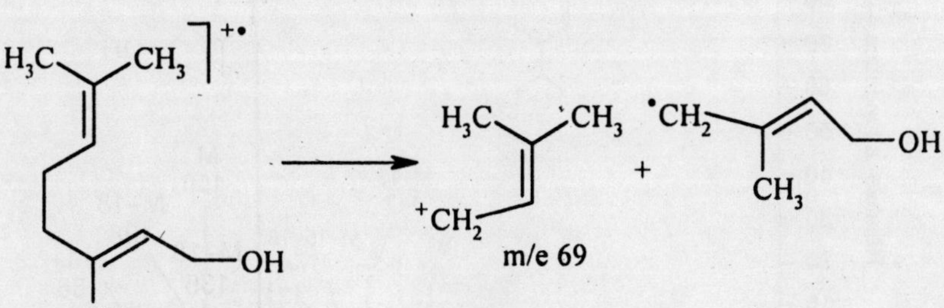

Geraniol ($M^{+\bullet}$)
m/e 154

Scheme 6.75. Fragmentation pattern for Geraniol.

(b) Aromatic

The mass spectra of thymol and carvacrol are given in Fig 6.75 and 6.76 respectively. These compounds are much more stable than the acyclic compounds as revealed by the presence of high concentration of ions with large m/e values. The strongest peaks in each case, i.e., m/e=M and M^+-15, indicate the firmness with which the hydroxyl group is bound (Scheme 6.77).

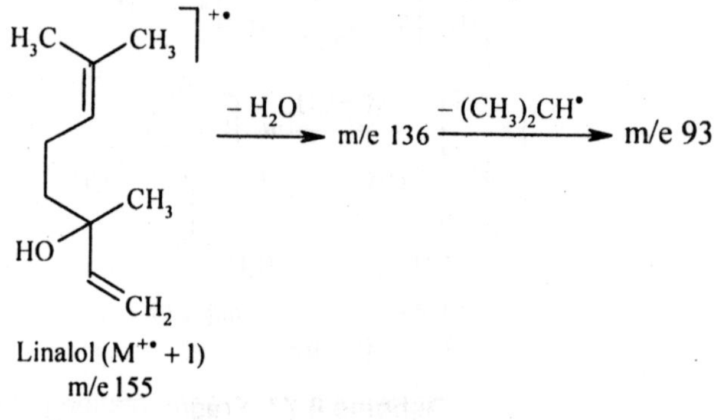

Scheme 6.76. Fragmentation pattern for Linalol.

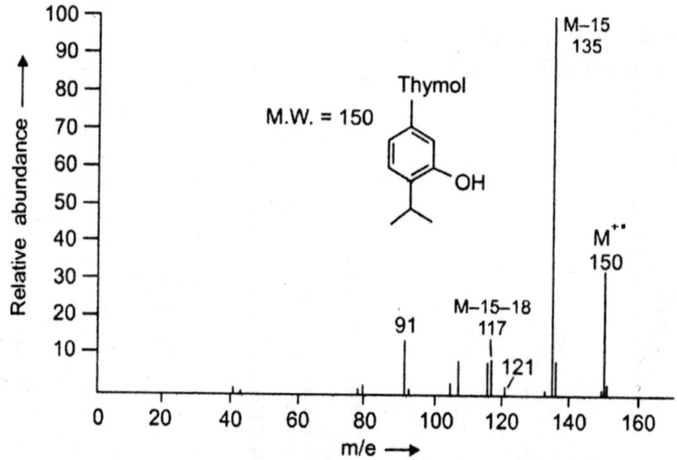

Fig. 6.75. Mass spectrum for Thymol.

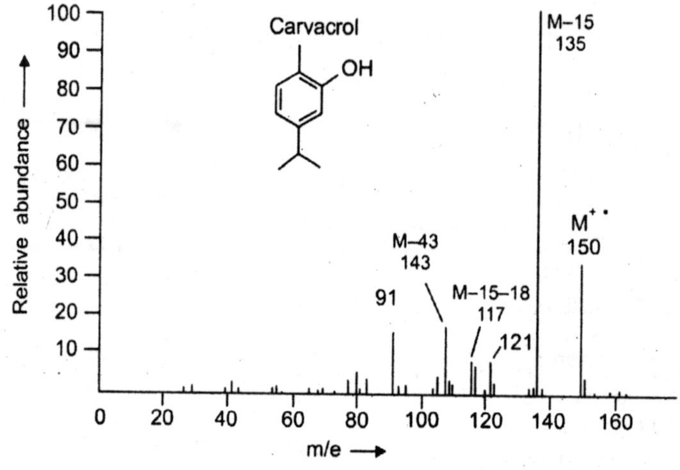

Fig. 6.76. Mass spectrum for Carvacrol.

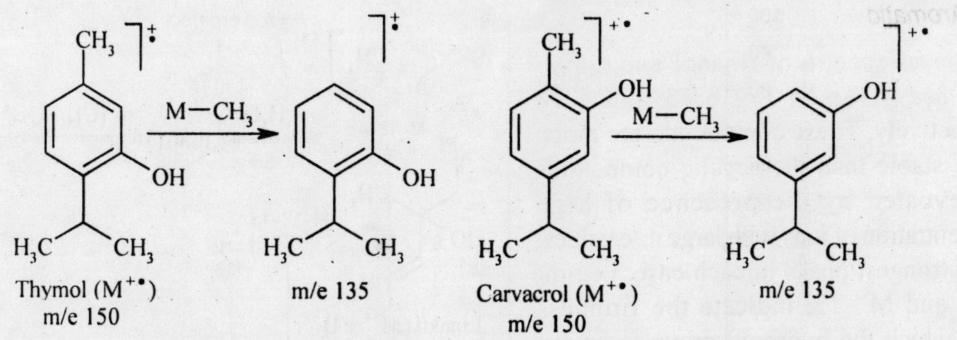

Scheme 6.77. Fragmentation pattern for Thymol and Carvacrol.

(c) Non aromatic

The mass spectra of alpha terpineol and menthol are given in Fig 6.77 and 6.78 respectively. The alpha terpineol is tertiary alcohol and so base peak at m/e 59 is due to tertiary cation (Scheme 6.78 and 6.79).

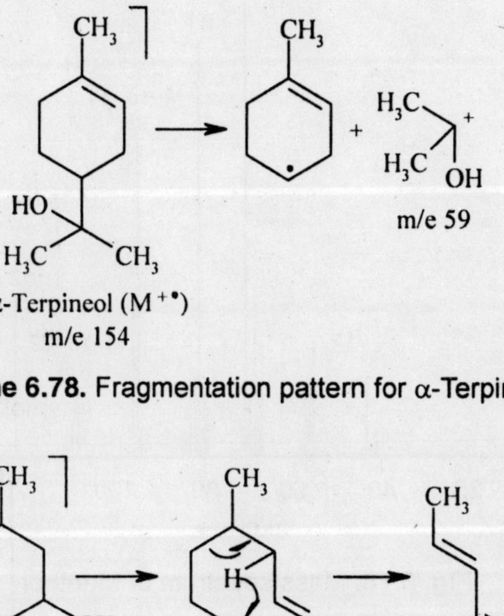

Scheme 6.78. Fragmentation pattern for α-Terpineol.

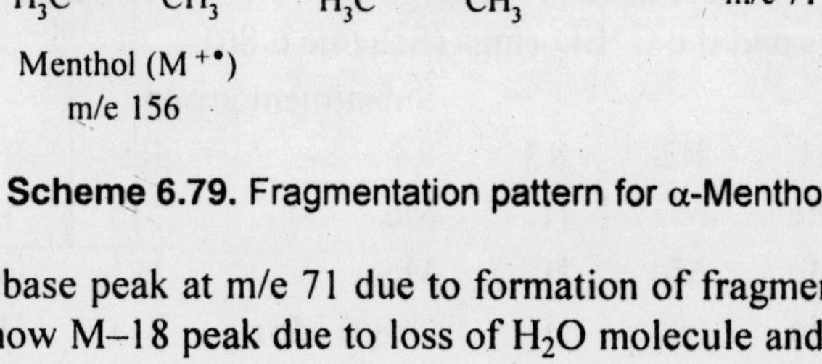

Scheme 6.79. Fragmentation pattern for α-Menthol.

Menthol shows the base peak at m/e 71 due to formation of fragment, CH_3–CH = CH–OH^+. Both the compounds show M–18 peak due to loss of H_2O molecule and M–18–43 due to loss of H_2O and isopropyl group.

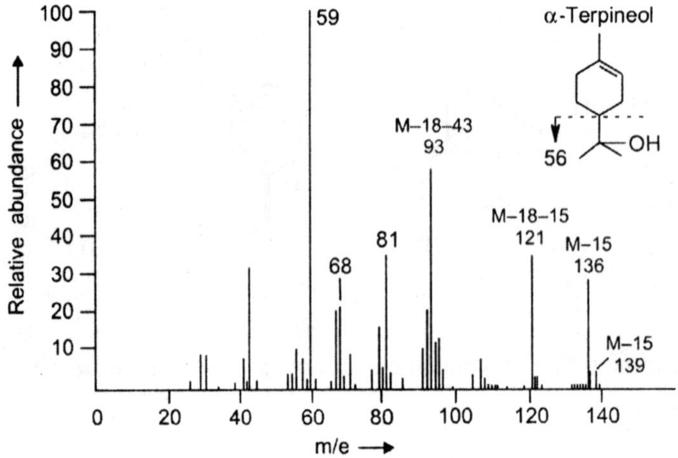

Fig. 6.77. Mass spectrum of α-Terpineol.

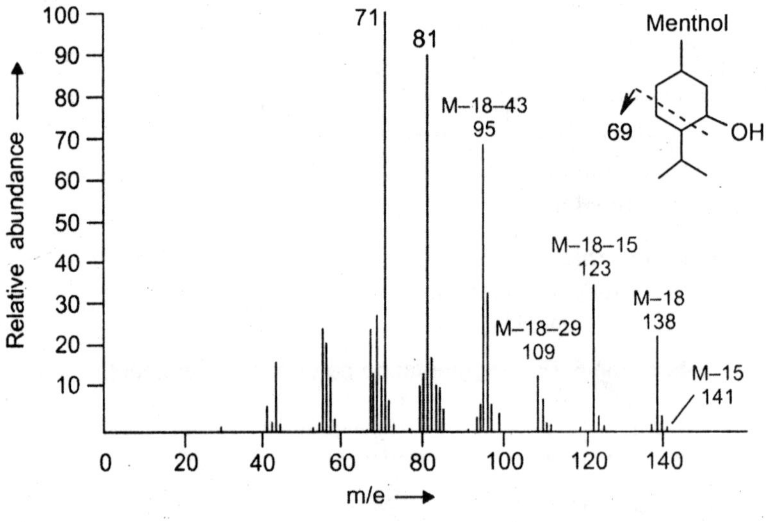

Fig. 6.78. Mass spectrum of Menthol.

6.16.4.2 Triterpenoids

Triterpenes that contain Δ^{12}–double bond (1) undergo a retro-Diels-Alder reaction to form fragments containing the ABC*-rings and the C*ED-rings (Scheme 6.80).

	Substituent group					
Compound	R1	R2	R3	R4	R5	R6
β-Amyrin	Me	Me	H	Me	Me	H
α-Amyrin	Me	Me	H	Me	H	Me
Oleanolic acid	Me	Me	H	COOTMSi	Me	H
Ursolic acid	Me	Me	H	COOTMSi	H	Me

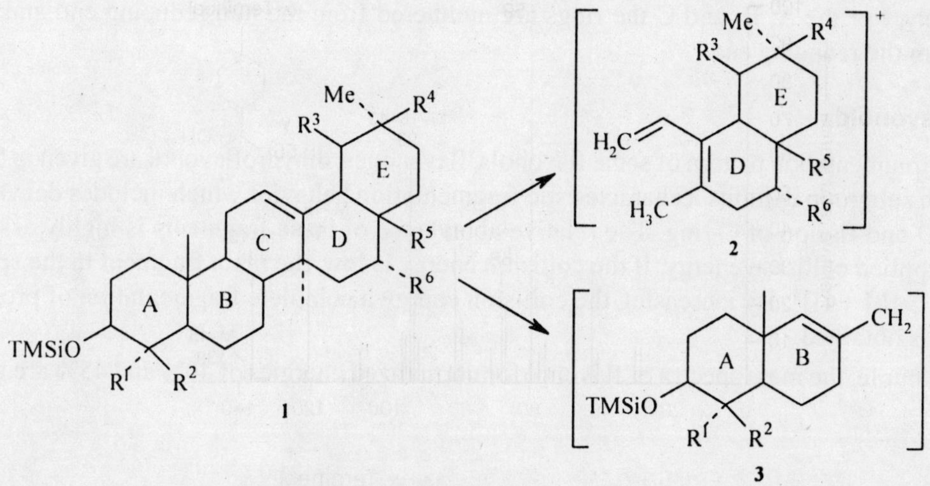

Scheme 6.80. Mass spectral fragmentation pattern of trimethylsilylated triterpenes.

6.16.5.2 Carbohydrates

Under different ionization conditions the fragmentation patterns are similar and depending on determining factors can be classified into two groups:

(i) Glycosidic cleavages of bond linking two sugar rings

(ii) Cross-ring cleavages – breaking of two bonds

The first group provides information about sequence and branching and the second group about linkage.

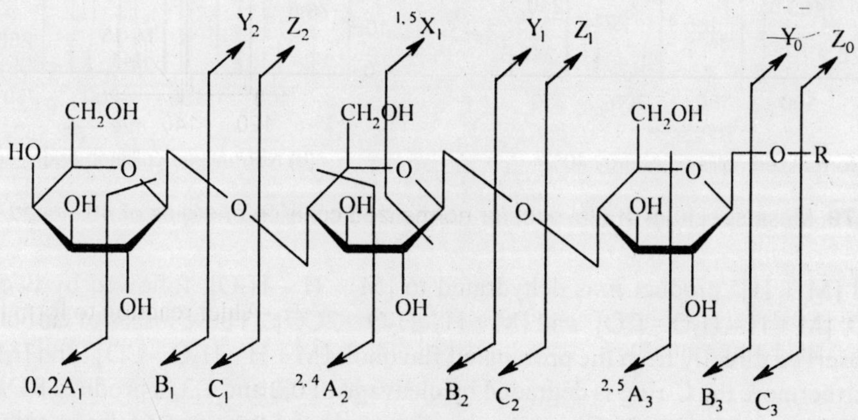

Scheme. 6.81. Schematic representation of the major fragment ions from Carbohydrates.

A schematic describing the fragmentation pattern for carbohydrates was introduced in 1988 by Domon & Costello and it is shown in Scheme 6.81. Ions that retain the charge at the reducing terminus are X (cross-ring), Y, and Z (glycosidic) and the complementary ions are A, B, and C respectively. For the A, B, and C the rings are numbered from the non-reducing end and for the others from the reducing end.

6.16.6 Flavonoids

The mass fragmentation pattern of some flavonols, flavanones, dihydroflavonol are given in Scheme 6.82. Each subgroup exhibits a characteristic fragmentation behavior which includes dehydration, loss of CO and fission of C-ring. The relative abundance of these fragments is highly associated with the applied collision energy. If the collision energy is low, the main fragment in the spectrum produced is $[M + H]^+$. By increasing the collision energy a complete fragmentation of protonated molecule is obtained.

For example, the mass spectra of flavonol for normalized energies of 40% and 45% are given in Fig. 6.79.

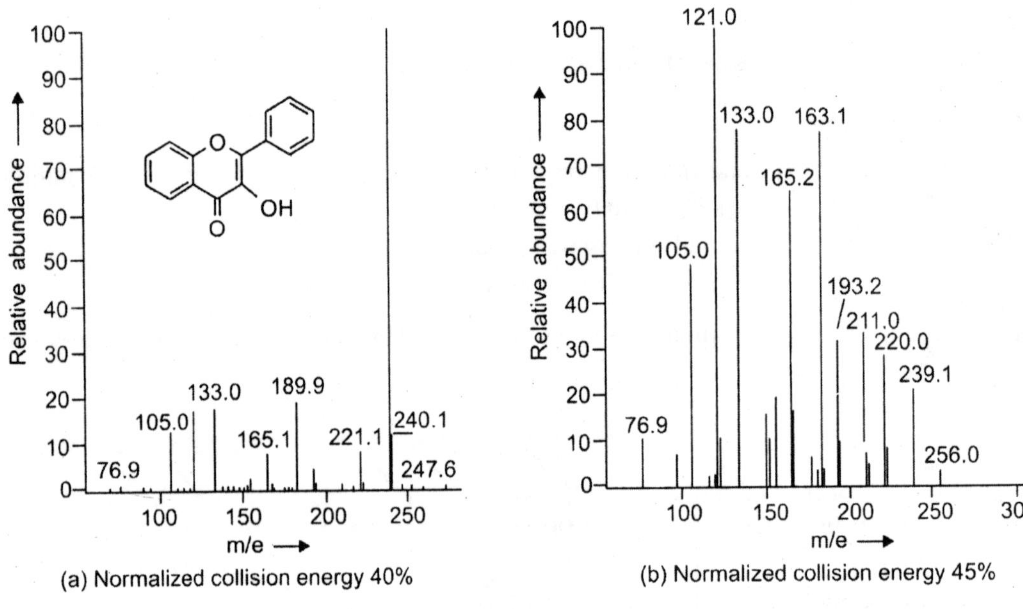

Fig. 6.79. Mass spectrum of Flavonol for normalized collision energies of 40 % and 45 %.

Flavonol $[M + H]^+$ product ions dehydrated to $[M + H - H_2O]$, followed by two sequential losses of CO: $[M + H - H_2O - CO]^+$ and $[M + H - H_2O - 2CO]^+$. These losses of carbon monoxide were also observed directly from the protonated flavonol: $[M + H - H_2O - CO]^+$ and $[M + H - H_2O - 2CO]^+$. Furthermore the C-ring is degraded by cleavage of 0,2 and 1,3 to produce RDA fragment. For example, Quercetrin due to C-ring fragment reveals the presence of fragmentation at m/e 165,153,149, and 137 by the cleavage of 0.2 & 1,3.

Flavones (e.g.. luteolin) exhibit the presence of fragments at m/e 153, 137, and 135 due to cleavage of bonds 0,2 and 1,3. There is also loss of water molecule followed by CO from protonated molecule.

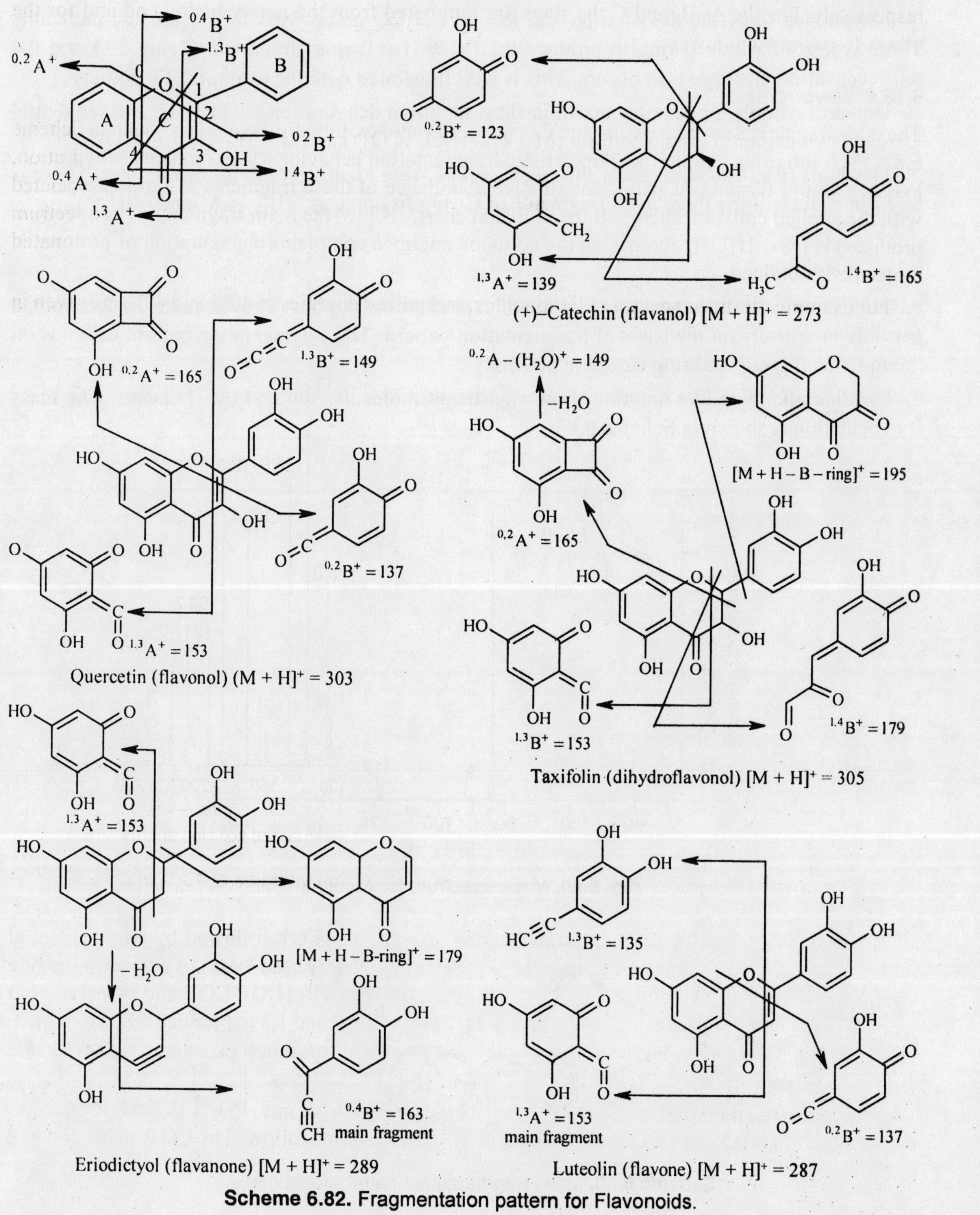

Scheme 6.82. Fragmentation pattern for Flavonoids.

Flavonones show the dehydration and loss of CH_2CO group from the protonated molecule. There is loss of whole B-ring to produce the [M + H – B-ring] fragment. C-ring 1, 3 and 0,4 retrocyclization cleavage also occurs. This is well illustrated with the example of Eriodictyol.

Dihydrofavonols for example taxifolin show an initial dehydration of $[M + H]^+$ and sequential losses of two carbonyl groups to form $[M + H - H_2O - CO]^+$ and $[M + H - H_2O - 2CO]^+$.

Flavanols (e.g. Catechin) show the cleavage of C-ring identical to those of flavones. There is high abundance of the three main fragments of C-ring fission e.g. $^{1,2}B^{+\cdot}$, $^{1,3}A^+$ and $^{1,4}B^+$.

6.16.7 Alkaloids

Alkaloids represent the largest single group of natural products whose structures can be determined partially or entirely on the basis of fragmentation pattern. The fragmentation pattern depends on the functional group and ring structure present.

Pyridine alkaloids like nicotine show significant molecular ion and (M–1) peaks. The mass fragmentation is shown in Scheme 6.83.

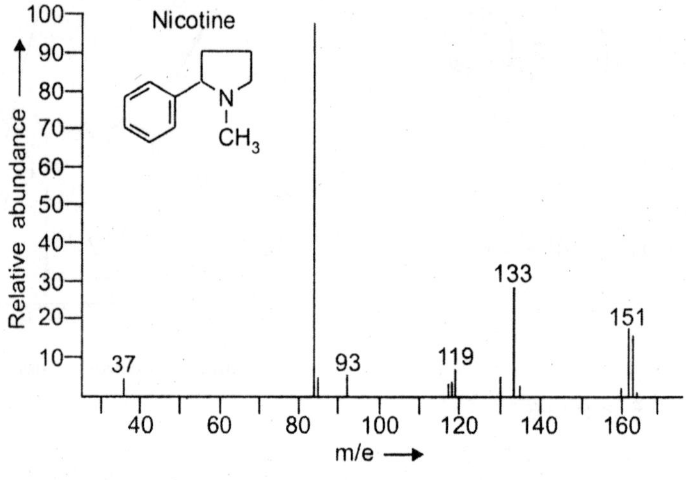

Fig. 6.80. Mass spectrum for Nicotine.

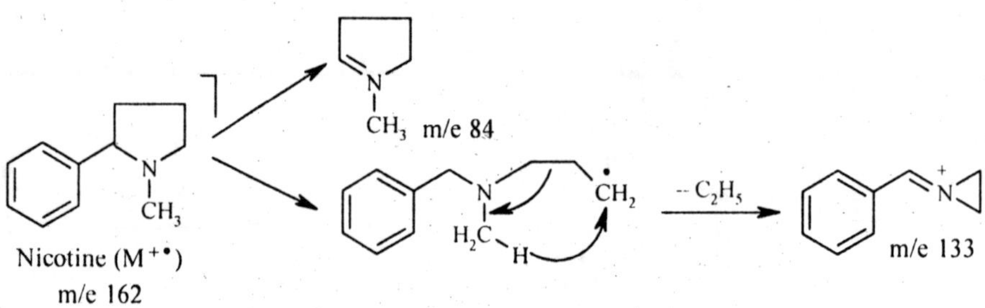

Scheme 6.83. Mass fragmentation pattern for Nicotine.

The quinoline alkaloids like quinine show major fragment at m/e 136 and 159 due to quinuclidine and quinoline moiety. There is also fragment at m/e 160 due to H-rearrangement.

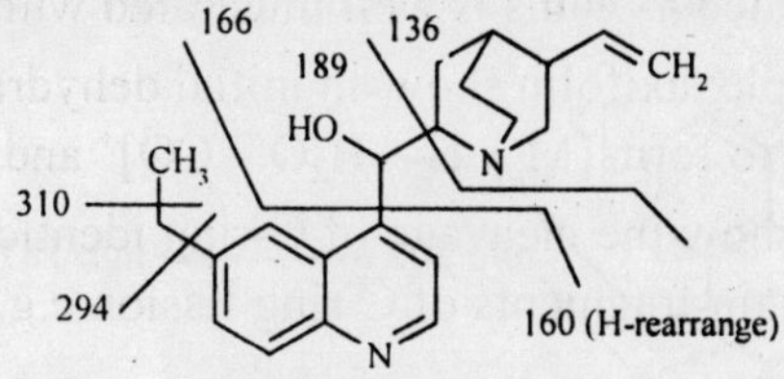

Quinine

The mass spectrum of Morphine is presented in Fig. 6.81. The spectrum shows a molecular ion peak at m/e 285 with a relative abundance 100%. Its fragmentation pattern is given in Scheme 6.84.

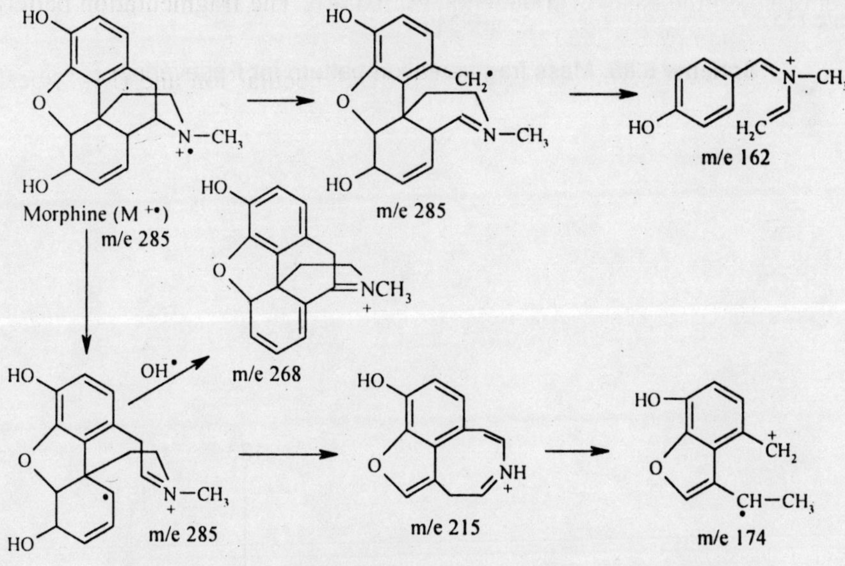

Scheme 6.84. Mass fragmentation pattern for Morphine.

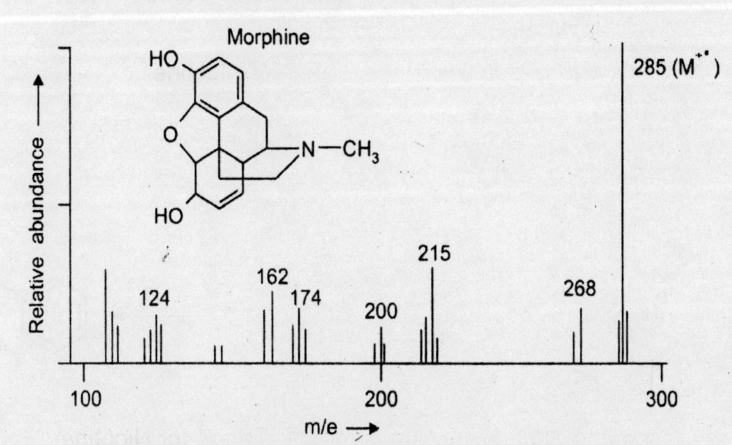

Fig. 6.81. Mass spectrum for Morphine.

Papaverine ($C_{20}H_{21}NO_4$, MW:339), a benzylisoquinoline alkaloid, revealed an apparent protonated molecular $(M + H)^+$ at m/e 340. The tandem MS analysis of MH^+ provided the MS/MS product ions at m/e 202, 187, 171, 151 and 135 (Scheme 6.85).

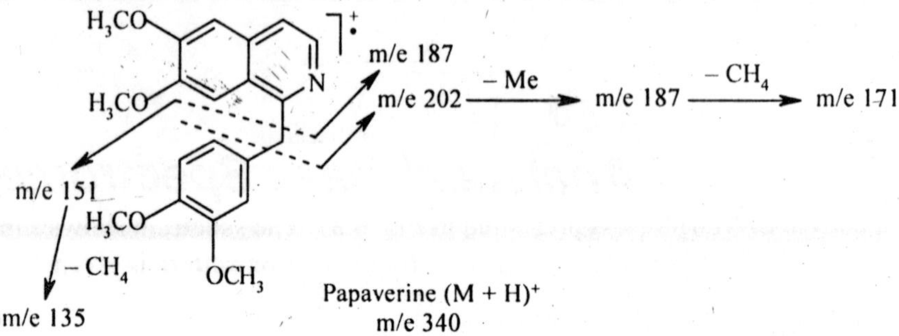

Scheme 6.85. Mass fragmentation pattern for Papaverine.

CHAPTER

7

Analytical Mass Spectrometry

Each organic compound has specific fragmentation process depending on the functional group present in it and ion source. Qualitative and quantitative analysis are done with the identification of fragments appeared in mass spectrum of particular compound.

7.1 QUALITATIVE ANALYSIS

The fundamental equation of a mass spectrometer is:

$$\frac{m}{e} = \frac{m^2R^2}{2V} \qquad \text{... (i)}$$

This equation expresses the relationship between the mass to charge ratio (m/e) of an ion, the magnetic field (H), the radius of the trajectories of the ions (R) and the applied accelerating voltage (V). This equation can also be modified as:-

$$m = \frac{k}{V}$$

where

$$k = \frac{1}{2}H^2R^2$$

The mass of the ion focussed on the collector of the mass spectrometer is therefore, inversely proportional to the applied accelerating voltage and this relationship suggests that the different ions can be focussed by varying the acceleration potential at constant magnetic field. By releasing appropriate values of the voltage, the specific ion (single ion detection) can be focussed. By suitably varying the accelerating voltage between certain fixed mass numbers, the ion corresponding to these prescribed values can be focussed, successively (multiple ion detection).

Some of the compounds like hallucinogens are active in the order of micrograms, quantities and therefore, their identification from tissues or biological liquids requires the use of a very sensitive method, such as mass spectrometry. It can be detected by either single or multiple ions detection technique. Similarly, the identification of performance enhancing compound in the blood or urine of an athlete prior to competition may alone be sufficient to ban the athlete from competing.

7.1.1 Single Ion Detection

Only one ion is focussed (generally an intense one). This technique can be used either by coupling with gas chromatograph or by using high resolution mass spectrometer.

In the first method, mass spectrometer is combined with gas chromatograph. Here, mass spectrometer is used as a selective gas chromatograph detector. This technique can increase the sensitivity of detection by a factor of between 1,000 and 10,000 with respect to normal gas chromatographic detectors like electron capture, flame ionization or thermal conductivity detector. An example of this application is the determination of 2,5–dimethoxy 4–methyl amphetamine. Its mass spectrum show prominent peak at m/e 166 (Fig. 7.1). Hence, acceleration potential corresponding to this mass is focussed and mass spectrum is recorded. Mass fragmentogram is a graph of total ion current versus time.

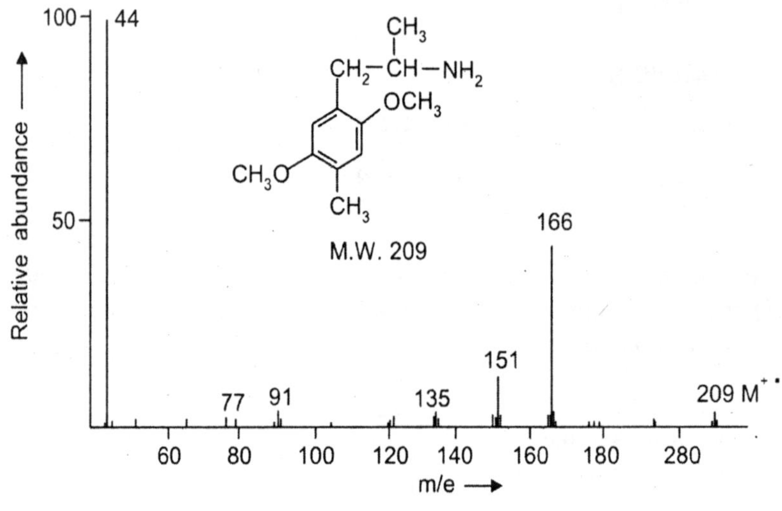

Fig. 7.1. Mass spectrum of 2,5–Dimethoxy–4–methyl-amphetamine.

By this method, it can be detected in quantities as low as 100 pg. DDT, in trace amounts as low as 10 pg, has been similarly determined. Similarly, testosterone is derivatized with N-methyl-N-trimethylsilyl-trifluoroacetamide (MSTFA), N-trimethylsilylimidazole (TMSI) and dithioerythritol, and subjected to MS analysis for qualitative identification.

In second method (high resolution mass spectrometry), it is possible to differentiate the ions that have the same nominal m/e ratio but have different elemental composition. This method can be applied for determination of p-tyramine, a precursor of catechol-amines, isolated from brain extract. The sample is introduced directly into the ion source and a doublet is observed at the nominal mass 108. The high resolution mass spectrometer is focussed on m/e 108.0575, an ionic fragment corresponding to lipid-hydrocarbon that have a peak at m/e 108.0939.

7.1.2 Multiple Ion Detection

When the mass spectrometer is employed as a multiple ion detector, it focuses on two or three ionic fragments within a 10-30% range of the magnetic scan of the instrument or on up to eight fragments over the whole field using a quadrupole mass spectrometer. For example, the mass spectrum of desmethyl chloropromazine trifluoro-acetate (DMCP-TFA) shows three prominent peaks at m/e 232, 234 and 246. The component separated by gas chromatograph (Fig. 7.2) is focussed on the three peaks at m/e 232, 234 and 246.

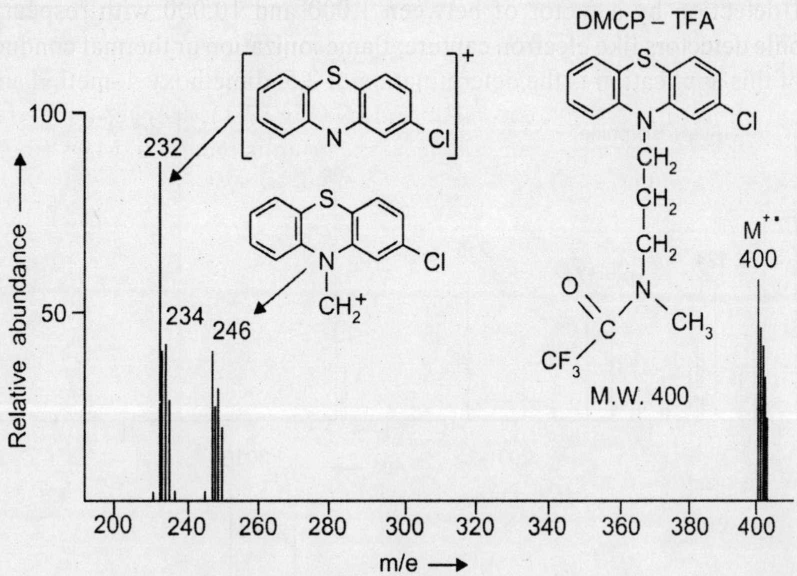

Fig. 7.2. Partial mass spectrum of desmethyl chlorpromazine trifluoro acetate (DMCP-TFA).

Similarly, drugs of abuse like morphine, 6–acetyl morphine, heroin, codeine, etc. can be determined in the urine sample in the Forensic analysis of criminals. To the urine sample sodium carbonate (10%) is added to adjust the pH 9.5 and then extraction is done with mixture of $CHCl_3$-isopropyl alcohol (3:1). Then sample is subjected to GC–MS analysis. The presence of suspected drugs of abuse can be detected by typical multiple ion detection, given in the Table 7.1.

Table 7.1. Typical fragment ions peaks (m/e) along with their % intensity

1.	Codeine	299(100), 229(24), 162(46),124(23)
2.	Morphine	285(100), 268(16), 162(58),124(20)
3.	Thebaine	311(100), 296(30), 242(11),2114(9)
4.	6-Acetyl morphine	327(100), 268(53), 162(11),124(13)
5.	Heroin	369(59), 327(100), 310(36),268(47),162(11)
6.	Desmethyl papaverine	325(77), 324(100), 310(30),266(13)

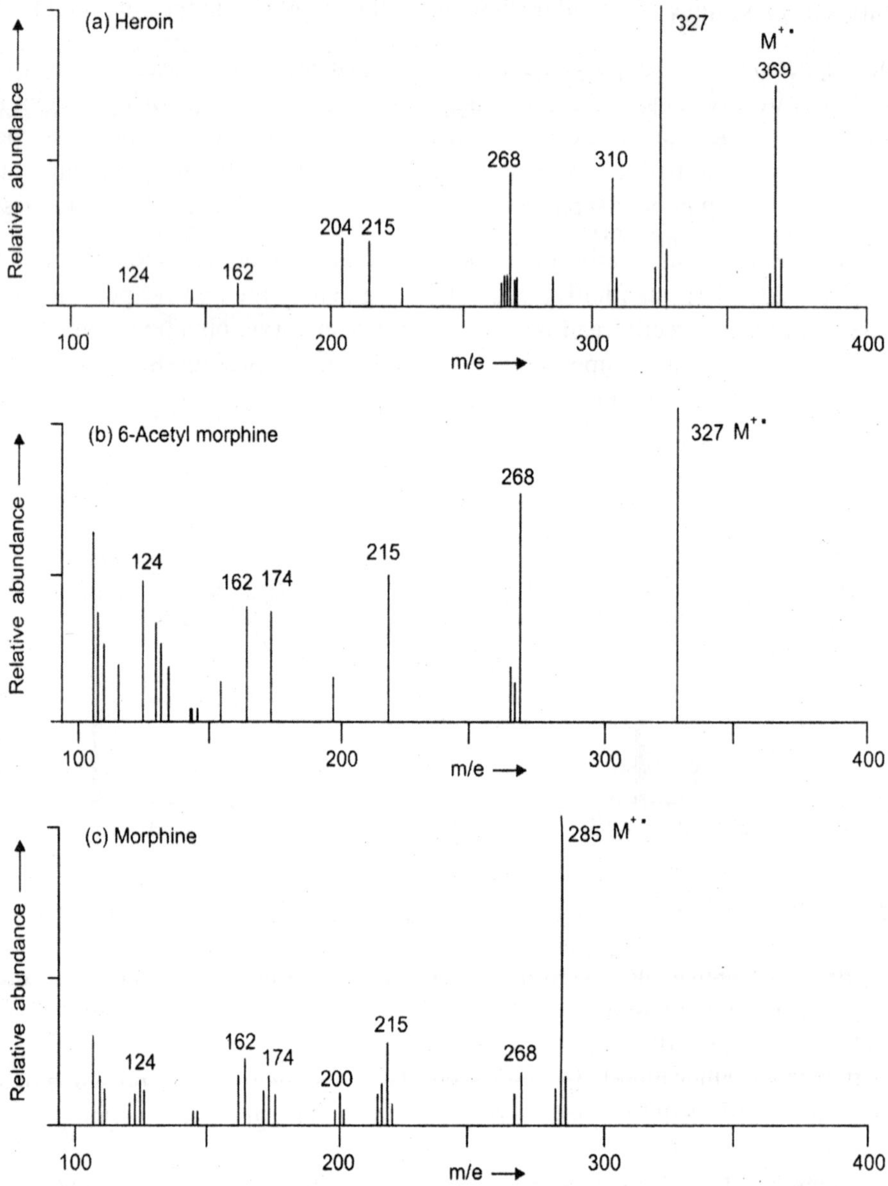

Fig. 7.3. Mass spectra of (a) Heroin, (b) 6-Acetyl morphine, (c) Morphine.

7.2 QUANTITATIVE ANALYSIS

This method is analogous to those illustrated above using the single ion detection method but has the additional advantage of greater specificity. This result is obtained by focussing on more than one characteristic ionic fragment of a molecule and this ensures the identity of compound displayed. For quantitative estimation, calibration curve is plotted with the help of internal standard, then from this calibration curve, quantity of unknown sample is determined. The internal standard has the same characteristics and is of a similar (though not the same) size to the compounds of interest. This ensures that the ionization and detection efficiencies of the internal standard and the compound under investigation are essentially identical. It is desirable to have the peak area under the ion signal rather than the height of an ion signal for quantitation because the latter is affected by mass resolution of measurement.

Example 1

This method is useful in the quantitative determination of imipramine. The spectrometer is focussed on fragment at m/e 235. The quantitative estimation is given by the relative peak areas of the ion fragment. The quantity is directly read out from calibration curve, obtained from standard. This method is useful to estimate the compound in the presence of complex mixtures as in extracts from biological fluids without interference.

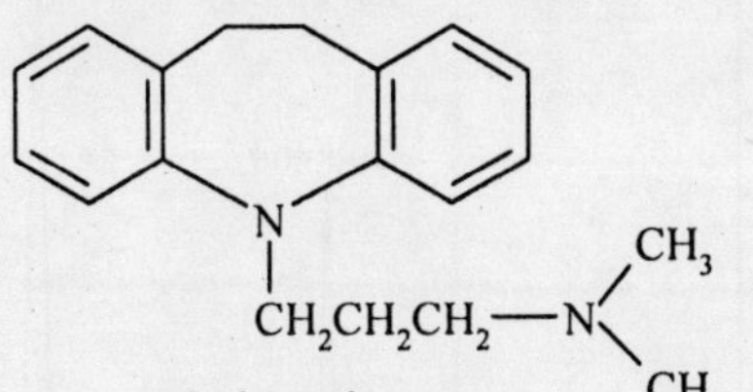

Imipramine

Example 2

A quantitative mass spectral analysis of the dimethyl derivative of 5–fluorouracil in blood plasma can also be done as illustrated in Fig. 7.4. In this analysis, the response from the substance of interest is measured relative to that from an internal standard added to the sample. The top trace shows the SIM profile of the molecular ion at m/e 158. The compound of interest produces the center peak. Two minor peaks arise from other sample components that also produce ions at m/e 158. The lower trace is the SIM profile of the same molecule having 15 N substituted for the normal 14 N at both nitrogen positions. Since both nitrogens are substituted, the signal from its molecular ion is observed at m/e 160(2 mass unit higher). Although both the sample and standard have the same retention time, they are detected separately by virtue of their different masses. Standards may be a closely related substance or may be chemically identical but synthesized by substituting a isotope of one of the elements as in this example.

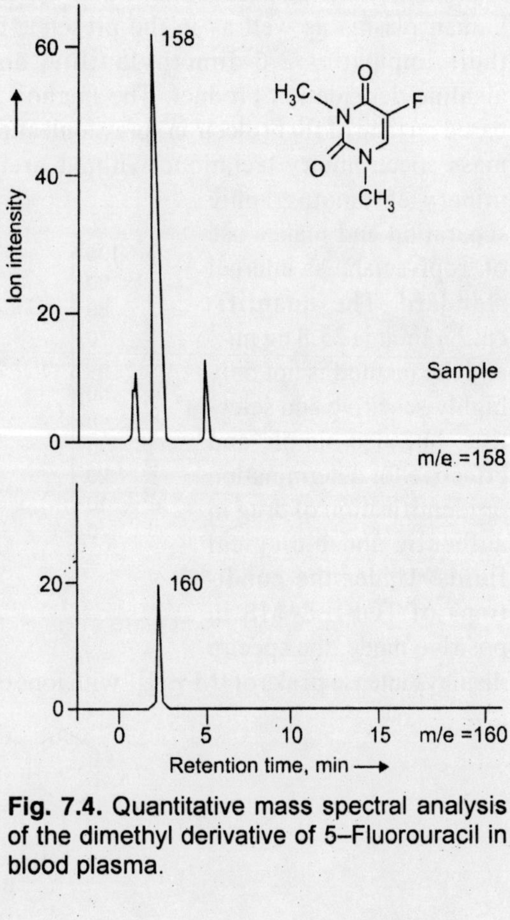

Fig. 7.4. Quantitative mass spectral analysis of the dimethyl derivative of 5–Fluorouracil in blood plasma.

Example 3

Cotinine is a metabolite of nicotine that has been detected in both smokers and non smokers by single (selected) ion technique in the blood, saliva and urine sample. The EI mass spectrum of cotinine exhibits a fragment ion at m/e 98 and molecular ion at m/e 176 (Fig. 7.5). Selected ion monitoring of the base peak at m/e 98 affords optimal sensitivity for its quantitative estimation. The internal standard, d^3-deutrocotinine is used for making calibration curve. Detection limit is 5–50 ng ml^{-1}.

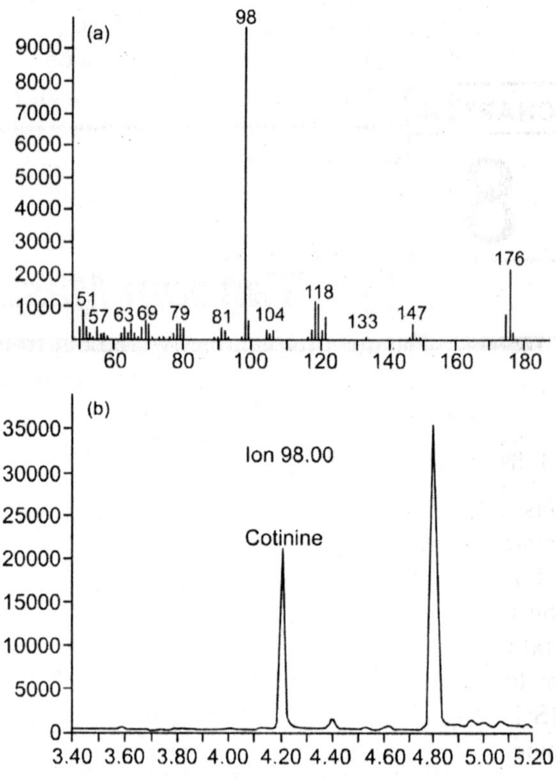

Fig. 7.5. EI mass spectrum of Cotinine.

Example 4

Mass spectrometry can be used for quantitative analysis of the local anesthetic drug, Nupivacaine in pharmaceutical and spiked human plasma as well as in the presence of their impurities 2,6-dimethylaniline and alkaline degradation product. The method is based on time of flight electron spray ionization mass spectrometry technique without preliminary chromatographic separation and makes use of ropivaciane as internal standard. The quantification limit is 23.8 ng ml^{-1} and the method is not only highly sensitive and selective, but also simple and effective for determination or identification of drug in authentic and biological fluids. Under the conditions of TOF ES–MS in positive mode, the spectra displays intense peaks of $[M + H]^+$ with ions of the highest mass to charge, 289.2226 for bupivacaine.

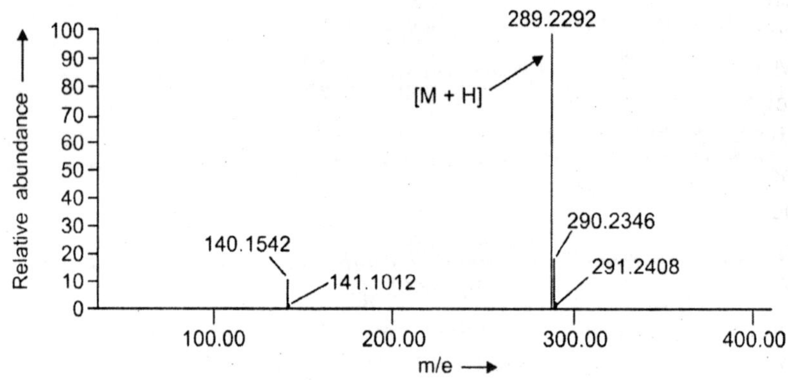

Fig. 7.6. Mass spectrum of Bupivacaine.

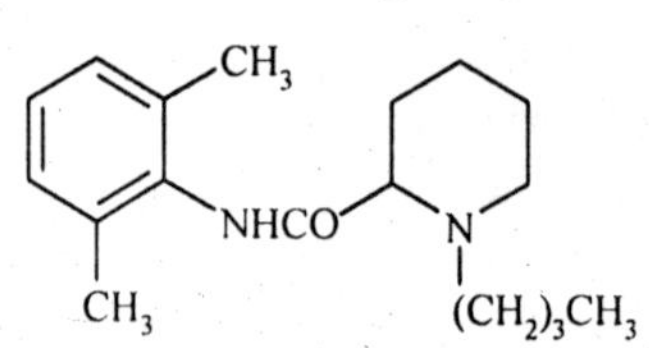

Bupivacaine

CHAPTER 8

Tandem Mass Spectrometry (MS/MS)

8.1 INTRODUCTION

Mass spectrometry is commonly combined with separation devices such as gas chromatograph (GC) and liquid chromatograph (LC) (Fig. 8.1). The GC or LC separates the components in a mixture and the each component is introduced, one by one into the mass spectrometer. The MS/MS is a analogous technique where first stage device is another mass spectrometer.

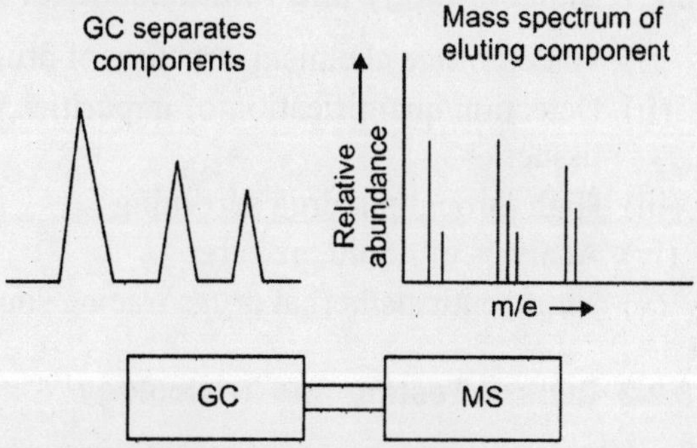

Fig. 8.1. Schematic representation of mass spectrometer interfaced to a GC.

Suppose that we analyze a mixture of components by soft ionization method. Each component produces a characteristic ionic species such as $[M + H]^+$. To keep the discussion simple, let's assume that each component has unique molecular weight. The first stage mass spectrum of a mixture contains peaks for component present in a mixture. Now suppose we would like to identify one of the mixture components. The second stage spectrums tell us the molecular weight but also represent the fragment ions that provide the structural information of component of interest.

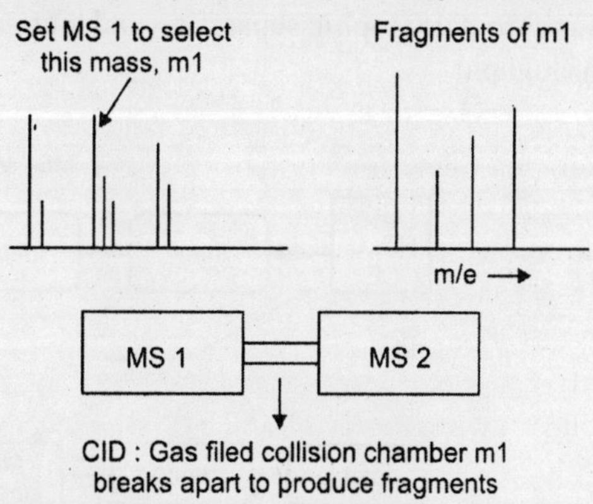

Fig. 8.2. Schematic representation of two mass spectrometers Tandem MS/MS.

The simplest form of tandem mass spectrometer combines two mass spectrometers (Fig. 8.2). The first mass spectrometer is used to select single (precursor) mass that is characteristic to the given analyte in a mixture. The mass selected ions pass through the region where they are activated in some way that causes them to produce fragment (product) ions. This is usually done by colliding the ions with a neutral gas in a process called collision activation (CA) or collision induced dissociation (CID). The second mass spectrometer is used to separate the fragment ion according to mass. The resulting MS/MS spectrum consists of only of product ions from the selected precursor. Chemical background and other mixture components are absent.

Basically, tandem mass spectrometry uses 2 (or more) mass analyzers in a single instrument. One purifies the analyte ion from a mixture using a magnetic field. The other analyzes fragments of the analyte ion for identification and quantification.

8.2 APPLICATIONS OF TANDEM MASS SPECTROMETRY

It is used in industry and academic for both routine assays and research purposes. Some applications are:

8.2.1 Biotechnology and Pharmaceutical

(i) To determine chemical structure of drugs and drug metabolites.
(ii) Detection/quantification of impurities, drugs and their metabolites in biological fluids and tissues.
(iii) High throughput drug screening
(iv) Analysis of liquid mixtures
(v) Nutraceuticals/herbal drugs/tracing source of natural products or drugs

8.2.2 Clinical Testing and Toxicology

To detect the inborn errors of metabolism, cancer, diabetes, various poisons, drugs of abuse, etc.

MS/MS used with or without chromatographic separation offers the advantage of (i) analytical sensitivity and (ii) selectivity for drug and drug metabolite analysis. These advantages are achieved through reduction in interferences from other sample components. This allows the development of analytical methods for complex mixtures that are fast, require less stringent sample preparation, less chromatographic separation and therefore consumes much less solvent, allowing higher sample throughput.

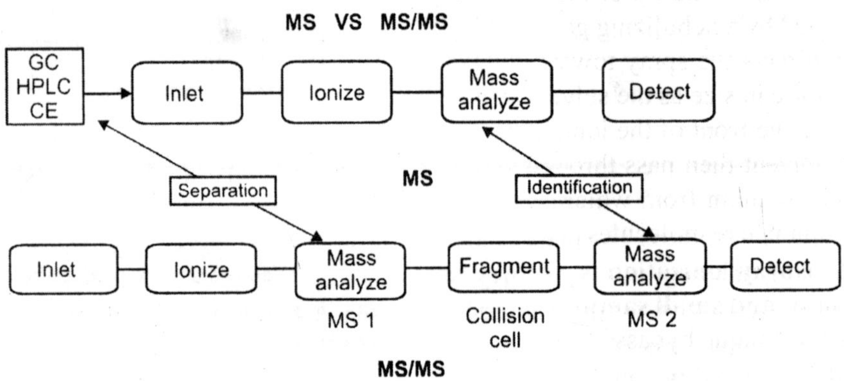

Fig. 8.3. Comparison of single mass spectrometer with MS-MS instrumentation.

8.3 MS-MS INSTRUMENTATION

Single stage mass spectrometry measures the molecular mass of a compound and/or its fragments. **MS/MS consists of two or more** mass spectrometer analyzers all in a single instrument. The Fig. 8.3 illustrates the comparison of Single mass spectrometer (MS) with MS-MS instrumentation.

Tandem mass spectrometers like other mass spectrometers have 4 main parts: (1) **ionization source**, (2) **Sample inlet system,** (3) **analyzer**, and (3) **detector.**

8.3.1 Ionization source

A sample introduced into the ionization source (typically by HPLC) becomes ionized. Ionization process makes the sample components easier to manipulate. The resulting ions are entered into the analyzer where they are separated according to their **mass -to-charge ratios (m/e)**. The separated ions are then fragmented. The fragments are detected and the signal created by the detected fragment ions is sent to a data system where the m/e ratios are stored together with their relative abundance. This data is presented in the format of **m/e spectrum.**

The analyzer and detector of the mass spectrometer, and sometimes the ionization source, are maintained under high vacuum to give the ions a reasonable chance of traveling from one end of the instrument to the other without any hindrance from air molecules. Most MS/MS the ionization sources use an **Atmospheric pressure ionization** (API) technique.

8.3.1.1 Methods of sample ionization

The choice of ionization method depends on the type of sample under investigation and the mass spectrometer. Ionization methods most commonly used in tandem mass spectrometry include:

The first 3 ionization techniques are commonly adapted for small molecular weight compounds.

(i) Electrospray Ionization (ESI) is an **API** technique suited for analysis of polar molecules ranging from less than 100 Da to more than 1,000,000 Da in molecular mass.

During electrospray ionization the sample is dissolved in a volatile polar solvent and pumped through a narrow stainless steel capillary (~100 μm diameter) at a flow rate between 1 μL/min and 1 ml/min. The "electrospray" is generated by applying a high voltage (~3000 V) to the tip of the capillary. This creates a strong electric field that causes the solvent and sample to elute from the tip of the capillary as **an aerosol of highly charged droplets.** This is assisted by a nebulizing gas (usually nitrogen) flowing around the outside of the capillary and directs the spray towards the analyzer part of the instrument. The charged droplets decrease in size as the solvent is evaporated by the flow of heated nitrogen gas that blows across the front of the ionization source. The charged ions eventually become freed from the solvent then pass through an orifice (called a sampling cone) into a chamber that is under vacuum from which it is then directed through a small aperture into the analyzer section where molecules are separated according to molecular mass.

Nanospray ionization is a special type of ESI that uses very **low flow rates (30 to 1000 nl/min) and small sample volumes** (1-4 μl) at concentrations of 1 to 10 μmol/l are used. This technique bypasses the need of a HPLC.

ESI is operated in 2 modes: In **positive ionization** mode, an organic acid like formic acid is often added in order to add a H^+ ion to the sample molecules; **protonated molecular**

ions have molecular weight of the formula $(M + H)^+$. In **negative ionization** mode a trace of ammonia solution or a volatile amine is added to aid in removal of an H+ ion from the sample molecules to give a molecular weight determined by the formula $(M - H)^-$.

If the sample has functional groups that readily accept a proton (H^+) then positive ion detection is used **e.g. amines $R\text{-}NH_2 + H^+ = R\text{-}NH_3^+$ as in proteins or peptides.** If the sample has functional groups that readily lose a proton then negative ion detection is used **e.g. carboxylic acids $R\text{-}CO_2H = R\text{-}CO_2^-$ and alcohols R-OH = R-O- as in saccharides or oligonucleotides.**

ESI is known as **a "soft" ionization method** as the sample is ionized by the addition or removal of a proton (H^+), with very little extra energy remaining to cause fragmentation of the sample ions. This is an advantage when analyzing drug metabolites and conjugates.

(ii) Atmospheric Pressure Chemical Ionization (APCI) uses heat to vaporize the column eluate and a corona discharge to ionize the solvent molecules and produce analyte ions by a variety of chemical ionization methods.

(iii) Atmospheric Pressure Photoionization (APPI) like APCI uses heat to vaporize the column eluate but uses UV light and chemicals added to the solvent to produce analyte ions through charge and proton transfer reactions.

(iv) Matrix assisted-laser desorption/ionization (MALDI) uses **laser** light to ionize the sample. Typically a sample is pre-mixed with a special matrix compound for consistent and reliable results. The matrix compound allows the laser light to excite the sample causing it to ionize and move from the surface of the mixture and into the mass spectrometer. This technique does not require a chromatography step.

MALDI is also a "soft" ionization method and is mainly adapted to high molecular weight compounds like proteins.

8.3.2 Sample inlet system

Sample can be inserted directly into the ionization source, or can undergo some type of chromatography en route to the ionization source. This latter method of sample introduction usually involves: high pressure liquid chromatography (HPLC), gas chromatography (GC) or capillary electrophoresis (CE) separation column.

8.3.3 Mass analyzers

The main function of the **mass analyzer** is to the **separate** ions, formed in the ionization source, according to their **m/e** ratios. More popular tandem mass spectrometers.(based on analyzers) include those of the **quadrupole-quadrupole type (also known as Triple Quadrupole instruments), or the hybrid types:** including magnetic sector/quadrupole, and more recently, the quadrupole/time-of-flight (Q-TOF) geometries.

8.3.3.1 Triple Quadrupole Mass spectrometer

The Fig. 8.4 is a schematic representation of Triple Quadrupole Mass Analyzer. As can be seen from Fig. 8.4 the analyzer consists of three single quadrupole mass analyzer in series. The first

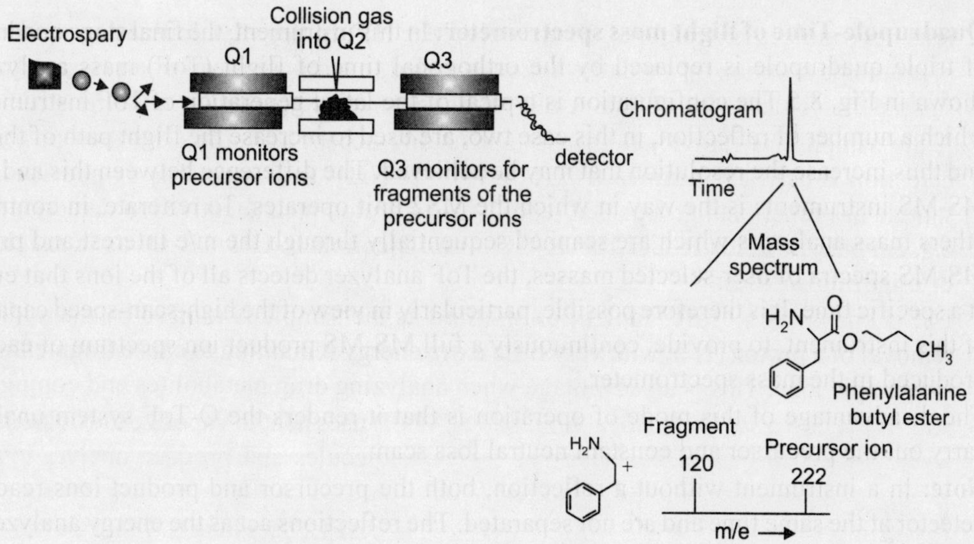

Fig. 8.4. Schematic representation of Triple Quadrupole Mass Analyzer.

Quadrupole acts like a mass filter, only those ions with specific m/e value can pass Q1; the second Quadrupole Q2 is not used as mass separation device. It acts as a collision cell where, the ions coming out from first quadrupole Q1 collides with some gas atoms and breaks into small fragments and focuses any product ions into the third Quadrupole Q3. Both sets of quadrupole may be controlled to allow the transmission of single m/e or range of m/e to give the desired analytical information. In the quadrupole Q2 or collision cell, an inert gas (typically argon or xenon) is admitted to collide with the selected sample ions to bring out their fragmentation. The process is known as collision induced dissociation (CID). The actual change in mass from a precursor molecule ion to a product molecule ion is referred to as a transition and is written as 315.1>109 for a molecule of mass M + 1 =315.1 producing a molecule of mass 109 following reaction in the collision cell.

8.3.3.2 Hybrid mass spectrometer

A **hybrid mass spectrometer** is a device for tandem mass spectrometry that consists of a combination of two or more m/e separation devices of different types.

(a) **Magnetic sector quadrupole mass spectrometer:** When the first quadrupole of the triple quadrupole is replaced by double focusing mass analyzers, the instrument is termed s hybrid (-hybrid of magnetic sector and quadrupole technologies). The advantage of this configuration is that the MS instrument can be used as high resolution condition to select the ion of interest. Despite the efficiency of modern chromatography, complete resolution of components, especially if mixtures are involved, is not possible and background signal may be observed. Low resolution mass spectrometers allow us to differentiate between components with similar retention properties but whose mass spectra contains ions at different m/e ratios while high resolution mass spectrometers allow us to do this but also to differentiates between components whose mass spectra contain ions with the same nominal mass but which have different atomic compositions. In this way, further specificity is conferred on the analysis.

(b) **Quadrupole-Time of flight mass spectrometer:** In this instrument, the final stage quadrupole of triple quadrupole is replaced by the orthogonal time of flight (ToF) mass analyzer as shown in Fig. 8.5 The configuration is typical of the latest generation of ToF instrument in which a number of reflection, in this case two, are used to increase the flight path of the ions and thus increase the resolution that may be achieved. The difference between this and other MS-MS instruments is the way in which the MS2 unit operates. To reiterate, in contrast to others mass analyzers which are scanned sequentially through the m/e interest and provide MS-MS spectra of user-selected masses, the ToF analyzer detects all of the ions that enter it at a specific time. It is therefore possible, particularly in view of the high-scan-speed capability of this instrument, to provide, continuously a full MS-MS product ion spectrum of each ion produced in the mass spectrometer.

The disadvantage of this mode of operation is that it renders the Q-ToF system unable to carry out the precursor and constant neutral loss scan.

Note: In a instrument without a reflection, both the precursor and product ions reach the detector at the same time and are not separated. The reflections act as the energy analyzer and product ion with different energies, after passage through the reflection, will have the different flight time to the detector and thus separated.

(c) **Tandem Mass Spectrometer on the ion trap:** In fact, the principle of Ion-Trap Mass Analyzer

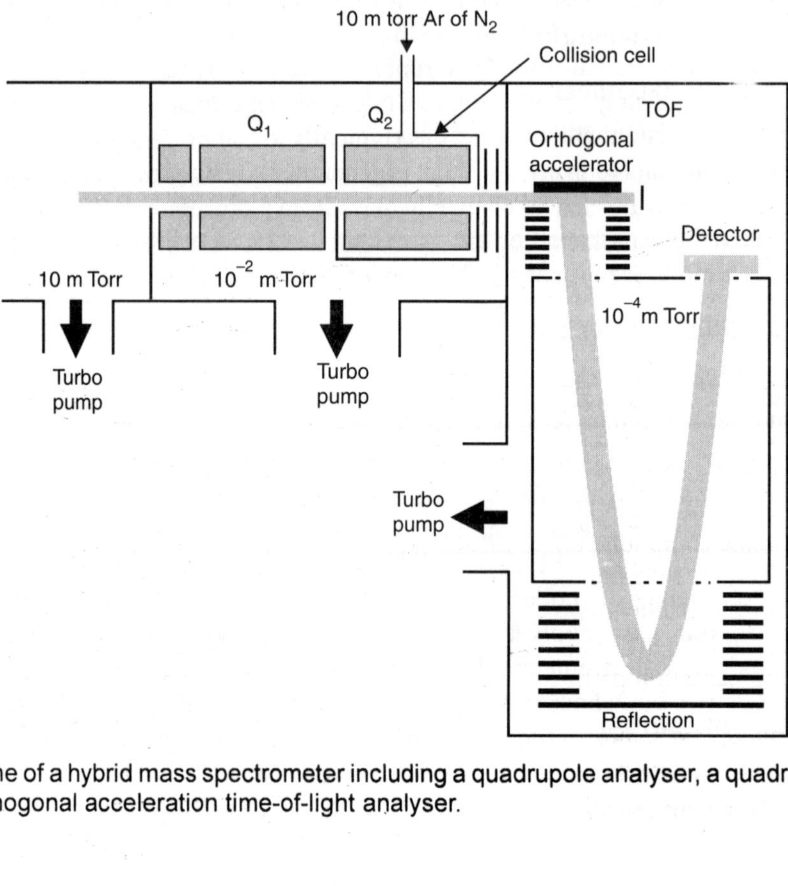

Fig. 8.5. Scheme of a hybrid mass spectrometer including a quadrupole analyser, a quadrupolar collision cell and an orthogonal acceleration time-of-light analyser.

is the same as the Triple Quadrupole Mass Analyzer. First, the trap selects some specific proteins with certain m/e values, all the other proteins will fly out of the trap; then the voltage is suddenly increased, which leads to the energy increase of the remaining ions, so the ions collide with the gas atoms and produce many fragments; like in Triple Quadrupole Mass Analyzer, the fragments are caught to produce the final mass spectrum.

8.3.3 Triple Quadrupole VS Ion-Trap

The similarity between Triple Quadrupole and Ion-Trap is the principle. Both types, first select some specific ion, then break this specific ion into small pieces and catch the fragments to yield the final mass spectrum.

One of the difference between these two analyzers is that they produce different fragments for the same protein ion. Trap-ion trends to fragment the ions more thoroughly. The net result is higher efficiency in fragmenting of molecule.

8.3.4 Detection and recording of sample ions

The **detector** monitors and amplifies the ion current and then transmits the signal to the data system where it is recorded in the form of a **mass spectrum**. The **m/e** values of the ions are plotted against their **intensities** to show the **number of components** in the sample, the **molecular mass** of each component, and the **relative abundance** of the various components in the sample.

The type of detector is supplied to suit the type of analyzer; the more common ones are the **photomultiplier**, the **electron multiplier** and the **micro-channel plate** detectors.

8.3.5 Types of MS/MS experiments

Consider a precursor ion m^{1+} that decomposes to produce product ion m^{2+} and a neutral loss N.

MS/MS experiments can be classified according to which of these species (precursor, product, neutral loss) is constant. Note that thee is no requirement that the product and precursor ion is positively charged; the terminology is identical to negative charged ions.

Here commonly used four types of experiments (using triple quadrupole) are shown in Fig 8.6.

8.3.5.1 Product (Daughter) ion scanning

The first mass analyzer selects a specified sample ion and so allows only that ion to pass. This ion is usually the molecular-related (i.e. $(M + H)^+$ or $(M - H)^-$) ions. These chosen ions pass into the collision cell, and are bombarded by gas molecules. This breaks up the molecule into fragments. These fragment ions are then separated according to their m/e ratios, by the second mass analyzer. All the fragment ions arise directly from the precursor ions specified. The result is a fingerprint pattern specific to the compound under investigation. This type of experiment is particularly useful for providing structural information. For example, the product ion spectrum of the [M + H]+ of buspirone in Fig. 8.7 displays two key fragment ions at m/e 122 and m/e 265. These ions are attributed to structurally informative product ions on each side of the buspirone molecule as highlighted in fragmentation pathway.

8.3.5.2 Precursor (Parent) ion scanning

The first mass analyzer allows all sample ions to pass through it. The second analyzer is set to monitor specific fragment ion that is generated in the collision cell. All precursor molecules that

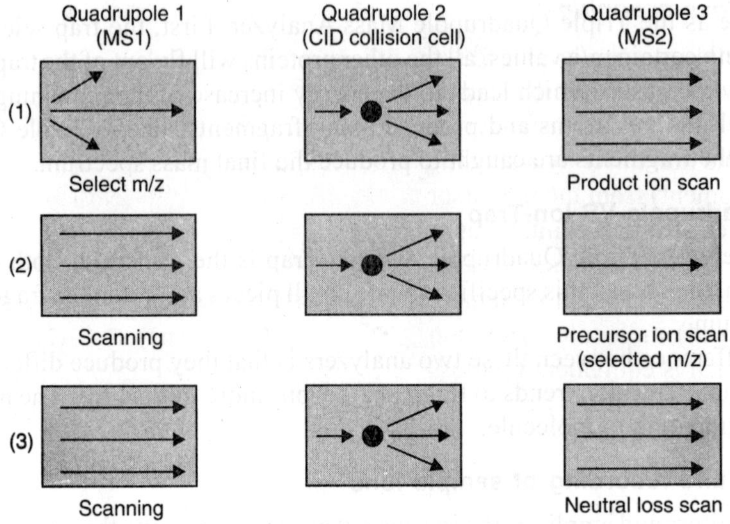

Fig. 8.6. Types of MS/MS experiments.

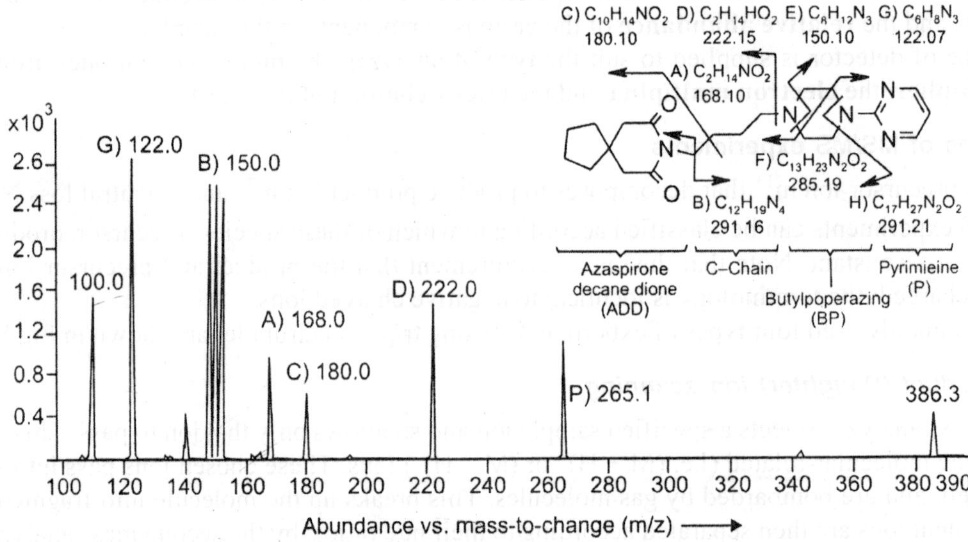

Fig. 8.7. MS/MS spectrum of buspirone by QQQ product ion scan and interpretation of the fragmentation pattern.

give rise to the specific fragment will be detected. This type of experiment is useful for monitoring groups of compounds contained within a mixture which fragment to produce common fragment ions. For example, all the acylcarnitine methyl ester cation exhibits a signal at m/e 99 (usually the base peak on CID). As shown in Fig. 8.8, this ion (m/e 99) is derived from the loss of triethylamino group and acyl group from acylcarnitine. In the precursor ion scan mode, quadrupole Q3 of the triple quadrupole transmits ion of m/e 99 while Q1 is scanned from m/e 200 to 450 generates a profile consisting of molecular cation of acylcarnitine with little chemical interferences.

8.3.5.3 Neutral loss scanning

Involves both analyzers collecting data, across the whole m/e range. But the second analyzer is set that it will only detect products fragments that differ by a specific mass (neutral fragment) from the precursor ion. This type of experiment could be used to monitor all of the carboxylic acids in a mixture. Carboxylic acids tend to fragment by losing a (neutral) molecule of carbon dioxide, CO_2, which is equivalent to a loss of 44 Da or atomic mass units. All ions pass through the first analyzer into the collision cell. The ions detected from the collision cell are those from which 44 Da have been lost. Precursor ion and neutral loss methods are useful to detect unknown metabolites or for screening for structurally related compounds.

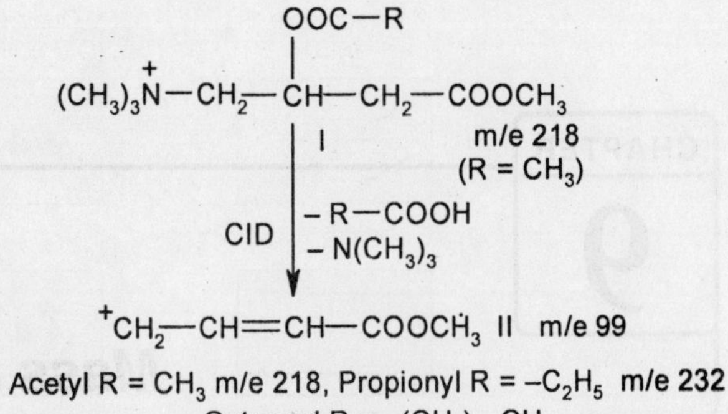

Fig. 8.8. Fragmentation of acyl carnitine methylester cation by CID in a triple quadrupole mass Spectrometer showing the origin of common fragment at m/e 99.

Similarly, neutral or acidic amino acids can be detected after derivatization with butyl alcohol. Neutral loss scanning only allow to pass the fragment ion to the detector which shows the loss of mass of 102 due to release of butyl formate (Fig. 8.9).

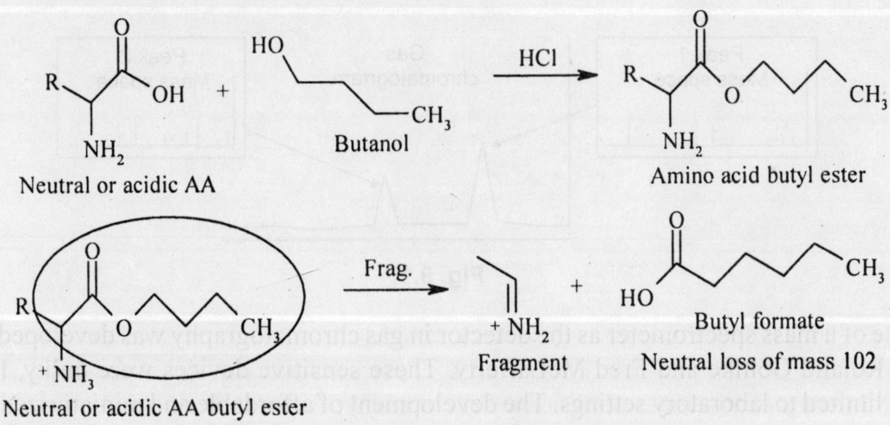

Fig. 8.9. Derivatization and neutral loss scanning.

8.3.5.4 Selected Reaction monitoring (SRM)

Involves setting both analyzers such that only ions of selected molecular weight are allowed to pass through the first analyzer and only specifically selected fragments arising from these are measured by the second analyzer. This method is widely used in drug testing in blood and urine samples. It is also very sensitive and specific.

CHAPTER

9

Gas Chromatography–Mass Spectrometry (GC–MS)

9.1 INTRODUCTION

A mixture of compounds to be analyzed, is initially injected into the GC where the mixture is vaporized in a heated chamber. The gas mixture travels through a GC column, where the compounds become separated as they interact with the column. The chromatogram (Fig. 9.1) shows peaks due to the individual component, resulting from the separation process. Those separated compounds then immediately enter the mass spectrometer for identification. Here, mass spectrometer serves the purpose of detector.

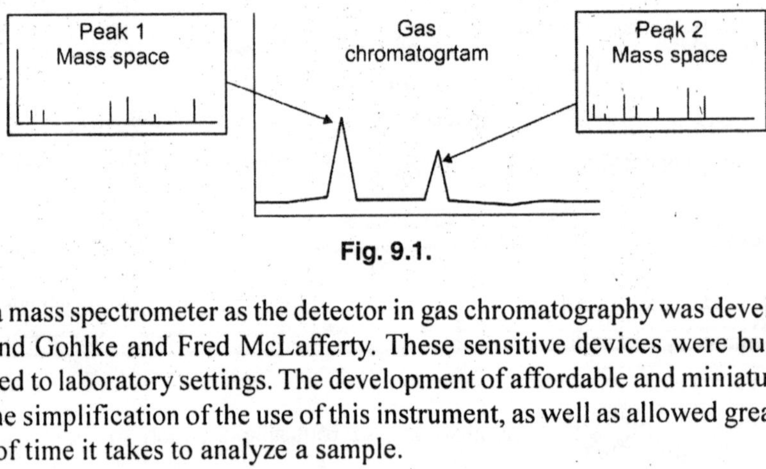

Fig. 9.1.

The use of a mass spectrometer as the detector in gas chromatography was developed during the 1950s by Roland Gohlke and Fred McLafferty. These sensitive devices were bulky, fragile, and originally limited to laboratory settings. The development of affordable and miniaturized computers has helped in the simplification of the use of this instrument, as well as allowed great improvements in the amount of time it takes to analyze a sample.

Gas chromatography-mass spectrometry (GC–MS) is a hyphenated (coupled) analytical technique that combines the features of gas-liquid chromatography and mass spectrometry to identify different substances within a mixture. The GC–MS is composed of two major building blocks: the gas chromatograph and the mass spectrometer. Gas chromatography separates the components of a mixture and mass spectroscopy characterizes each of the components individually. By combining the two techniques, an analytical chemist can both qualitatively and quantitatively evaluate a solution

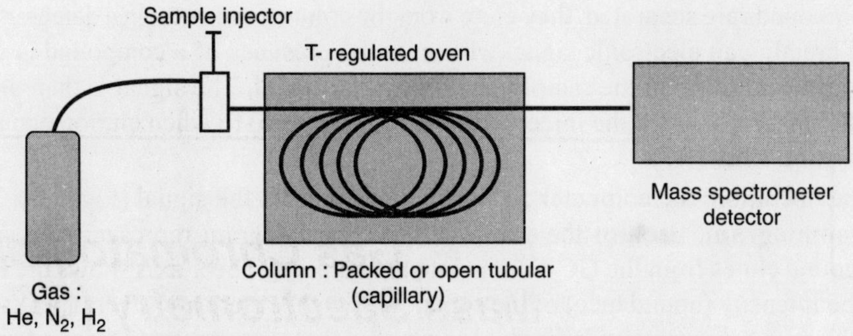

Fig. 9.2. Diagrammatic representation of GC–MS.

containing a number of components. The uses for GC–MS are numerous. They are used extensively in the medical, pharmacological, environmental, and law enforcement fields.

9.2 GAS CHROMATOGRAPHY

In general, chromatography is used to separate mixtures of chemicals into individual components. Once isolated, the components can be evaluated individually.

In all chromatography, separation occurs when the sample mixture is introduced (injected) into a **mobile phase**. In liquid chromatography (LC), the mobile phase is a solvent. In gas chromatography (GC), the mobile phase is an inert gas such as helium.

The mobile phase carries the sample mixture through what is referred to as a **stationary phase.** The stationary phase is a usually chemical that can selectively attract components in a sample mixture. The stationary phase is usually contained in a tubular device. This tube is referred to as a column. Columns can be glass or stainless steel of various dimensions.

The mixture of compounds in the mobile phase interacts with the stationary phase. Each compound in the mixture interacts at a different rate. Those that have least affinity with stationary phase will exit (elute from) the column first. Those that have most affinity with the stationary phase will exit the column last. By changing characteristics of the mobile phase and the stationary phase, different mixtures of organic compounds can be separated. Further refinements to this separation process can be made by changing the temperature of the stationary phase or the pressure of the mobile phase.

GC has a long, thin column containing a thin interior coating of a solid stationary phase (5% phenyl, 95% dimethylsiloxane polymer). This 0.25 mm diameter column is referred to as a capillary column. This particular column is used for semi volatile and non-polar organic compounds. These organic compounds must be in solution for injection into the gas chromatograph. The solvent must be volatile and organic (for example, hexane or dichloromethane).

The capillary column is held in an oven that can be programmed to increase the temperature gradually (or in GC terms, ramped). This helps in separation process. As the temperature increases, those compounds that have low boiling points elute from the column sooner than those that have higher boiling points. Therefore, there are actually two distinct separating forces, temperature and stationary phase interactions mentioned previously.

As the compounds are separated, they elute from the column and enter in a detector. The detector is capable of creating an electronic signal whenever the presence of a compound is detected. The greater is the concentration in the sample, the bigger the signal. The signal is then processed by a computer. The time from when the injection is made (time zero) to when elution occurs is referred to as the **retention time** (RT).

During the operation, the computer generates a graph from the signal (Fig. 9.3). This graph is called a **chromatogram**. Each of the **peaks** in the chromatogram represents the signal created when a compound elutes from the GC column into the detector. The x-axis shows the RT, and the y-axis shows the intensity (abundance) of the signal. In Fig. 9.3, there are several peaks labeled with their RTs. Each peak represents an individual compound that was separated from a sample mixture. The peak at 4.97 minutes is from dodecane, the peak at 6.36 minutes is from biphenyl, the peak at 7.64 minutes is from chlorobiphenyl, and the peak at 9.41 minutes is from hexadecanoic acid methyl ester.

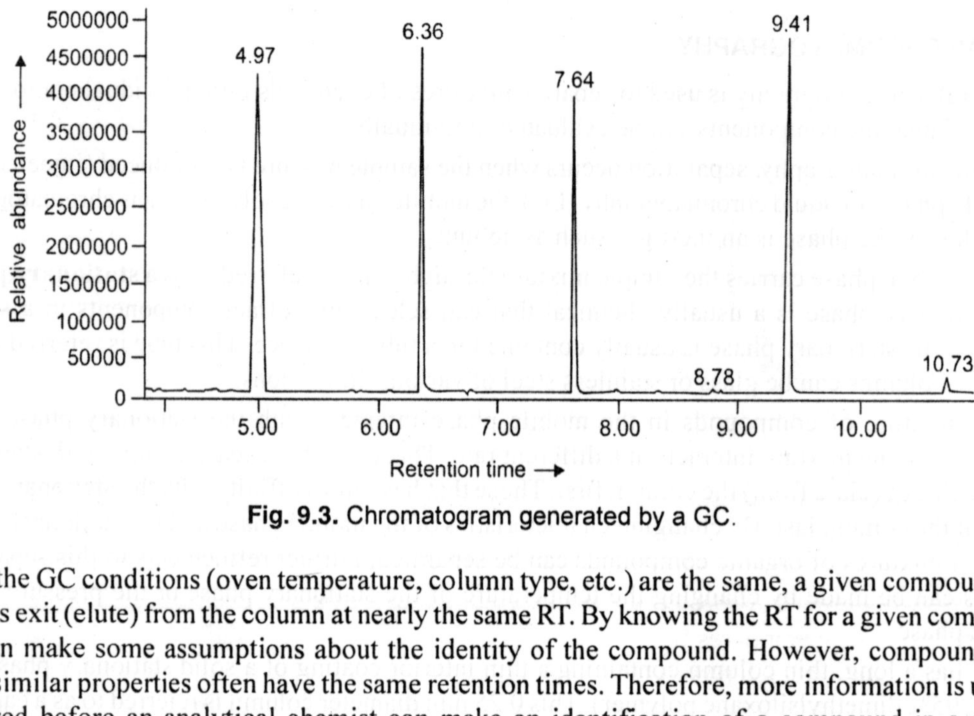

Fig. 9.3. Chromatogram generated by a GC.

If the GC conditions (oven temperature, column type, etc.) are the same, a given compound will always exit (elute) from the column at nearly the same RT. By knowing the RT for a given compound, we can make some assumptions about the identity of the compound. However, compounds that have similar properties often have the same retention times. Therefore, more information is usually required before an analytical chemist can make an identification of a compound in a sample containing unknown components.

9.3 MASS SPECTROSCOPY

As the individual compounds elute from the GC column, they enter into the ionization source. There, they are bombarded with a stream of electrons causing them to break apart into fragments. These fragments can be large or small pieces of the original molecules depending on the type of ionization source.

The fragments are actually charged ions with a certain mass. The mass of the fragment divided by the charge is called the mass to charge ratio (m/e). Since most of the fragments are singly charged (+1), m/e usually represents the mass (molecular weight) of the fragment.

The mass analyzer (usually a **quadrapole**), focuses each of the fragments through a slit into the detector. The quadrapoles are programmed by the computer to direct only certain m/e fragments through the slit. The rest bounce away. The computer has the quadrapoles cycle through different m/e's one at a time until a range of m/e's are covered. This occurs many times per second. Each cycle of ranges is referred to as a **scan**.

The computer records a graph for each scan. The x-axis represents the m/e ratios. The y-axis represents the signal intensity (abundance) for each of the fragments detected during the scan. This graph is referred to as a **mass spectrum** (Fig. 9.4).

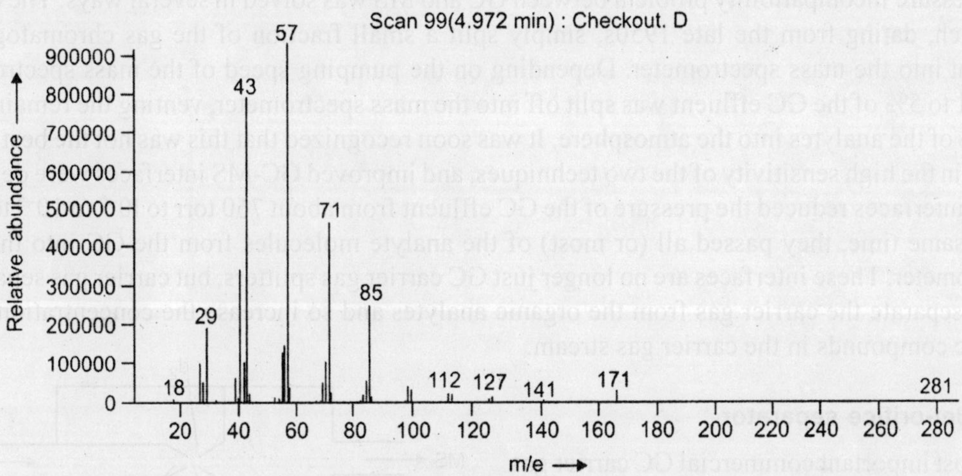

Fig. 9.4. Mass-spectrum generated by an MS.

The mass spectrum produced by a given chemical compound is essentially the same every time. Therefore, the mass spectrum is essentially a fingerprint for the molecule. This fingerprint can be used to identify the compound. The mass spectrum in Fig. 9.4 is produced by dodecane. The computer on GC–MS has a library of spectra that can be used to identify an unknown chemical in the sample mixture. The library compares the mass spectrum from a sample component and compares it to mass spectra in the library. It reports a list of likely identifications along with the statistical probability of the match.

9.4 GC–MS

When GC is combined with MS, a powerful analytical tool is created. GC can separate volatile and semivolatile compounds with good resolution but it cannot identify them. MS can provide detailed structural information on most compounds that can be exactly identified but it cannot readily separate them. Gas chromatography and mass spectrometry are, in many ways, highly compatible techniques. In both techniques, the sample is in the vapor phase, and both techniques deal with about the same amount of sample (typically less than 1 ng). Unfortunately, there is a major incompatibility between the two techniques: The compound exiting the gas chromatograph is a trace component in the GC's carrier gas at a pressure of about 760 torr, but the mass spectrometer operates at a vacuum of about 10^{-6} to 10^{-5} torr. This difference in pressure of 8 to 9 orders of magnitude, creates a considerable problem. For satisfactory performance, the mass spectrometer analyser housing has to be maintained at a very low pressure, typically about 10^{-6} to 10^{-7} Torr, otherwise analyte ions will not reach the ion detector owing to collisions with other neutral atoms and molecules. For this reason, the introduction of a sample from the atmosphere must be accompanied by some kind of interface/restrictor to keep the total mass (solvent/gas) entering in the mass spectrometer low enough to be compatible with the pumping capacity of the vacuum system.

9.5 INTERFACE USED IN GC-MS

The pressure incompatibility problem between GC and MS was solved in several ways. The earliest approach, dating from the late 1950s, simply split a small fraction of the gas chromatographic effluent into the mass spectrometer. Depending on the pumping speed of the mass spectrometer, about 1 to 5% of the GC effluent was split off into the mass spectrometer, venting the remaining 95 to 99% of the analytes into the atmosphere. It was soon recognized that this was not the best way to maintain the high sensitivity of the two techniques, and improved GC-MS interfaces were designed. These interfaces reduced the pressure of the GC effluent from about 760 torr to 10^{-6} to 10^{-5} torr, but at the same time, they passed all (or most) of the analyte molecules from the GC into the mass spectrometer. These interfaces are no longer just GC carrier gas splitters, but carrier gas separators. These separate the carrier gas from the organic analytes and so increase the concentration of the organic compounds in the carrier gas stream.

9.5.1 Jet-orifice separator

The most important commercial GC carrier gas separator is called the jet separator (Fig. 9.5). This device works on the basis of the differences in diffusibility between the carrier gas and the organic compound. The carrier gas is almost always a small molecule such as helium (mass 4) or hydrogen (mass 2) with a high diffusion coefficient, whereas the organic molecules (higher mass) have much lower diffusion coefficients. In operation, the GC effluent (the carrier gas with the organic analytes) is sprayed through a small nozzle, indicated as d^1 in Fig. 9.5, into a partially evacuated chamber (about 10^{-2} torr). Because of its high diffusion coefficient, the helium is sprayed over a wide solid angle (tremendous expansion of gases), whereas the heavier organic molecules are sprayed over a much narrower angle and tend to go straight across the vacuum region. By collecting the middle section of this solid angle with a skimmer (marked d^3 in Fig. 9.5) and passing it to the mass spectrometer, the higher-molecular-weight organic compounds are separated from the carrier gas, which is removed by the vacuum pump. Most jet separators are made from glass by drawing down a glass capillary,

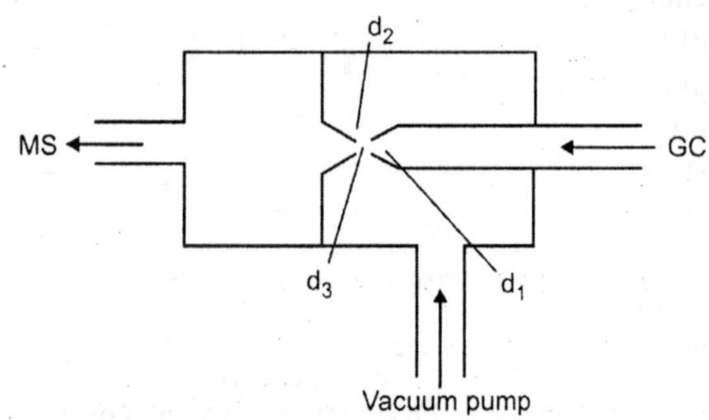

Fig. 9.5. The jet separator, a device for interfacing a packed column GC with an MS. The three distances are typically d_1, 100 μm; d_2, 300 μm; and d_3, 240 μm.

sealing it into a vacuum envelope, and cutting out the middle spacing (marked d^2 in Fig. 9.5). It is important that the spray orifice and the skimmer be perfectly aligned.

These jet separators work well at the higher carrier gas flow rates used for packed GC columns (10 to 40 ml/min); however, there are certain disadvantages. Packed GC columns are an almost infinite source of small particles upstream of the jet separator. If one of those particles escapes from the column, it can become lodged in the spray orifice and stop (or at least severely reduce) the gas flow out of the GC column into the mass spectrometer. Part of this problem can be eliminated with a filter between the GC column and the jet separator, but eventually a particle will plug up the orifice. In fact, sometimes it is not a particle at all, but rather tar (mostly pyrolyzed GC stationary phase) that has accumulated in the spray orifice over time. Clearly, these devices require maintenance.

9.5.2 GC-MS interface (for fused silica capillary GC columns)

Currently, the most common strategy, which is ideally suited for capillary GC columns, is to pass all of the carrier gas flow into the ion source of the mass spectrometer. This works only if the GC gas flow is sufficiently small and the pumping speed of the mass spectrometer's vacuum system is sufficiently high to handle the gas flow. For most capillary GC columns, the gas flow is 1 to 2 ml/min, and for most modern mass spectrometers, the pumping speed is at least 300 L/sec. The development of flexible, fused silica capillary columns has made this approach routine.

In practice, most GC-MS interfacing is now done by simply inserting the capillary column directly into the ion source. Fig. 9.6 is a diagram of one such system. The fused silica column runs through a 1/16-in.-diameter tube directly into the ion source. Other gases, such as methane for chemical ionization, are brought into the ion source by a T joint around the capillary column. One of the other two lines into the ion source is used for a thermocouple vacuum gauge tube so that the pressure in the ion source can be roughly measured. The remaining line into the ion source is for the delivery of the mass spectrometer calibration standard, perfluorotributylamine (to take the standard spectrum). Most joints are welded together to avoid leaks when this inlet system is thermally cycled or vented. The only removable (Swagelok) fitting is at the junction of the GC column and the far end of the inlet tube (marked with an asterisk in Fig. 9.6). This fitting uses Vespel ferrules. Once the ferrules are on the GC column and it is in the ion source, it is desirable to cut off a few centimeters of the column, if possible. This eliminates the possibility offine particles partially occluding the end of the column.

Note: *Fittings are used to connect the various components of an GC system together while maintaining a leak-free flowpath. Using the correct fitting eliminates dead volume that can contribute to peak broadening, decreased resolution, split peaks, sample carry-over and gas collection. No matter how sophisticated the instrumentation, it can not compensate for poor fittings. Stainless steel compression fittings consist of an external threaded nut and a tapered ferrule that compresses onto the outer wall of the tubing as the nut is tightened inside a tapered port. The nut provides the driving force that compresses the ferrule enough to grip the tubing.*

If the end of the column cannot be placed directly in the ion source, the material in the GC–MS interface becomes important. The interface is held at 250 to 280°C; thus, it should not include a reactive metal (such as copper). In some interfaces, glass-lined stainless steel tubing has been used, even though this tubing is difficult to bend properly.

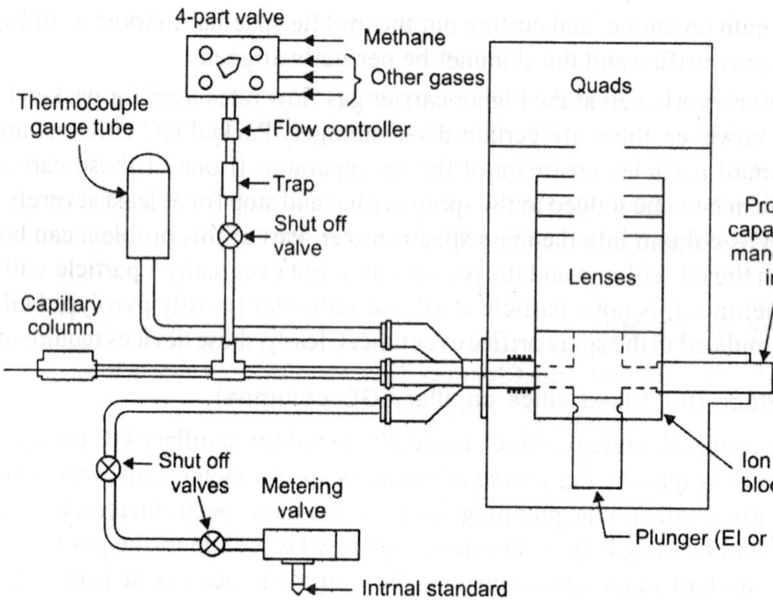

Fig. 9.6. A typical GC-MS interface for fused silica capillary GC columns. The end of the GC column enters the ion source of the mass spectrometer.

9.5.3 Membrane separator

The membrane separator operates preferen-tially on organic analyte. It is thin membrane (a few square millimeter) typically made of silicone elastomer, used as interface between GC and MS. The membrane is a sandwich (Fig. 9.7) between spiral channels, column effluent on one side under pressure, MS on other side under vacuum – relies on differen-tial permeability of carrier gas vs analyte molecules. For one type interface, using a silicone membrane, the selectivity for organic molecules (the analyte) over helium (the carrier gas) is 50,000. The effluent from chromatograph is directed onto this membrane. The membrane is organic in nature and so absorbs and dissolves the organic constituents from gas stream. The inert carrier gas, such as helium, argon, or hydrogen, is not soluble in the organic membrane; thus it is discharged through the exit of the separator. Those organic compounds that dissolve in the elastomer diffuse rapidly through the very thin membrane into vacuum of the ion source. In this way, the separator preferentially allows the passage of organic constituents across the membrane into mass spectrometer with an enrichment factor of approximately 100. Despite being a very effective enrichment procedure, it also suffers from discrimination effects with more polar analytes and produces significant band broadening of their chromatographic peaks.

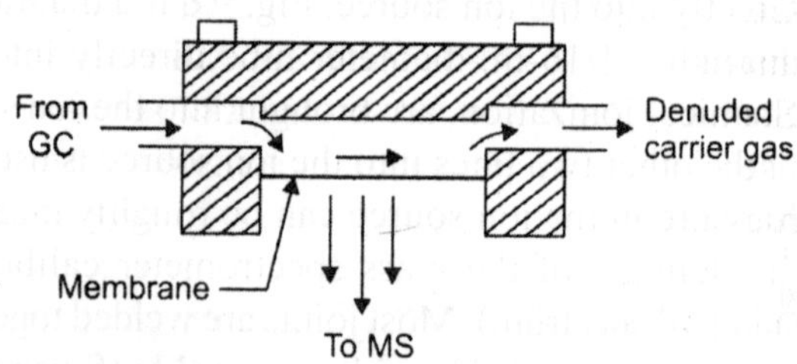

Fig. 9.7. Schematic diagram of Membrane separator.

9.6 LIMITATIONS OF GC-MS

Although GC/MS is considered to be excellent technique in scientific analysis, GC/MS does have some limitations. Because great faith is maintained in GC/MS analysis, erroneous results are not expected and hard to dispute. However, false positives and false negatives are possible.

Some problems with GC/MS originate in improper conditions in the GC portion of the analysis. If the GC instrument does not separate the specimen's compounds completely, the MS feed will be impure. This usually results in background "noise" in the mass spectrum. If the carrier gas in the GC process is not correctly deflected from entering the MS instrument, similar contamination may occur.

Only compounds with vapour pressure succeeding 10^{-10} torr can be analyzed by GC–MS. Many compounds that have lower pressures can be analyzed if they are chemically derivatized (for example, as trimethylsilyl ethers).

9.7 APPLICATIONS OF GC-MS

9.7.1 Environmental Monitoring and Cleanup

GC-MS is becoming the tool of choice for tracking organic pollutants in the environment. The cost of GC-MS equipment has decreased significantly, and the reliability has increased at the same time, which has contributed to its increased adoption in environmental studies. There are some compounds for which GC-MS is not sufficiently sensitive, including certain pesticides and herbicides, but for most organic analysis of environmental samples, including many major classes of pesticides, it is very sensitive and effective.

9.7.2 Criminal Forensics

GC-MS can analyze the particles from a human body in order to help link a criminal to a crime. The analysis of fire debris using GC-MS is well established, and there is even an established American Society for Testing Materials (ASTM) standard for fire debris analysis. GCMS/MS is especially useful here as samples often contain very complex matrices and results, used in court, need to be highly accurate.

9.7.3 Law Enforcement

GC-MS is increasingly used for detection of illegal narcotics, and may eventually supplant drug-sniffing dogs. It is also commonly used in forensic toxicology to find drugs and/or poisons in biological specimens of suspects, victims, or the deceased.

9.7.4 Food, Beverage and Perfume Analysis

Foods and beverages contain numerous aromatic compounds, some naturally present in the raw materials and some forming during processing. GC-MS is extensively used for the analysis of these compounds which include esters, fatty acids, alcohols, aldehydes, terpenes etc. It is also used to detect and measure contaminants from spoilage or adulteration which may be harmful and which is often controlled by governmental agencies, for example pesticides.

9.7.5 Medicine

In combination with isotopic labeling of metabolic compounds, the GC-MS is used for determining metabolic activity. Most applications are based on the use of ^{13}C as the labeling and thus measurement of $^{13}C/^{12}C$ ratios with an **isotope ratio mass spectrometer (IRMS)**; have made the pharmacokinetic studies easier.

CHAPTER

10

Liquid Chromatography–Mass Spectrometry (LC–MS)

10.1 INTRODUCTION

Liquid chromatography/Mass Spectroscopy (LC/MS) is a technique which combines liquid chromatography HPLC, (powerful analytical separation technique) with mass spectroscopy, (powerful analysis & detection technique). The separation power of modern chromatography combined with the selectivity and very low detection limits of modern mass spectrometers enables us to analyze very complex samples with a high degree of confidence.

There are three major problems while combining the liquid chromatography with mass spectrometry.

(i) There is a need to eliminate the elution solvent. Suppose, for example, this solvent is water and the column being used has a very small diameter that allows the flow rate to be limited to 0.1 ml min^{-1}. This corresponds to 0.1 g min^{-1} of water or 5.6 mmol min^{-1}, which yields a flow rate of 135 cm^3 min^{-1} of gas at atmospheric pressure, which is still too much to be injected in a source under vacuum in mass spectrometer.

(ii) There is incompatibility with mobile phase composition as a result of frequent use of non volatile additives in liquid chromatography separation.

(iii) Liquid chromatography normally is used for compounds that are not volatile and are not suitable for gas chromatography. Hence, there is need of non volatile/thermally labile analytes to be analyzed by LC–MS technique.

Different methods are used to tackle these problems. Some of these coupling methods, such as moving-belt coupling or the particle beam (PB) interface, are based on the selective vaporization of the elution solvent before it enters the spectrometer source.

Other methods such as direct liquid introduction (DLI) or continuous flow FAB (CF-FAB) rely on reducing the flow of the liquid that is introduced into the interface in order to obtain a flow that can be directly pumped into the source. In order to achieve this it must be reduced to one-twentieth of the value calculated above, that is 5 μl min^{-1}.

These flows are obtained from HPLC capillary columns or from a flow split at the outlet of classical HPLC columns. Finally, a series of HPLC/MS coupling methods such as thermospray

(TSP), electrospray (ESI), atmospheric pressure chemical ionization (APCI), and atmospheric pressure photoionization (APPI) can tolerate flow rates of about 1 ml min^{-1} without requiring a flow split. Introducing the eluent entirely into the interface increases the detection sensitivity of these methods. ESI can accept flow rates from 10 nl min^{-1} levels to 0.2 ml min^{-1}. As it is more dependent on concentration than on the total quantity injected, there is little advantage of using it at high flow rates.

10.2 INTERFACES USING DESORPTION TECHNIQUES

The interfaces in this category are based on the selective vaporization of the elution solvent before it enters the spectrometer source.

10.2.1 Moving Belt Interface

The principle of the technique is shown in Fig. 10.1. The effluent of the LC is directed onto the surface of a belt made from pure nickel or polyimide. It runs through a series of vacuum stages into the ion source of the mass spectrometer. Infrared heaters and washing are included to minimize the memory effects and to clean the belt. Considerable effort has been directed towards spraying process, since the integrity of the chromatography is highly dependent on the efficiency and the precision of the transfer; thermally assisted spraying, thermospray and frit systems with contact to the belt have been developed to cover the surface of the belt smoothly and evenly.

The interface has an unusual advantage among the LC/MS interfaces in that it achieves the complete separation of chromatography and mass spectrometry, therefore permitting the independent optimization of chromatographic and mass spectrometric conditions. HPLC using reversed and

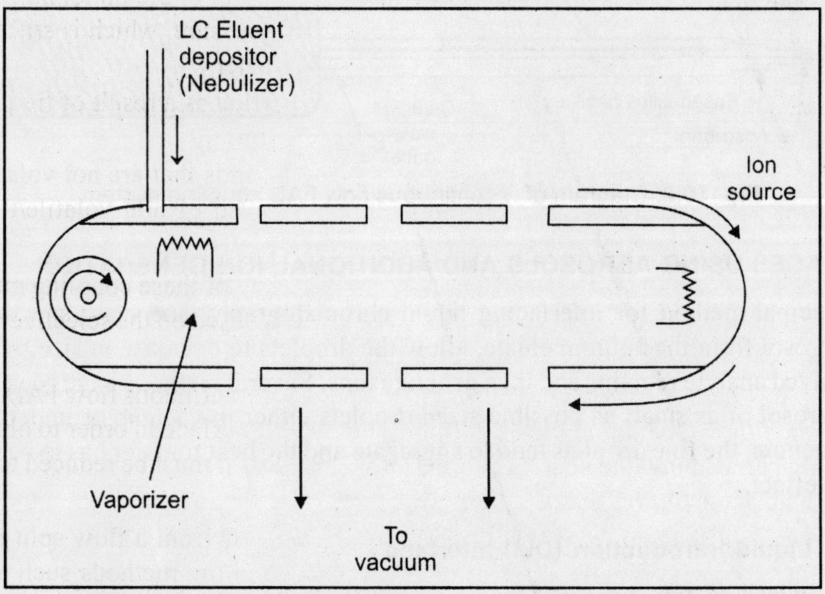

Fig. 10.1. The moving belt interface for LC-MS coupling.

normal phases, in normal and micro versions and supercritical fluid chromatography have been used with EI, CI, SIMS, FAB and laser desorption.

However, severe background problems and, at least when used with thermal desorption, the limitations due to vaporization in addition to the elaborate technical requirements (including further vacuum systems, maintenance of the belt and consequently the rather high costs) have limited the number of devices used in routine analysis.

10.2.2 Continuous Flow FAB Coupling

The continuous flow FAB coupling invented by Caprioli *et al.* consists of linking the end of a capillary chromatographic column with the end of an FAB nozzle by a capillary which passes through the introduction nozzle. The glycerol (1–5%) is added to the chromatographic solvent. The flow rate varies from 1 to 5 μl min^{-1}, which is pumped easily. The solvent evaporates but the glycerol stays at the nozzle surface with the eluted compounds and serves as a FAB matrix. Fig.10.2 shows a diagram of such a coupling.

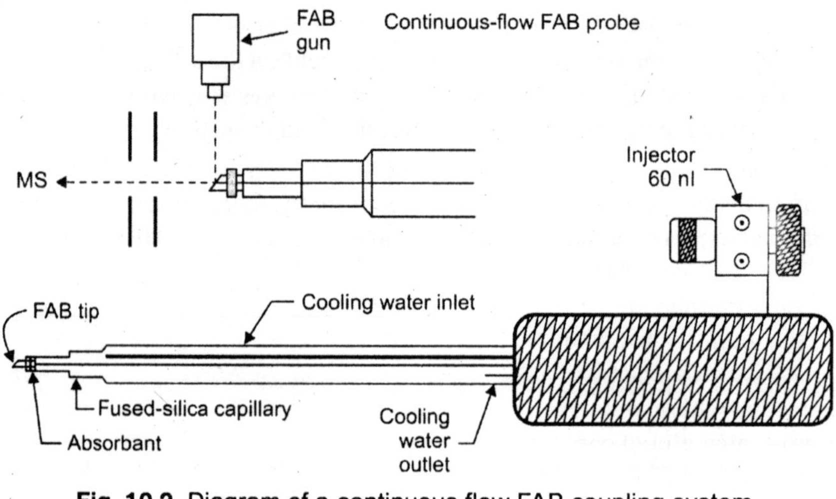

Fig. 10.2. Diagram of a continuous flow FAB coupling system.

10.3 INTERFACES USING AEROSOLS AND ADDITIONAL ION GENERATION

A second principal method for interfacing liquid chromatography and mass spectrometry is to produce an aerosol from the column eluate, allow the droplets to decrease in size by evaporation until the dissolved analyte remains and then generate ions. Several methods have been employed to produce an aerosol of as small as possible sized droplets either in vacuum or under atmospheric pressure. In vacuum, the fine droplets tend to aggregate and the heat transfer has to be optimized to minimize this effect.

10.3.1 Direct Liquid Introduction (DLI) Interface

The direct liquid introduction, proposed by Tal'roze in 1968 and again by Baldwin. They introduced the eluent directly into mass spectrometer through the capillary at flow rates below 1 ml min^{-1} (Fig.

10.3). Inside the source, volatile compounds were ionized by electron ionization. The low flow rate employed was the limitation. McLafferty in 1973 revived the idea of liquid introduction through a capillary and this led to development of direct introduction interfaces. In this, a flow of typically 10-20 ml/min is allowed to enter the vacuum chamber of the spectrometer without any separation of eluent and analyte. This can be achieved by using a micro HPLC, a narrow capillary or a diaphragm with a typically 5 mm hole, splitting 1–4% from the main stream; the latter approach was used in a first commercial version. The construction is relatively simple. The main disadvantage can be seen in the inflexibility with respect to the ionizing method (CI only using the eluent as reactant gas) and limitations in compounds amenable to analysis, which were not substantially different from those possible by GC/MS. In addition, only volatile buffers can be used. Although this interface demonstrated the feasibility of LC/MS in organic analysis and several attempts have been made to improve the performance by adding makeup gas streams to the liquid, the disadvantages were so problematic that today it is rarely in use.

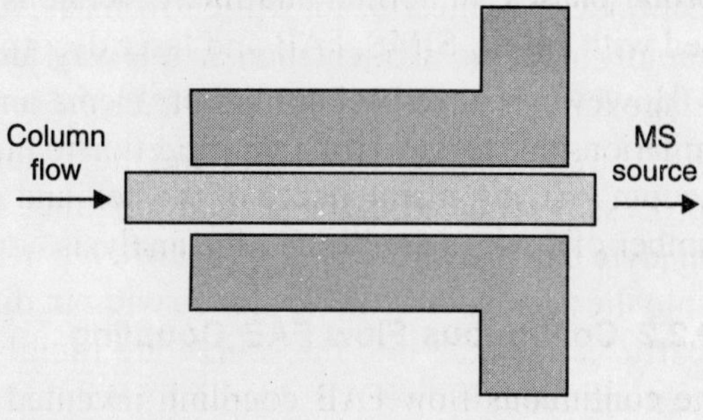

Fig. 10.3. Direct liquid introduction interface.

10.3.2 Particle Beam Interface Coupling

The particle beam interface is a device that allows the separation of solvent rapidly and efficiently from the eluent coming from a liquid chromatographic column. The chromatographic eluent is pumped through the capillary up to a glass concentric nebulizer (Fig.10.4). The eluent then is transformed into a cloud of droplets that are scattered by a helium concentric flow. The spray passes through a desolvation chamber, the walls of which are heated and the pressure of which is slightly lower than atmospheric pressure. During this travel the droplets undergo partial desolvation and yield slightly solvated eluted compound droplets. The resulting entrained mixtures of analyte particles in residual solvent molecules and helium atoms is drawn through a small orifice into a pumped chamber (at approximately 10 torr). It causes a rapid expansion of gases. The relatively massive solid analyte particles gain substantial momentum during this expansion of gases and

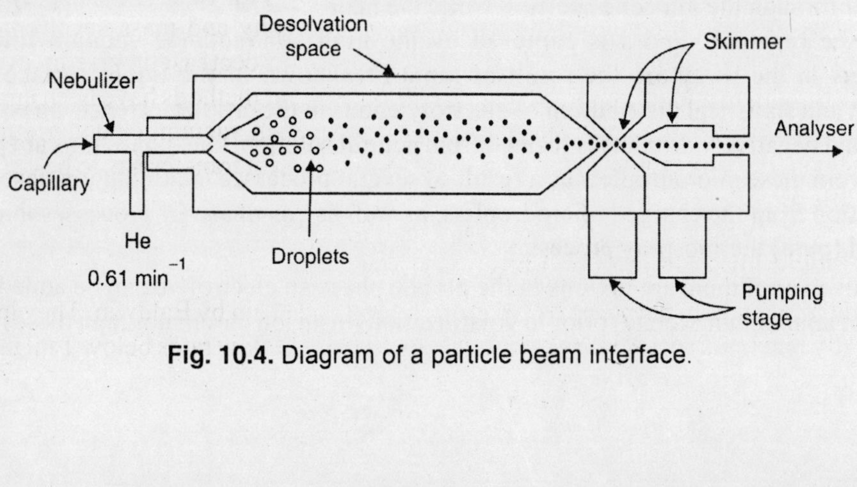

Fig. 10.4. Diagram of a particle beam interface.

continue in a linear beam while low mass, relatively solvent molecules and helium atoms expand rapidly in the radial orientation. In this way, analyte particles travel directly into the next concentration stage for enrichment of the analyte in the residual solvent through the skimmer.

The skimmed solvent vapor and the helium are mechanically pumped out of the apparatus. This process is repeated in the second pumping stage (about 500mTorr). Finally, the flow enriched in analyte particles consisting of a narrow particle beam with a diameter smaller than 100 nm is sent into the mass spectrometer source without disturbing the vacuum. In the EI or CI mode, the analyte particles injected into the source are rapidly vaporized before ionization. In the FAB mode, the particle beam is directed onto an FAB nozzle covered by a matrix. Thus, the particles collide with the matrix surface and are trapped in it.

10.4 INTERFACES USING AEROSOLS INCORPORATING ION GENERATION

In this section, two important LC/MS techniques, thermospray and electrospray, are described. Both techniques have the common feature that the generation of ions is an integrated part of the interface, which therefore dictates the ionization mode. But the success of both techniques depends largely on the processes of ion generation.

10.4.1 The Thermospray Interface Ion Source

Thermospray, pioneered in 1980 by Vestal and coworkers is to date the most widely used LC/MS technique for routine applications in the chemical industry, although electrospray is moving in very fast. The technique is sketched in Fig.10.5.

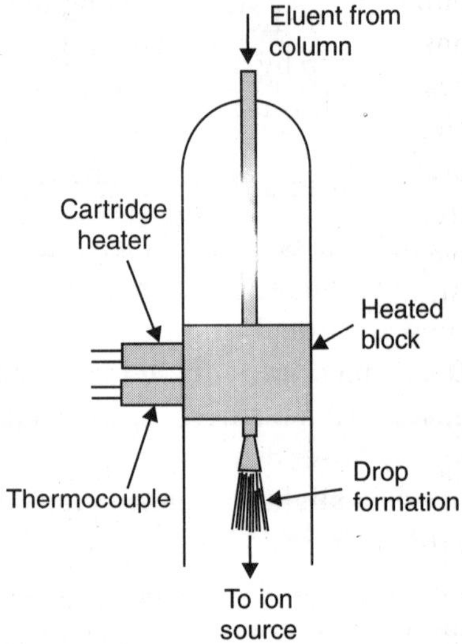

Fig. 10.5. Thermospray Ion Source.

The thermospray interface can be considered as a natural extension of the direct inlet system. It is comprised of a heated probe, a desolvation chamber, an ion skimmer and a vacuum line. The probe is made of a resistively heated capillary tube connecting the column with the MS ionization source. The liquid flowing through the hot capillary is partially evaporated so that an ultrasonic spray of vapor and charged microdroplets is obtained at the probe exit. Ions present in the source are transferred into the mass spectrometer through the ion cone aperture while the main portion of the residual vapors is captured by the high conductance vacuum line. Charged microdroplets in the spray are the result of rapid breakdown of the liquid surface during the vaporization and statistical distribution of electrolyte ions in the droplets. Hence, an equal mixture of positive and negatively droplets is formed from neutral solution. Gas-phase ions are produced in the source from these microdroplets as a result of several processes including ion desolvation and ion evaporation from the charged microdroplets, as well as gas-phase CI processes that constitute the so called (pure) thermospray process.

Note: However, if there are no ions in the mobile phase an electrolyte can be added (e.g., a 0.1 M solution of ammonium acetate) prior to volatilization (in an ion chromatograph these may already be present).

10.4.2 Electrospray Interface

An early report describing an *electrospray* interface was that of Whitehouse *et al* and this type of interface is probably the one most commonly used in contemporary LC/MS instruments.

A diagram of the electrospray interface is shown in Fig. 10.6. The electrospray interface differs from the thermospray in that it is *operated at atmospheric pressure* whereas the thermospray usually functions at a *reduced pressure* (1 to 10 torr). The sample solution is sprayed from the end of a stainless steel capillary usually situated about 1 cm from the ion sampling orifice. A potential of 3–5 kV is applied between the jet and the orifice plate and the gradient may be positive or negative. The ions are formed by the potential between the capillary jet and the plate. The ionizing efficiency of the electrospray depends on the ionizing potential. Increasing the potential difference first increases the drop size but initially no ions are formed. Increasing the voltage further results in an expanding mist of droplets. Under these conditions, the droplets are charged and ions are formed. The flow rate is restrained to a few micro liters/min, because the volume of liquid that can be drawn from the jet by electrical sheer forces is also limited. In many electrospray interfaces, solvent-evaporation is aided by a warm stream of nitrogen that flows counter current to the spray. In addition, any uncharged droplets are swept away from the orifice by this nitrogen stream. Further increase in the voltage initiates a corona discharge that interferes with the ion productions and should be avoided.

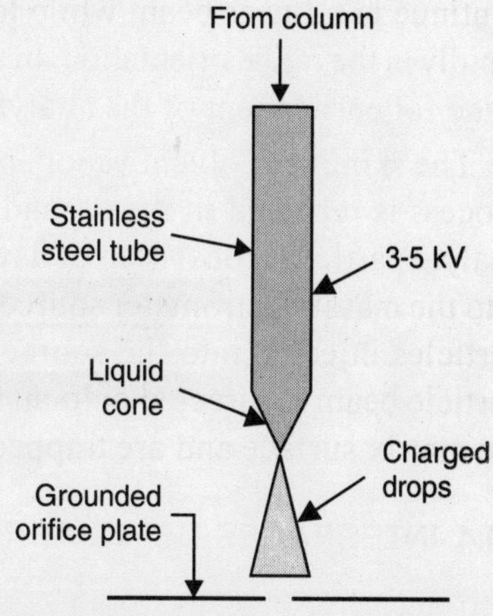

Fig. 10.6. The Electro spray Interface.

10.4.3 Atmospheric Pressure Chemical Ionization

Modern APCI sources for LC/MS coupling is originally developed by Horning and co-workers. The original source consisted on an atmospheric pressure vaporization chamber in which 1-2 μl of a liquid sample was injected through the septum. A hot carrier (N_2) was introduced into the chamber to help vaporization and to transport the analyte to an area close to beta source(63 Ni) (Fig. 10.7). In this area gas ionization, primary electrons interact with nitrogen carrier gas and solvent molecule which in turn ionize the analyte molecule through ion molecule reactions. Ions are then transferred through a small aperture and mass analyzed.

Modern APCI interfaces use some kind of heated pneumatic nebulizer probe for nebulization and a high voltage needle to produce a corona discharge responsible of inducing the ionization of nitrogen carrier gas and solvent molecule which in turn ionize the solvent molecule.

10.5 APPLICATIONS OF LC/MS

10.5.1 Pharmacokinetics

LC-MS is very commonly used in pharmacokinetic studies of pharmaceuticals. These studies give information about how quickly a drug will be cleared from the hepatic blood flow, and organs of the body. MS is used for this due to high sensitivity and exceptional specificity compared to UV (as long as the analyte can be suitably ionized), and short analysis time.

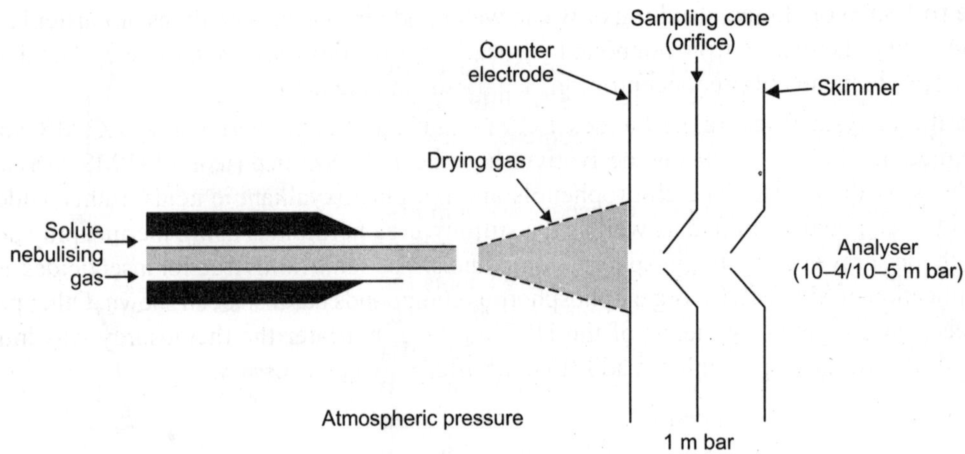

Fig. 10.7. APCI technique.

The major advantage MS has is the use of tandem MS–MS. The detector may be programmed to select certain ions to fragment. The process is essentially a selection technique, but is in fact more complex. The measured quantity is the sum of molecule fragments chosen by the operator. As long as there are no interferences or ion suppression, the LC separation can be quite quick. It is common now to have analysis times of 1 minute or less by MS-MS detection, compared to over 10 mins with UV detection.

10.5.2 Proteomics

LC-MS is also used in the study of proteomics where again components of a complex mixture must be detected and identified in some manner. The bottom-up proteomics LC-MS approach to proteomics generally involves protease digestion and denaturation (usually trypsin as a protease, urea to denature tertiary structure and iodoacetamide to cap cysteine residues) followed by LC-MS with peptide mass fingerprinting or LC-MS/MS (tandem MS) to derive sequence of individual peptides. LC-MS/MS is most commonly used for proteomic analysis of complex samples where peptide masses may overlap even with a high-resolution mass spectrometer. Samples of complex biological fluids like human serum may be run in a modern LC-MS/MS system and result in over 1000 proteins being identified, provided that the sample was first separated on an SDS-PAGE gel or HPLC-SCX.

10.5.3 Drug development

LC-MS is frequently used in drug development at many different stages including Peptide Mapping, Glycoprotein Mapping, Natural Products Dereplication, Bioaffinity Screening, In Vivo Drug Screening, Metabolic Stability Screening, Metabolite Identification, Impurity Identification, Degradant Identification, Quantitative Bioanalysis, and Quality Control.

10.5.4 Environmental analysis

The examples from application in environmental analysis have to be very divers, because the matrices and the analytes span over a wide range of physically and chemically different materials. Matrices can be soil, sand or sludge, drinking or waste water and air (gaseous analytes or particulates). The analytes range chemically from nonpolar hydrocarbons to ionic organometallic species, all requiring an appropriate means of preconcentration, separation and detection.

For the analysis of several herbicides, LC/MS and in particular thermospray LC/MS, appears to be the method of choice. Triazine derivatives have been determined (using LC/MS/MS) and their photolysis products also. The chlorophenols and the phenoxyalkanoic acids, rather widely used herbicides, can be determined as well as the sulfonylurea herbicides using thermospray and CZE/MS with ion spray and organophosphorus compounds. The same holds true for insecticides, although the application of SFC/MS for organophosphorous compounds has also been shown. Other pesticides have been investigated by means of the DLI interface, but later the themospray was introduced successfully, although postcolumn addition of buffer may be necessary.

CHAPTER

11

Biological Mass Spectrometry

11.1 INTRODUCTION

The application of mass spectrometry (MS) to biology began in the 1940s, when heavy stable isotopes were used as tracers to study processes such as CO_2 production in animals. Since that time, advances in technology have increased the range of sample types that can be ionized and the range of masses that can be measured, which has diversified the applications of MS. The biological applications of MS currently encompass such diverse areas as screening newborns for metabolic disorders, comparing protein expression levels between cells grown in different media, determining the bioavailability of minerals in food, and studying how pharmaceutical drugs are metabolized *in vivo*. The wide varieties of sample types that can now be analyzed, and the breadth of information that can be obtained, have helped MS to permeate into an extensive range of research areas. The result is that MS has become an essential analytical tool in biological research. The current importance of MS to biological research is highlighted by the 2002 Nobel Prize in Chemistry, which was awarded to John Fenn and Koichi Tanaka "for their development of soft desorption ionization methods for mass spectrometric analysis of biological macromolecules.

The goal of this review is to familiarize the reader with MS and some of its current applications to biological research. The total number of applications is too large to cover in a single review, so we provide a general overview with an emphasis on protein characterization, one of the newest and most widespread applications of biological MS.

11.2 APPLICATIONS OF MS IN BIOLOGICAL RESEARCH

The range of MS applications to biology is extensive. Here we divide them into three basic categories: isotope ratio MS, small organic molecule MS, and macromolecular MS. For each of these groups we discuss common applications.

11.2.1 Isotope-Ratio MS

Isotope-ratio MS (IRMS) is a technique that measures the relative stable isotopic abundance of elements. The elemental isotope ratio can be analyzed for a complex system (bulk IRMS), for a specific compound within a mixture, or for a specific position within a compound. As an example, the $^{13}C/^{12}C$ ratio can be measured for a tissue sample, for a specific fatty acid within the tissue, or for a specific carbon position within the fatty acid. IRMS can reveal information regarding the origin or state of a complex system. For instance, the ratio of $^{13}C/^{12}C$ in apple juice can indicate if the juice has been adulterated with corn syrup. The ratios of $^{13}C/^{12}C$, $^{15}N/^{14}N$, and $^{87}Sr/^{86}Sr$ can pinpoint the geographic origin of ivory, which can help conservationists prevent future poaching.

In biomedical research, IRMS is frequently used with projects involving stable isotopic tracers. For these experiments, compounds containing elements with abnormal stable isotope ratios are introduced into a system of interest (e.g. by feeding or by injection). The change in the isotopic ratio of the element in the system is then recorded with IRMS. Stable isotope tracers can be used to study the absorption, retention, and utilization of a nutrient *in vivo*. Stable isotope tracers can also be used to study energy expenditure or as a clinical tool for disease diagnosis. IRMS uses magnetic sectors as the mass analyzers and Faraday cups as the ion detectors. The ion source is usually an electron impact or thermal ionization source. An article by Davidsson and coworkers describes an experiment to test the effectiveness of two different iron absorption enhancers (Na_2 EDTA and ascorbic acid) to increase the iron absorbed by children in school meal program. On the first day, children were fed a breakfast "shake" containing one of the enhancers and $^{57}FeSO_4$. The next day, the same children were fed a breakfast "shake" containing either the original enhancer at a different concentration or a second enhancer and $^{58}FeSO_4$. Blood samples were taken before the first meal was given and 2 weeks after the second meal was consumed. The ratio of $^{58}Fe/^{57}Fe$ in the blood was measured to determine which meal allowed more iron absorption. It was found that ascorbic acid at a concentration of 70 mg/meal increased the iron absorbed to 115% of the daily requirement. This double stable isotope technique is useful because two variables can be tested in the same patient at the same time.

11.2.2 Small Organic Molecules

The mass spectrometric analysis of organic compounds gives information on the molecular mass, chemical formula, chemical structure, or quantity of the analyte. Based on the measured *m*/e and their peak intensities, the formula and chemical structure can be determined manually and/or by comparison with a reference database of spectra. As an example, Lavermicocca et al. used MS to identify novel antifungal compounds produced by *Lactobacillus plantarum* strain 21B (a bacterium used in making sourdough bread). Components of a culture filtrate were separated and tested for antifungal activity. Those that showed the highest activity were then characterized using gas chromatography-MS. The spectra were compared with those in a MS spectra library, and the compounds present were identified.

MS is also a valuable tool in the high-throughput analysis of compounds created in combinatorial libraries, such as those created to discover new drugs. If the mass spectrometer is connected to an LC system with appropriate columns, both structural information and information regarding the binding affinity of a molecule can be obtained MS can also be used to study drug metabolism by identifying the primary metabolites from *in vitro* studies and by measuring them *in vivo* to determine pharmacokinetic parameters. An example of this type of experiment is a study done by Oo et al. In this study, researchers administered oseltamivir (a treatment for influenza) to healthy patients between

1 and 12 years of age. The concentrations of oseltamivir and one of its metabolites were then monitored over time in the urine and plasma using MS. The pharmacokinetic data obtained allowed appropriate dosing schedules for children to be developed. For instrumentation, small organic molecule MS often uses an electron impact or chemical ionization ion source. A wide variety of mass analyzers are used, and tandem MS is often employed to increase the structural information obtained.

11.2.3 Macromolecules

MS analysis of macromolecules includes the study of proteins, peptides, oligonucleotides, oligosaccharides, and lipids. We defer a discussion of applications to the study of proteins and peptides to "Protein Characterization". The research on the analysis of oligonucleotides has focused on studying modified oligonucleotides that may not be compatible with the current enzymatic techniques used to sequence DNA. McLafferty and coworkers were able to sequence oligonucleotides up to 100 nucleotides in length using an ESI source coupled to a Fourier transform-ion cyclotron resonance analyzer. MS can also be used to analyze DNA modifications such as methylation. The characterization of oligosaccharides is more difficult than that of proteins and oligonucleotides because of the isomeric nature of the subunit and its ability to form branched structures. However, the structures of a wide variety of oligosaccharides have been determined by using tandem MS.

Many classes of molecules within the "lipid" category, including fatty acids, acylglycerols, and steroids, have been characterized by MS. The characterization of fatty acylcarnitines in blood can be used to screen newborns for hereditary fatty acid oxidation disorders. MS is used to measure the chain length and abundance of fatty acylcarnitines present in the blood. By comparing the resulting spectrum to that of a normal infant, doctors can diagnose if a fatty acid oxidation disorder is present, and in some cases they can determine the exact enzyme in which the newborn is deficient.

Most macromolecular research relies on the use of ESI or MALDI as an ionization source. A variety of mass analyzers, including the ion trap and TOF, are used. Tandem MS is often employed to elucidate structural details or sequence information.

11.3 PROTEIN CHARACTERIZATION

MS has become a vital tool in proteomic research. It can give information on the identity of a protein, the amount of the protein that is present, and the modifications the protein contains.

11.3.1 Protein Identification

The most commonly used MS method to identify proteins is a combination of peptide mass fingerprinting and amino acid sequencing via tandem MS (see Fig. 11.1). Using these methods, sensitivity is routinely in the femtomole range. The amino acid sequence of each protein is unique, and therefore the set of peptide masses resulting from proteolytic cleavage provides a "fingerprint" of the protein. In the peptide mass fingerprinting technique, an unknown protein is reduced and alkylated (to break any disulfide bonds) and then digested enzymatically using a sequence-specific proteolytic enzyme such as trypsin. Next, the masses of the resulting peptides are measured using MS. For the spectra in Fig. 11.1, a MALDI ion source was used, which results in almost all of the ions being singly charged (see "Ion Sources"). The list of peptide masses from the spectra is entered into a search program, such as Mascot or ProFound, along with information about the enzyme used, accuracy of the mass measurement, and possible protein modifications that may be present. The software then searches through databases of amino acid sequence information, (e.g. Swiss-Prot or NCBInr. For each protein entry in the database, the software uses the amino acid sequence to predict the peptide masses that would result from digestion with the user-specified enzyme. The software then compares the list of peptide masses measured (using MS) to the list of predicted peptide masses and calculates the probability of a match. The result is a list of possible protein identifications and the probability that each identification is correct.

The probability that the match is correct can be increased by performing tandem MS on one or more of the original peptides. In tandem MS, peptides of a specific m/e, selected from the peptide mass fingerprint, are isolated from peptides of all other m/e. The isolated peptides are then fragmented by collisions with a gas such as helium that has been introduced into the mass spectrometer.

The new peptide pieces formed by the CID are then measured. The weakest bond in a peptide is the one between the amino acids. Therefore, for low-energy CID, the resulting MS/MS spectrum is a series of peaks that represent peptides that differ only in the number of amino acids they contain. By measuring the mass difference between each peak, one can determine the amino acid sequence of the original peptide. High-energy CID also causes side-chain fragmentation. This information can be useful to differentiate between amino acids of the same molecular mass (e.g. leucine and isoleucine). In Fig. 11.1 the peptide with an m/e of 2574.30 was chosen for tandem MS analysis. The peptide was isolated and fragmented and the mass spectrum of the resulting fragments is shown. The partial amino acid sequence can be found by calculating the difference in mass between peaks. For example, the mass difference between the peaks with m/e = 1577.80 and m/e = 1449.76 is 128.04.

This is within error of the mass of glutamine (Q), which is 128.06 Da. The probability of fragmentation, however, is not the same for all of the amide bonds. This is evident by the wide range of peak intensities in the tandem MS data and the fact that some peaks are missing. For instance, due to the structure of proline, fragmentation at the C-terminal end of proline is rare. This is why in Fig. 11.1, we do not see a peak at m/e = 2020.94, which is equal to m/e = 2117.99 minus the mass of proline.

Although some work has been done to identify simultaneously all the proteins in a complex mixture, protein separation prior to enzymatic digestion is often performed.

Proteins are separated using LC or gel electrophoresis (either one- or two-dimensional gel electrophoresis). If separated by gel electrophoresis, the protein band or spot is excised, the proteins within are digested "in-gel", and the resulting peptides are extracted for MS analysis.

A plug is excised from an electrophoresis gel, and the protein in the gel plug is digested and extracted. The masses of the peptides in the extract are then measured by MS to obtain the peptide mass fingerprint. Next, peptides can be selected to undergo fragmentation via tandem MS. Here, the peptide with m/e = 2574 (labeled with an **arrow**) has been selected and fragmented. Finally, both the MS and tandem MS data are searched against protein sequence databases to determine the protein that was present in the gel spot.

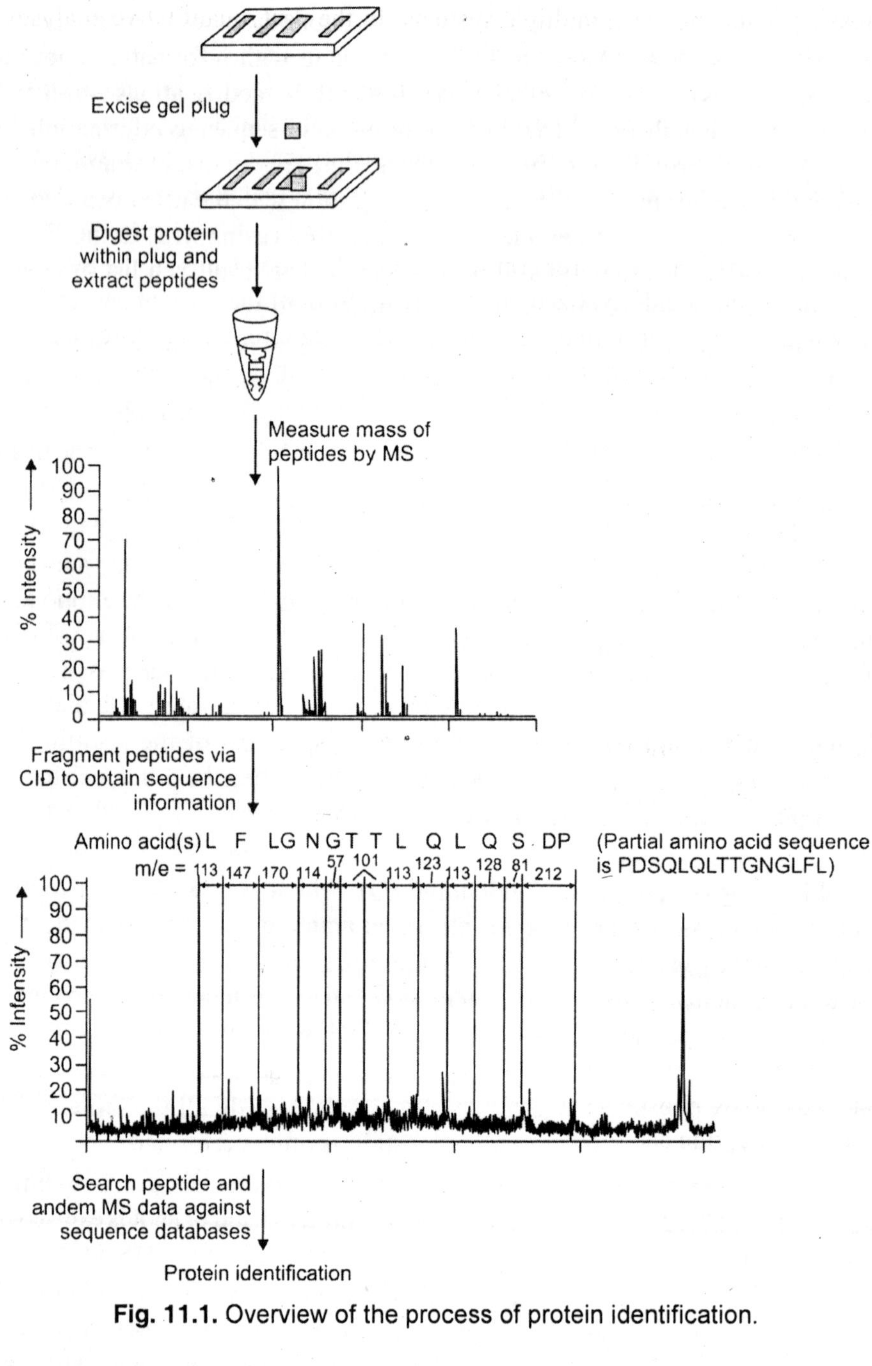

Fig. 11.1. Overview of the process of protein identification.

11.3.2 Protein Quantification

Proteomic research often requires knowing not only what proteins are being expressed by an organism, but also the level of protein expression. A common research technique is to compare the protein expression levels between multiple systems. In the past, quantitative analyses of protein levels using MS have been done by the metabolic labeling of the proteins in one system (e.g. cell lysates) with a heavy isotope such as 15 N. However, this procedure is limited to cells and tissues compatible with metabolic labeling. A new method for labeling that does not have this limitation is the isotope-coded affinity tags (ICAT) method. Note: Quantification of proteins in simple mixtures using the ICAT labeling approach requires the presence of several highly reactive cysteine residues in the targeted proteins.

In the ICAT approach, the ICAT reagent derivatizes the side chains of the cysteinyl residues. Proteins from one system are derivatized with a "light" form of the reagent and proteins from the other system with a "heavy" form. In the original ICAT procedure, the heavy form contained eight 2H atoms; however, in the current method, the heavy form includes nine ^{13}C atoms. The ICAT reagent has four parts: an affinity tag (biotin), a thiol specific reactive group for covalent attachment to cysteine side chains, a linker, and an isotope tag (which contains ^{13}C in the heavy form) (see Fig. 11.2). The tagged protein mixtures are combined and enzymatically digested. The digest is fractionated using cation exchange chromatography, which also removes any neutral species from the tryptic peptides. The tagged peptides (those that contain a cysteine) in each fraction are then separated from the others on an affinity column, and the biotin portion of the tag is cleaved off. The peptides are then separated using LC and analyzed by MS. The ratio of the intensities of the light- and heavy-labeled peptides gives a measurement of the ratio of protein expression in the two systems. The peptide is then analyzed with tandem MS to identify the parent protein.

11.3.3 Proteins with Post-translational Modifications

The function and activity of a protein is determined in part by any post-translational modifications that may be present. Over 200 distinct types of covalent modifications have been reported; the most common of these include phosphorylation, glycosylation, and ubiquitination. Here the use of MS to study phosphorylation will be reviewed. It is estimated that over 30% of proteins are phosphorylated. The conventional biochemical approach to studying phosphopeptides requires the use of radioactive labels and Edman sequencing, but a variety of approaches have been developed to study phosphorylation using MS. If the amino acid sequence of the protein is already known, the sample is digested and the peptides analyzed with MS. The *m*/e of the peptides measured with MS is compared with the predicted values. An increase in a peptide mass by 80 or 160 Da indicates covalent modification by phosphate (HPO_3) (mono- and diphosphorylated species, respectively). The phosphorylated peptide can then be analyzed using MS/MS to determine the exact position of the modification. If the protein is unknown, the sample is divided after digestion, and one portion is treated with a phosphatase. This step removes any phosphate groups, and a comparison of spectra before and after phosphatase treatment will indicate which peptides are modified. The modified peptides can be analyzed with MS/MS to identify the parent protein and the site of phosphorylation. The presence of phosphorylation can also be determined using different scanning modes on the mass spectrometer. In "neutral loss scanning," the mass spectrometer scans for an ion that when fragmented results in a specified neutral loss (change in mass but not in charge). When searching for phosphorylated peptides, the tandem MS spectra are searched for a fragment that has a mass 98 Da lower than the original peptide mass (with no change in charge).

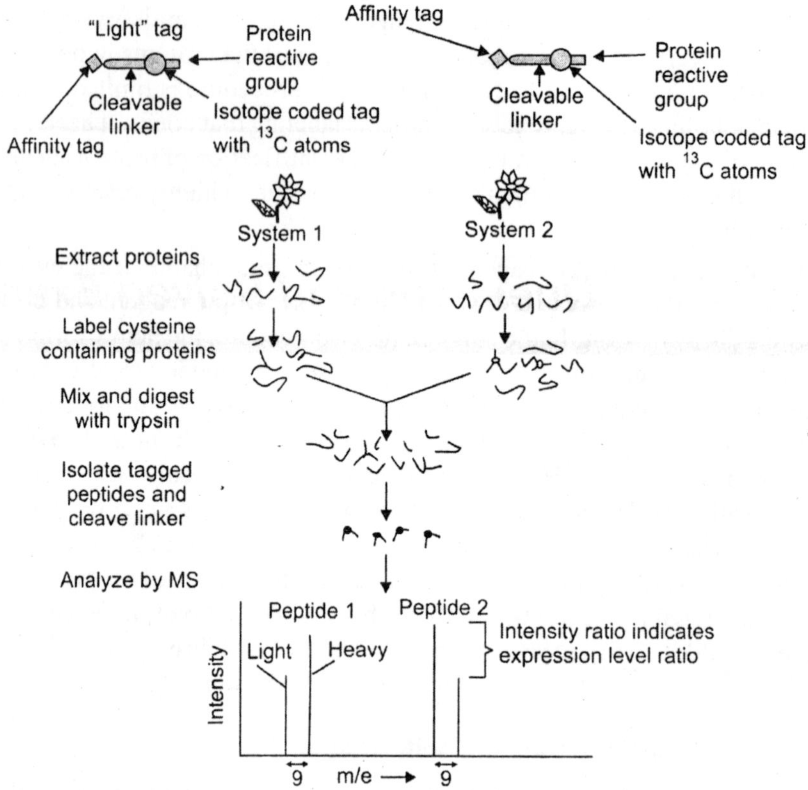

Fig. 11.2. Relative protein quantification using ICAT.

The ICAT reagents contain four main components: an affinity tag, a cleavable linker, an isotope tag (which contains zero or nine ^{13}C atoms for the "light" and "heavy" tags, respectively), and a group that reacts with cysteines. The proteins from one system are labeled with the "light" tag and the proteins from another system with the "heavy" tag. The proteins are mixed and digested with trypsin. The fragments containing cysteine residues are then isolated, the linker is cleaved to remove the affinity group, and the resulting peptides are analyzed with MS. The ratio of the "light" to "heavy" peaks in the spectra gives a measure of the ratio of protein expression between the systems.

This neutral loss indicates a loss of H_3PO_4 due to beta elimination. This process cannot detect phosphotyrosines, however, due to stability of the beta protons in the benzene ring. In "precursor ion scanning," the mass spectrometer scans for a specific product ion after fragmentation. For phosphotyrosines, the peptides are fragmented using CID and scanned for a positive fragment ion with 216 m/e (phosphotyrosine immonium ion). For other phosphorylations, the peptides are fragmented using CID and scanned for a negative ion with 79 m/e due to the release of PO_3^-. MS has been used to study a multitude of post-translational modifications, often employing the same approaches discussed here for phosphorylation: treatment with an enzyme to remove the modification (with subsequent spectra comparison), neutral loss scanning, or precursor ion scanning. It should be noted that for modifications by heterogeneous molecules (such as glycans), the structure of the modification could also be analyzed with MS.

Questions and Solved Exercise

1. What is the basic principle of mass spectrometry?
2. Discuss and sketch the basic components of a mass spectrometer?
3. What does m/z mean?
4. Define the term 'mass spectrum'..
5. What are (i) base peak, (ii) molecular ion peak, and (iii) fragment ion peak. Assign these in the below given mass spectrum.

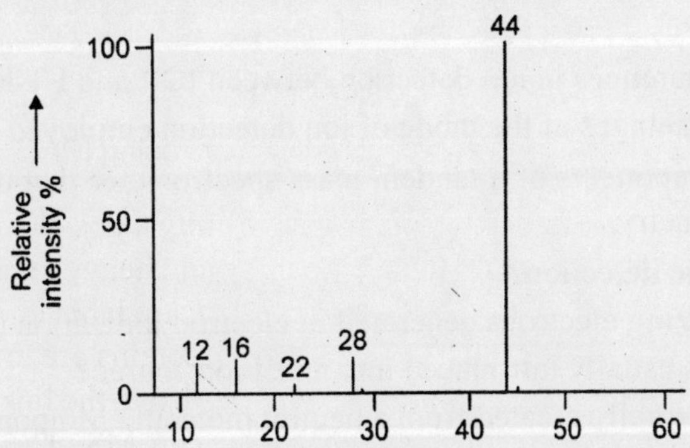

Can you identify the unknown compound from its spectrum?

6. a. What is the unit for atomic mass?
   b. What is m/z, Thomson, u and Dalton apart?
7. a. What is the difference between *nominal mass*, *isotopic mass*, and *relative atomic mass*?
   b. How do you calculate the relative atomic mass (atomic weight) from isotopic masses and abundance values?
8. What is the difference between low resolution and high resolution mass spectrometer? Discuss the importance of high resolution mass spectrometer.

9. Calculate the *accurate mass* of the following ions:
   a.. $HI^{+\cdot}$
   b. $H_2O^{+\cdot}$
   c. $C_6H_{12}^{+}$
10. Is a *resolution* setting of $R = 5000$ sufficient to separate $C_5H_9^+$ from CF_3^+ ions?
11. Do you recognize mass analyzers from their acronym? Specify the following analyzers:
    1. TOF
    2. B
    3. Q
    4. LIT
    5. QIT
    6. ICR
12. Explain the term "double-focusing magnetic sector instrument"?
13. Briefly describe the setup of a *linear quadrupole analyzer*. What advantages do *triple quadrupole* mass spectrometers offer in addition to *single quadrupole* instruments?
14. Briefly describe the setup of a *quadrupole ion trap*. Give a short explanation of the working principle of a quadrupole ion trap.
15. a. Explain the basic principle of *ion cyclotron resonance* (ICR).
    b. What is FT-ICR?
    c. What are the differences in ion detection between ICR and FT-ICR?
    d. Name major advantages of the mode of ion detection employed in FT-ICR.
16. Outline the key components of a tandem mass spectrometer that distinguish it from single stage mass spectrometry.
17. a. What is cryogenic detection?
    b. How are the ionizing electrons generated in electron ionization (EI)?
    c. How are samples usually introduced into an EI ion source?
    d. What ions are normally created from a neutral molecule M upon EI?
    e. Do EI spectra in general exhibit a high or a low degree of ion fragmentation?
18. Write down the structures of some molecular ions. Locate the charge at the most preferable position.
    - 1–Butene
    - Ethyl-isopropylether
    - Pyridine
    - Ethyl acetate
    - 2–Dimethylamino-diethylsulfide
    - Trifluoroethanol
19. a. What is the statement of the even-electron rule?
    b. What is the statement of Stevenson's rule?

c. Where will the charge reside according to Stevenson's rule? Write down the structures of the prefered fragment ions upon cleavage of the bonds indicated below:

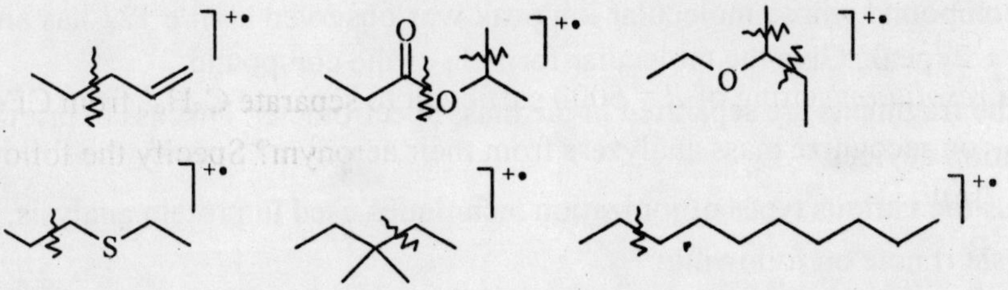

20. What is mass spectrometry (MS)? What information does mass spectrometry provide?
21. a. Explain the nitrogen rule.
    b. Apply the nitrogen rule to the compounds below. Do not calculate molecular weights. Simply fill "even" or "odd" into the second column.

Molecular composition	Monoisotopic mass is ...
C_3H_8	
$C_6H_{12}O_2$	
$C_6H_{11}NO$	
$C_{32}H_{25}N_3O_2S$	
$C_8H_{20}N_2$	
C_7H_9N	
C_3H_6BrN	
$C_9H_{11}ClN_4O_2$	
$C_{17}H_{32}Cl_2$	

22. What is the IHD of the following molecular formulae?
    (i) C_6H_{10}, (ii) C_6H_6, (iii) C_4H_8O, (iv) C_4H_8N, (v) C_2Cl_2
23. Calculate the IHD for each of the following.

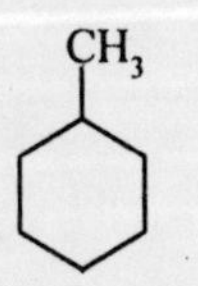

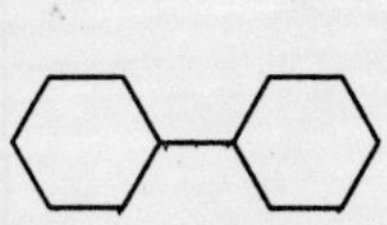

24. Write down the alpha-cleavages of butanone molecular ion.
25. a. How is ionization achieved in field ionization (FI)?
    b. In field desorption (FD), the analyte is supplied on the surface of an activated wire emitter. What advantage does this offer compared to FI?
26. Write short note on following:
    a. Maclafferty rearrangement
    b. Soft sources of ionization

26. a. Distinguish between 3-methyl cyclohexene and 4-methyl cyclohexene
    b. Show the fragmentation of cyclohexane at m/e 69, 56,55 and 41.
    c. A compound whose molecular ion peak was observed at m/e 122 has an equally intense (M + 2) peak. Give the molecular formula of the compound.
27. How the fragments are separated in the mass spectrometer. Discuss in brief various types of separation devices.
28. Discuss the various types of ionization techniques used in protein analysis.
29. Write short note on following:
    a. Types of detector used in mass spectrometry
    b. MALDI Technique
    c. Electron spray ionization technique
30. Compare the following:
    a. EI and CI methods for ionization
    b. FI and FD methods for ionization
31. Predict the fragmentation pattern for following:-
    a. Cyclohexanone
    b. Ethyl benzene
    c. Isobutyl benzene
    d. Butanal
    e. Acetaldehyde
32. How two compounds,pentan-2-one and pentan-3-one can be differentiated on the basis of mass fragmentation pattern.
33. The mass spectra of 1-pentanol (B)and ethyl acetate (A)are shown below. Match each spectrum with the correct molecule. Assign at least 2 of the fragments (not including the parent ion peak) for each molecule.

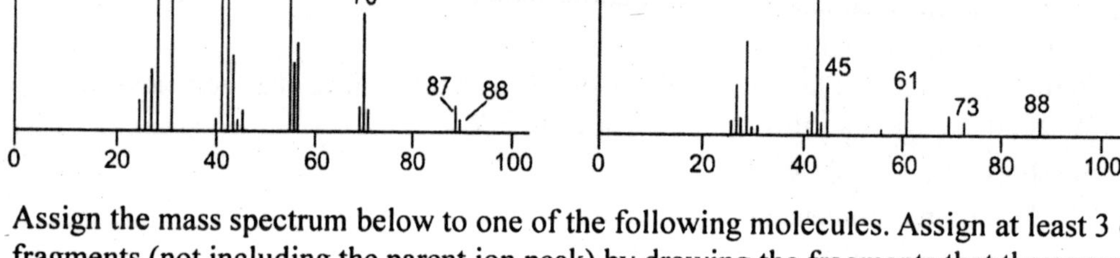

34. Assign the mass spectrum below to one of the following molecules. Assign at least 3 of the fragments (not including the parent ion peak) by drawing the fragments that they represent.

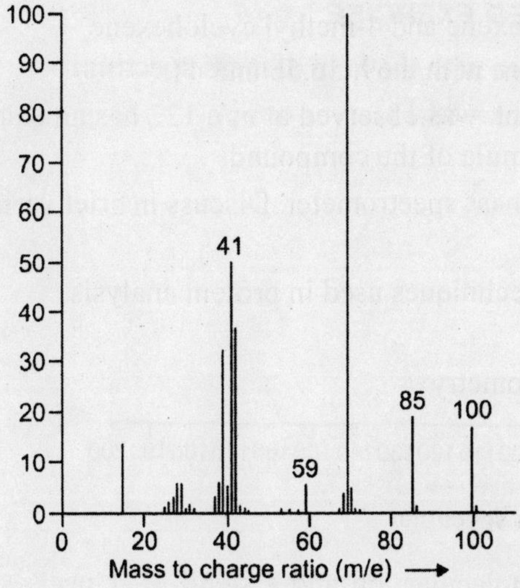

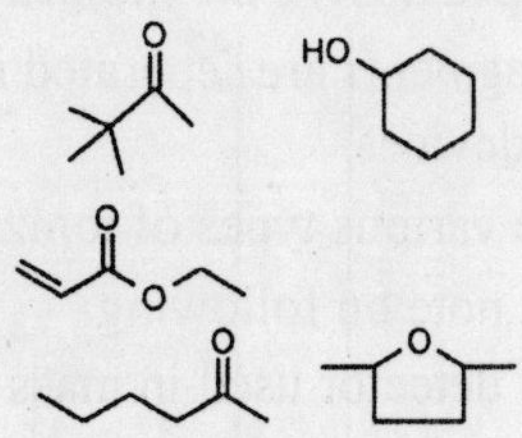

35. How the molecular formula can be determined with the help of mass spectrometry. Discuss with examples.
36. Write note on following:
    a. Diels alder rearrangement
    b. Metastable ion peaks
    c. Double charged ions
    d. Importance of Isotopic ions peaks in mass spectrometry
37. Discuss the applications of mass spectrometry.
38. Why vacuum is required in mass spectrometer. How it is maintained.
39. Discuss in brief the applications of mass spectrometry in medical Science.
40. How can you distinguish between the spectrum of n-butyraldehyde and that of iso-butyraldehyde?
41. To enhance resolution in a magnet sector type mass spectrometer, why is it necessary to add an electrostatic analyzer to create a double focusing type instrument?
42. Briefly describe the processes and instrumentation involved in the following ionization techniques used in mass spectrometry: a) chemical ionization; b) field desorption; c) fast atom bombardment; d) themospray.
43. Explain the presence of peaks at m/e 88, 71 and 60 in the mass spectrum of Ethyl butanoate.
44. A Hydrocarbon with a molecule formula C_7H_{12} (M^+ at m/e 96) shows large peak due to (M–15) and at m/e 54. Assign the structure to the hydrocarbon.
45. If in a tertiary amine $R_1CH_2NR_2R_3$, $R_1 > R_2 > R_3$ if $R_2 = C_2H_5$ and $R_3 = CH_3$, explain the formation of an ion with m/e 44 in its fragmentation pattern.

SOLVED EXERCISE

Exercise 1. Find out the chemical structure with the help of mass spectrum.
Mol. Formula = $C_5H_{12}O$, molecular weight = 88.15

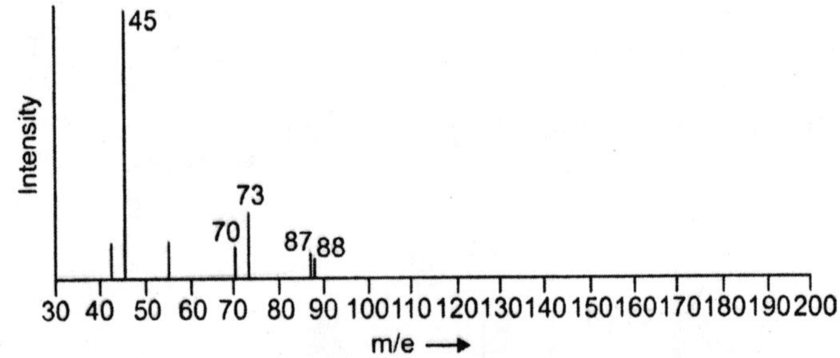

Mass spectrum

Answer. The spectrum shows a small molecular ion and a small M–1 peak, suggesting the presence of an alcohol (it cannot be an aldehyde since there are no degrees of unsaturation). The M–15 peak represents loss of a methyl group and the M–17 is consistent with loss of a hydroxy radical. For an alcohol, the base peak is often formed by expulsion of an alkyl chain to give the simple oxonium ion $R'CR''{=}OH^+$; to generate the observed m/e = 45, R′ must be CH_3 and R′ a H.

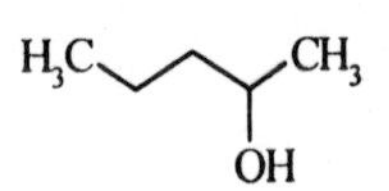

Chemical structure:
Chemical name: 2-pentanol
MS Fragments:

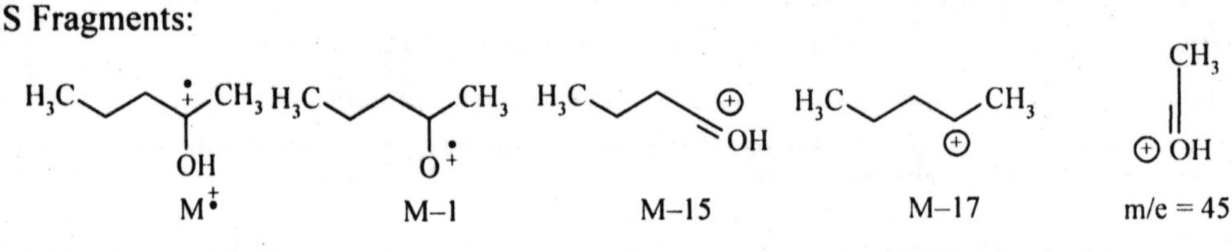

Exercise 2. Give the structure to the compound, possessing molecular formulae, $C_7H_{12}Br$ and molecular weight, 171.04. The mass spectrum is given below.

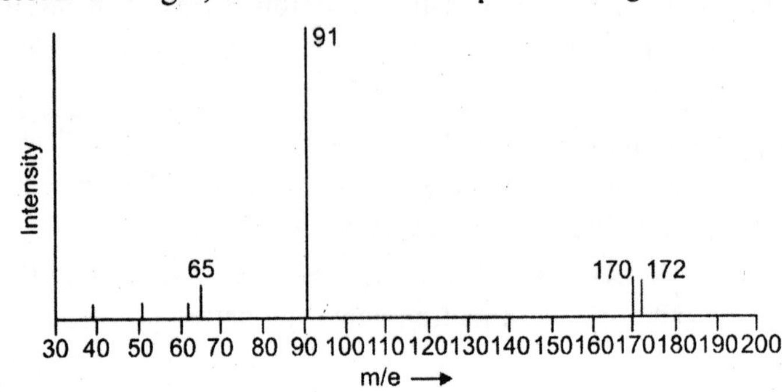

Mass spectrum

Answer. The spectrum shows two small peaks of equal intensity in the molecular ion region, strongly suggesting that the molecule contains bromine (equal concentrations of the ^{79}Br and ^{81}Br isotopes). The base peak represents loss of this bromine to give the peak at m/e = 91, which is highly suggestive of a benzyl fragment.

Chemical structure: 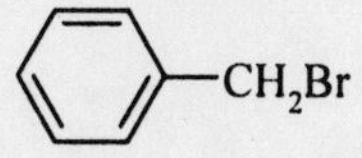

Chemical name: Bromomethyl benzene (benzyl bromide)

MS Fragments:

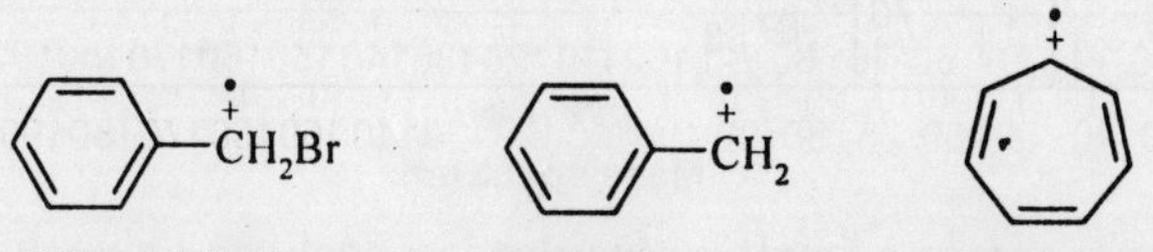

m+ (170 and 172) m/e 91 Tropylium ion

Exercise3. Give the structure to the compound having molecular formulae, $C_9H_{10}O$ and molecular weight, 134.18. The mass spectrum is given below.

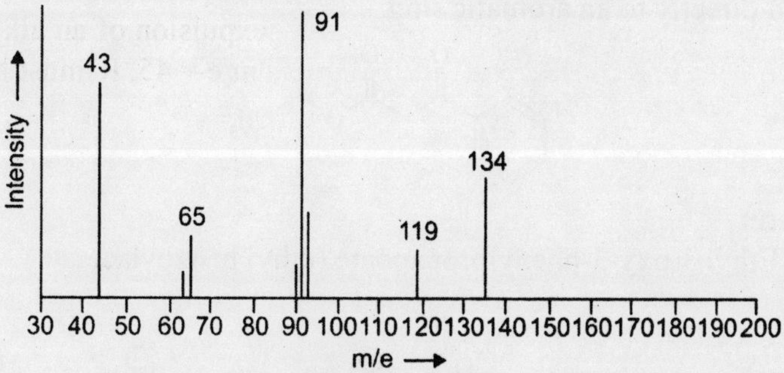

Mass spectrum

Answer. The spectrum shows a moderate molecular ion peak, and a peak at m–15, strongly suggesting the presence of a labile methyl group. The base peak occurs at m/e 91, which is highly suggestive of a benzyl fragment. The presence of an intense peak at m/e 43 is also suggestive of the presence of a methyl ketone, which can fragment to form the acylium ion.

Chemical structure: 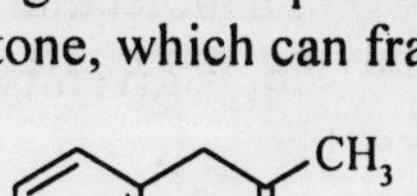

Chemical name: Benzyl methyl ketone

MS Fragments:

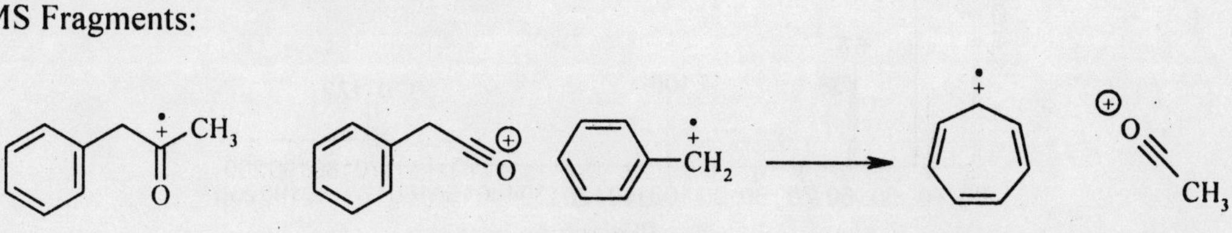

m^+ m–15 m/e 91 Tropylium ion m/e 43

Exercise 4. Give the structure to the compound having molecular formulae, $C_{11}H_{12}O_3$ and molecular weight, 192.21.The mass spectrum is given below.

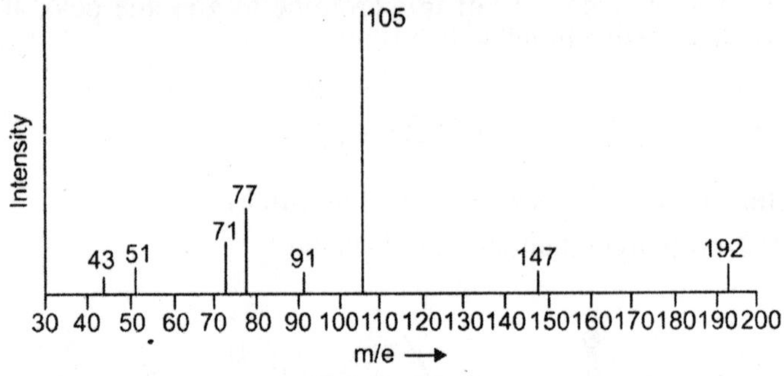

Mass spectrum

Answer. The spectrum shows a small molecular ion peak, and a peak at M–45, suggesting the presence of an ethoxy group (–O–CH_2CH_3). The very minor peaks at 91 and 43 suggest that the molecule does not contain a benzyl unit or a methyl ketone. The base peak occurs at m/e 105, and results from loss of a unit of m/e 73, which is also observed. The molecular ion at 105 is characteristic of a carbonyl bonded directly to an aromatic ring.

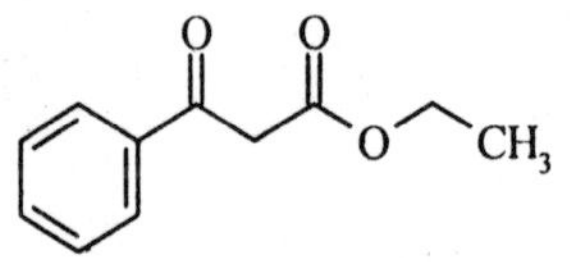

Chemical structure:
Chemical name: Ethyl 3-oxy-3-phenylpropanoate (ethyl benzoylacetate)
MS Fragments:

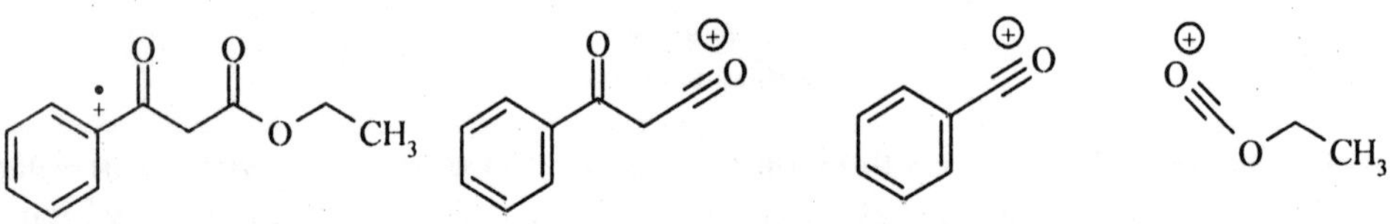

M⁺ M–45 m/e 105 m/e 73

Exercise 5. Give the structure to the compound having molecular formulae, $C_5H_8O_2$ and molecular weight, 100.12.The mass spectrum is given below.

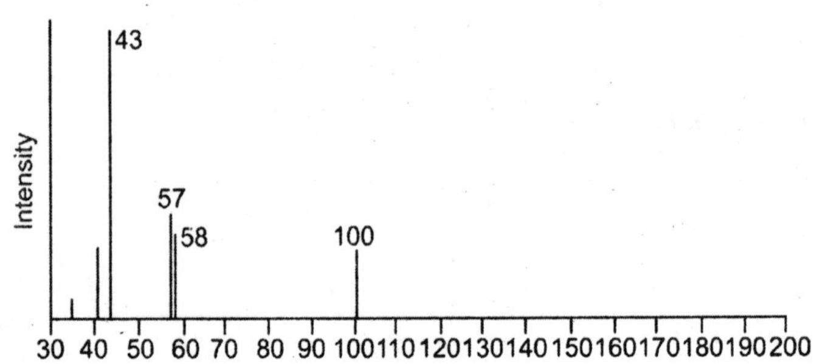

Mass spectrum

The spectrum shows a small molecular ion peak, and a pair of peaks at m/e = 57 and 58. The peak at m/e = 57 corresponds to loss of m/e = 43, which is the base peak and corresponds to the acylium ion ($CH_3C–O^+$). The m/e = 57 fragment corresponds to C_3H_5O, suggesting the original compound was an ester with this molecular formula.

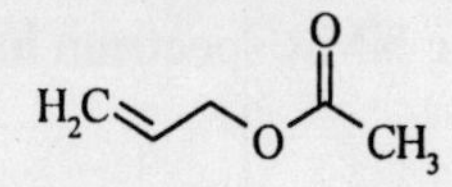

Chemical structure:

Chemical name: 2-propenyl ethanoate (allyl acetate)

MS Fragments:

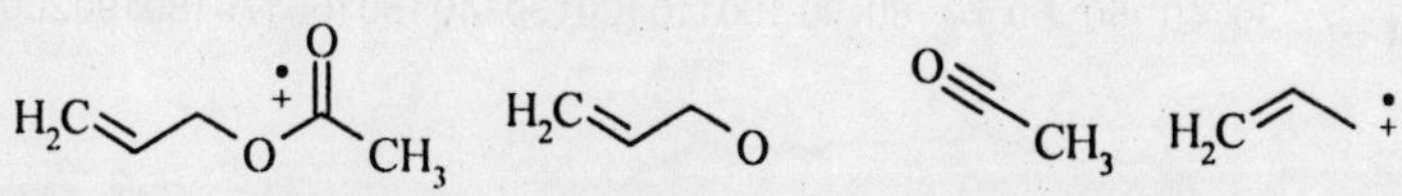

M^+ m/e 57 m/e 43 m/e 41

Exercise 6. One compound C_8H_8O gives the Mass spectra presented in the following figure. Deduce the structure and the cleavage processes of main fragment ions.

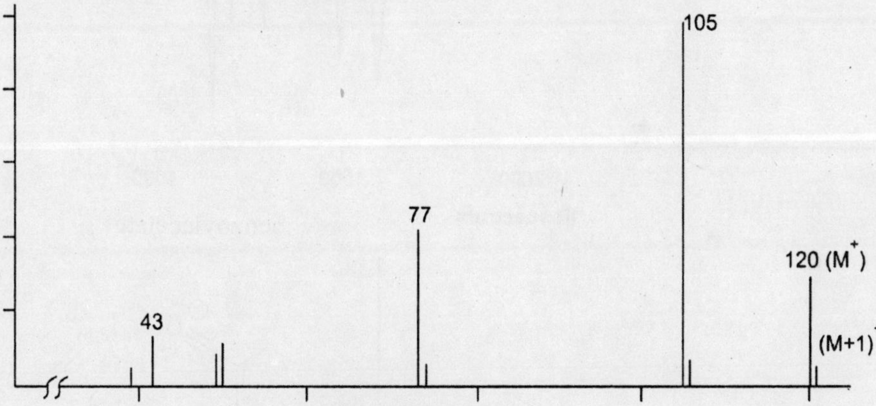

Mass spectrum

Answer. Acetophenone

Exercise 7. Compound C_7H_8O, has important bands in its UV absorption shows typical of the absorption a benzene ring. Its IR at 3400cm^{-1} (s), Its NMR has bands at δ4.3, δ5.1, and δ7.3(s), the true ratios are 2:1:5. Assign a structure to the compound that is compatible with spectral data given above.

Answer. Benzyl alcohol.

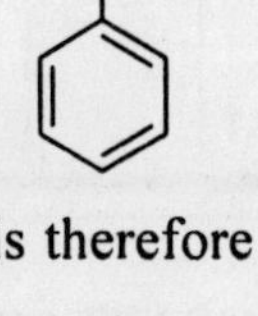

(i) The formula is CH_7O_8, and there is therefore four double-bands equivalent, suggest the formation of the benzene ring.

(ii) The UV spectrum has λ_{max} 240–290 nm, the absorption is middle, and typical of the benzene ring group, the presence of an benzene ring group is immediately apparent in the UV.

(iii) The IR spectrum with its very strong band at 1600 cm^{-1}, is shown by C=C conjugated aryl group.

(iv) From low-field to high-field, the NMR spectrum has five aromatic protons, one hydroxyl protons , two methane protons.

Exercise 8. Deduce the structure

Compound $C_7H_8O_2$

NMR Solvent: $CDCl_3$

IR Solvent: neat

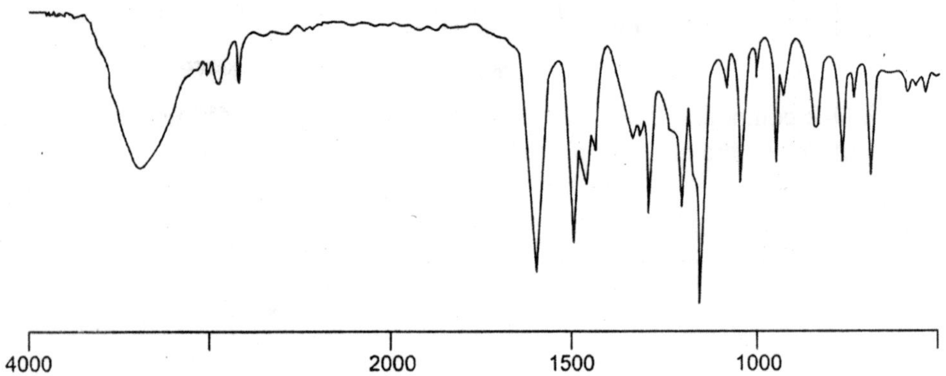

IR spectrum

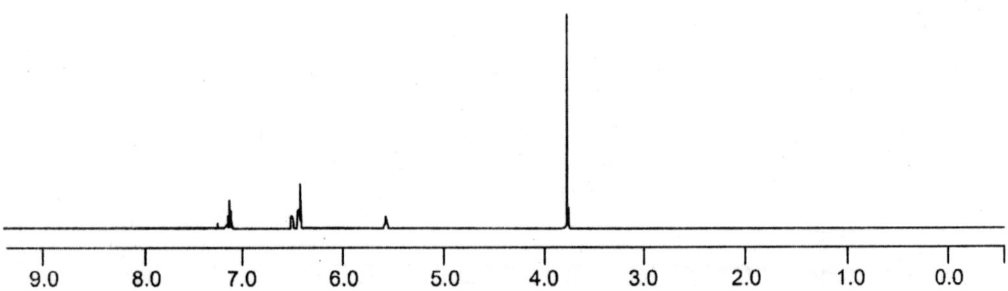

1H-NMR spectrum

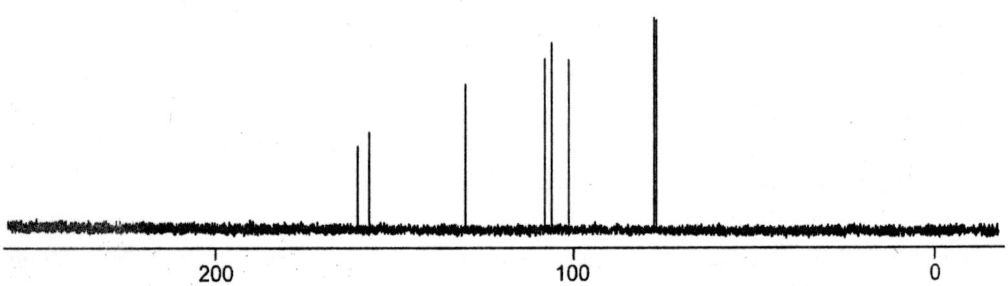

13C-NMR spectrum

Answer. 3-methoxyphenol.

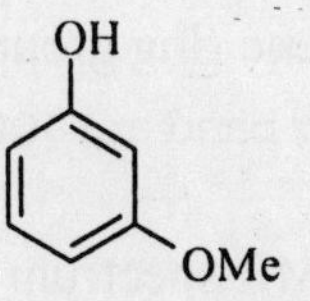

Exercise 9. The mass spectra of two constitutional isomers are shown here. Both are gases at room temperature. The molecular ion is the small peak at m/e 102.

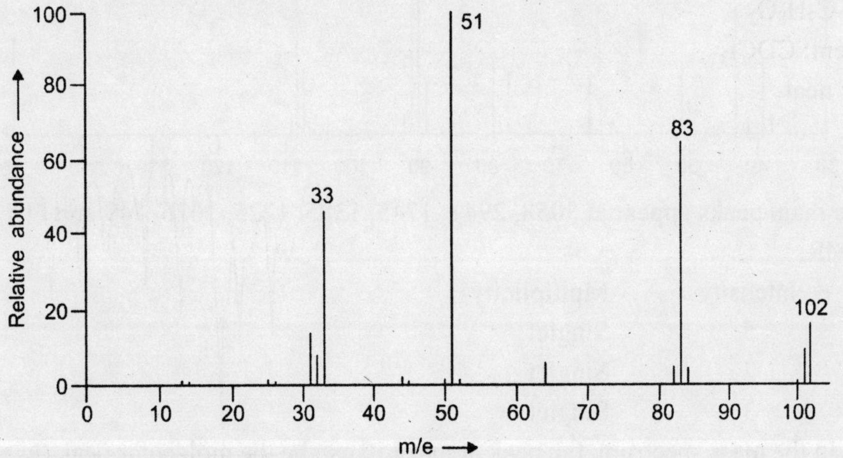

Isomer 1

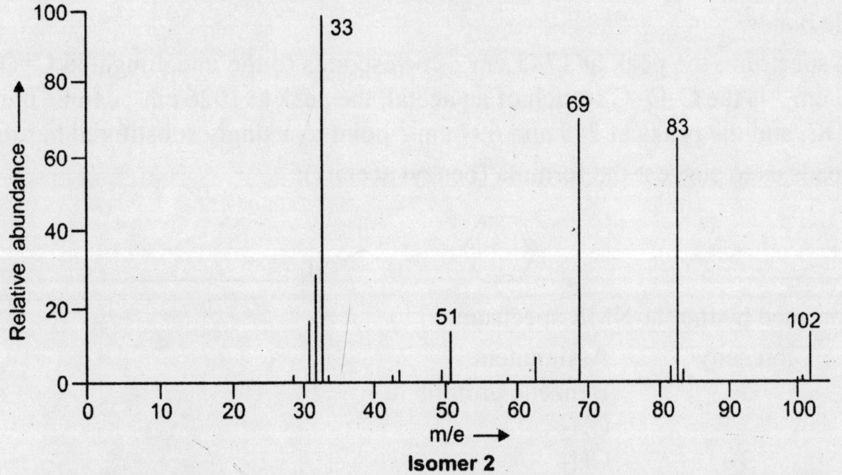

Isomer 2

Isomer 1: 1,1,2,2–tetrafluoroethane. The nearest large fragment ion to the small molecular ion is at m/z 83, a loss of 19 mass. This suggests loss of fluorine. The m/e 51 ion represents half the molecule. A hydrogen shift is necessary to explain the m/e 33 ion.

Isomer 2: 1,1,1,2–tetrafluoroethane. Important differences from isomer 1 are that the m/e 51 ion is much smaller, m/z 33 is much larger, and a new strong ion at m/e 69 has appeared. Since fluorine is present, this may be assigned as a trifluoromethyl cation.

Exercise 10. Identify the organic compound that yields the following mass spectrum:

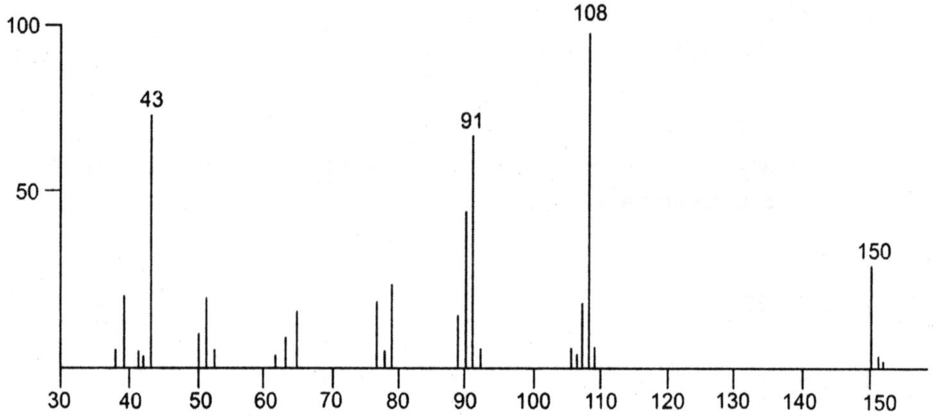

In IR, the main peaks appear at 3058, 2941, 1745, 1385, 1225, 1026, 749 and 697 cm^{-1}.

In ^1H-NMR:

δ	Intensity	Multiplicity
7.22	5	Singlet
5.00	2	Singlet
1.96	3	Singlet

Answer. In the mass spectrum, the peak at m/e 150 can be the molecular peak (even number of nitrogen atoms). The isotopic cluster suggests $C_9H_{10}O_2$ as the most probable formula with ve rings and/or double bonds.

In the IR spectrum, the peak at 1745 cm^{-1} corresponds to the unconjugated C=O stretch, the peak at 1225 cm^{-1} is the C–O–C stretch of an acetal, the peak at 1026 cm^{-1} can be the asymmetric stretch of COC, and the peaks at 749 and 697 cm^{-1} point to a singly substituted benzene.

All this leads us to suggest the formula (benzyl acetate):

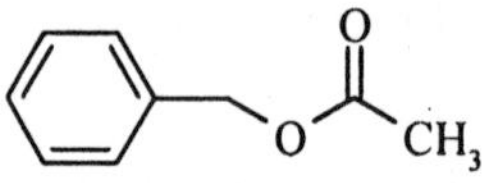

This is conrmed by the ^1H-NMR spectrum:

δ	Intensity	Assignment
7.22	5	Benzene protons
5.00	2	CH_2
1.96	3	CH_3

The main peaks in the mass spectrum are easily ascribed to the suggested formula:

150	molecular peak
108	$COCH_3$ loss with H transfer
91	tropylium ion
77, 78	benzene ions
43	CH_3CO^+

Exercise 11. Identify the organic compound that yields the following mass spectrum:

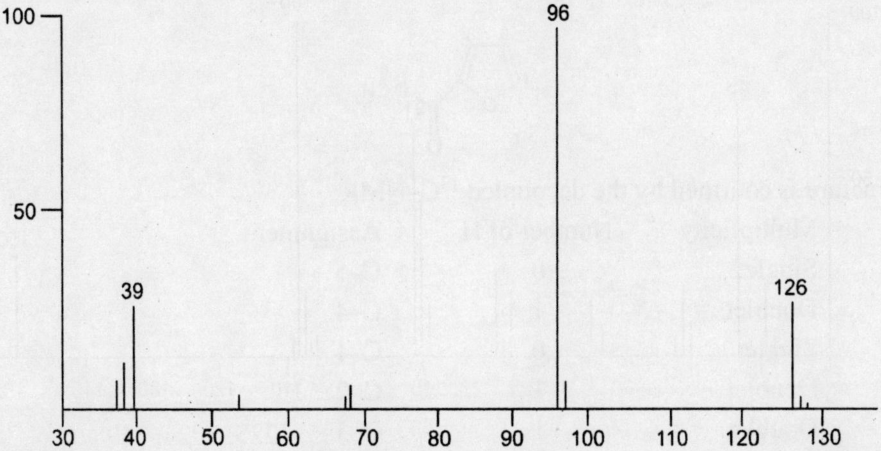

In IR, the main peaks appear at 3106, 2941, 1730, 1587, 1479, 1449, 1393, 1299, 1205, 1121 and 758 cm^{-1}.

In ^{1}H-NMR:

δ	Intensity	Multiplicity
7.51	1	Quadruplet
7.02	1	Quadruplet
6.45	1	Quadruplet
3.80	3	Singlet

In off-resonance decoupled ^{13}C-NMR:

δ	Multiplicity
160	Singlet
146	Doublet
144	Singlet
118	Doublet
112	Doublet
51	Quadruplet

Answer: The mass spectrum shows a peak at m/z 126 which can be the molecular peak (even number of nitrogen atoms); the isotopic cluster corresponds to $C_6H_6O_3$ (the exact mass can be conrmed by high resolution) with four rings and two double bonds. The base peak at m/e 95 corresponds to M–OCH_3.

The IR spectrum shows a peak at 1730 cm^{-1} that can be ascribed to a conjugated C=O, peaks at 1205 and 1121 cm^{-1} that can be ascribed to an ester C–O stretch, the peak at 758 cm^{-1} indicates the presence of an aromatic ring, and the same is true for the peaks at 3106, 1587 and 1479 cm^{-1}.

The ^{1}H-NMR spectrum conrms the presence of six protons and the ^{13}C-NMR conrms the presence of six Carbons. All this leads us to suggest the formula (carboxymethylfuran):

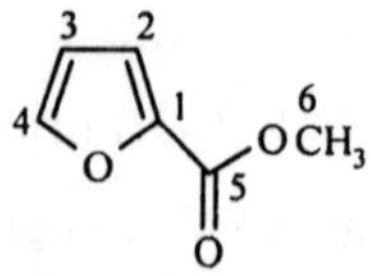

This structure is conrmed by the decoupled ^{13}C–NMR:

δ	Multiplicity	Number of H	Assignment
160	Singlet	0	C–5
146	Doublet	1	C–4
144	Singlet	0	C–1
118	Doublet	1	C–2
112	Doublet	1	C–3
51	Quadruplet	3	C–6

Exercise12. Identify the organic compound that yields the following mass spectrum:

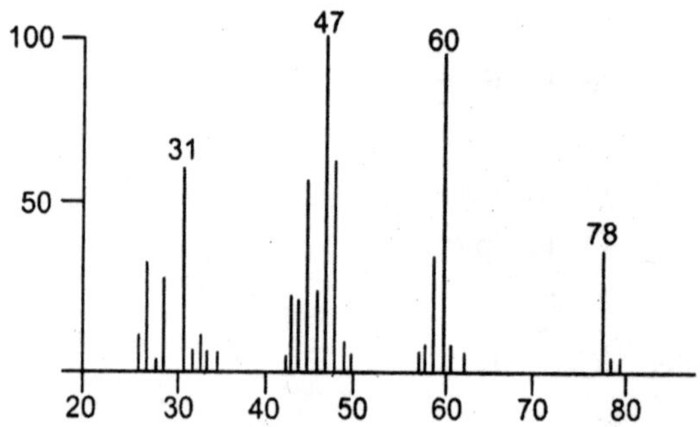

In IR, the main peaks appear at 3367, 3030, 2558, 1429, 1298, 1050 and 1020 cm^{-1}.
In off-resonance decoupled ^{13}C-NMR:

δ	Multiplicity
28	Triplet
64	Triplet

Answer: The molecular peak at m/e 78 indicates a molecule with an even number of nitrogen atoms. The intensity of the M + 2 peak indicates the presence of S; the remainder (46) could be due to C_2H_6O.

The crude formula that is suggested is thus C_2H_6OS, with no ring or double bond.

The decoupled ^{13}C-NMR spectrum conrms the presence of two C; in the off-resonance spectrum, the triplets indicate that four out of the six hydrogens belong to neighbouring methylene groups. The structure that is proposed is thus 2-hydroxyethanethiol:

$$HOCH_2CH_2SH$$

The IR spectrum conrms such a structure:

3367 cm^{-1}: OH stretch
2558 cm^{-1}: SH stretch
1050 cm^{-1}: CH_2OH primary alcohol

The main peaks in the mass spectrum are easily assigned:

78: molecular peak
60: H_2O loss
47: CH_2SH^+
31: CH_2OH^+

Appendices

Appendix 1

WEB SITES ON MASS SPECTROMETRY

Resources

i-mass: *http://www.i-mass.com*
Ion source: *http://www.ionsource.com*
Spectroscopy (incorporating Base Peak): *http://www.spectroscopynow.com*

Societies

American society for mass spectrometry: *http://www.asms.org*
Australian & New zealand for mass spectrometry: *http://www.anzsms.org/index.htm*
British Mass mass spectrometry society: *http://www.bmss.org.uk*
Mass spectrometry society of Japan: *http://www.mssj.jp*

Chemical and Biological Online Tools

Isotope Pattern Calculator: *http://www.shef.ac.ukl~chem/chemputer/isotopes.html*
FindMod tool: *http://au.expasy.org/tools/findmod/*
GlycoSuite at Proteome Systems: *http://tmat.proteomesystems.com/glycosuite/*
Mascot Search-Matrix Science: *www.matrixscience.com/search_form_select.html*
Peptide Search at EMBL: *http://vsites.unb.br/cbsp/paginiciais/peptsrcseqtag.htm*
Protein Prospector at UCSF: *http://prospector.ucsf.edu/*
PROWL at Rockefellar: *http://prowl.rockefellar.com/*
Web Elements Periodic Table: *http://www.webelements.com/*

Tutorials

Mass spectrometric tutorial: *http://www.astbury.leeds.ac.uk/facil/MStut/mstutorial.htm*

ASMS-What is Mass spectrometry: *www.asms.org/whatisms/*

Mass Spectrometry Tutorial: *www.chem.arizona.edu/massspec/*

BMSS What is Mass Spectrometry?: *http://www.bmss.org.uk/what_is/whatisframeset.html*

Cambridge University tutorial: *http://www-methods.ch.cam.ac.uk/meth/ms/theory/*

i-mass guides: *http://www.i-mass.com/guide/*

the mass spectrometer - *how it works*
www.chemguide.co.uk/analysis/masspec/howitworks.html

Mass spectrometry
www.cem.msu.edu/~reusch/.../Spectrpy/MassSpec/masspec1.htm

Appendix 2

ISOTOPE MASSES AND ABUNDANCES

Isotope	*Nominal mass*	*Mass*	*Relative abundance*	*Isotope*	*Nominal mass*	*Mass*	*Relative abundance*
^{1}H	1	1.007825	99.985(1)	^{35}Cl	35	34.968852	75.78(4)
^{2}H; D	2	2.014101	0.015(1)	^{37}Cl	37	36.965902	24.22(4)
^{3}H;T	3	3.016049	<0.0001	^{36}Ar	36	35.967546	0.3365(30)
^{4}He	4	4.002603	~100	^{38}Ar	38	37.962732	0.0632(5)
^{6}Li	6	6.015122	7.5(2)	^{40}Ar	40	39.962383	99.6003(30)
^{7}Li	7	7.016004	92.5(2)	^{39}K	39	38.9637069	93.2581(44)
^{9}Be	9	9.012182	~100	^{40}K	40	39.963998	0.0117(1)
^{10}B	10	10.012937	19.9(2)	^{41}K	41	40.961826	6.7302(44)
^{11}B	11	11.009305	80.1(2)	^{40}Ca	40	39.962591	96.941(156)
^{12}C	12	12.000000	98.93(8)	^{42}Ca	42	41.958618	0.647(23)
^{13}C	13	13.003354	1.07(8)	^{43}Ca	43	42.958766	0.135(10)
^{14}N	14	14.003074	99.632(7)	^{44}Ca	44	43.955481	2.086(110)
^{15}N	15	15.000108	0.368(7)	^{46}Ca	46	45.953693	0.004(3)
^{16}O	16	15.994914	99.757(16)	^{48}Ca	48	47.952533	0.187(21)
^{17}O	17	16.999131	0.038(1)	^{45}Sc	45	44.955910	~100
^{18}O	18	17.999160	0.205(14)	^{46}Ti	46	45.952630	8.25(3)
^{19}F	19	18.998403	~100	^{47}Ti	47	46.951764	7.44(2)
^{20}Ne	20	19.992440	90.48(3)	^{48}Ti	48	47.947947	73.72(3)
^{21}Ne	21	20.993846	0.27(1)	^{49}Ti	49	48.947871	5.41(2)
^{22}Ne	22	21.991385	9.25(3)	^{50}Ti	50	49.944792	5.18(2)
^{23}Na	23	22.989769	~100	^{50}V	50	45.947163	0.250(4)
^{24}Mg	24	23.985041	78.99(4)	^{51}V	51	50.943964	99.750(4)
^{25}Mg	25	24.985837	10.00(1)	^{50}Cr	50	49.946050	4.345(13)
^{26}Mg	26	25.982593	11.01(3)	^{52}Cr	52	51.940512	83.789(18)
^{27}Al	27	26.981538	~100	^{53}Cr	53	52.940653	9.501(17)
^{28}Si	28	27.976926	92.22(2)	^{54}Cr	54	53.938885	2.365(7)
^{29}Si	29	28.976494	4.69(1)	^{55}Mn	55	54.938049	~100
^{30}Si	30	29.973770	3.09(1)	^{54}Fe	54	53.939615	5.845(35)
^{31}P	31	30.973761	~100	^{56}Fe	56	55.934942	91.754(36)
^{32}S	32	31.972070	94.93(31)	^{57}Fe	57	56.935398	2.119(10
^{33}S	33	32.971458	0.76(2)	^{58}Fe	58	57.933280	0.282(4)
^{34}S	34	33.967866	4.29(28)	^{59}Co	59	58.933200	~100
^{36}S	36	35.967080	0.02(1)	^{58}Ni	58	57.935348	68.0769(89)

(Contd.)

Isotope	*Nominal mass*	*Mass*	*Relative abundance*	*Isotope*	*Nominal mass*	*Mass*	*Re abun*
^{60}Ni	60	59.930790	26.2231(77)	^{87}Sr	87	86.908882	7.
^{61}Ni	61	60.931060	1.1399(6)	^{88}Sr	88	87.905617	82.
^{62}Ni	62	61.928348	3.6345(17)	^{89}Y	89	88.905849	~
^{64}Ni	64	63.927969	0.9256(9)	^{90}Zr	90	89.904702	51.
^{63}Cu	63	62.929601	69.17(3)	^{91}Zr	91	90.905643	11.
^{65}Cu	65	64.927794	30.83(3)	^{92}Zr	92	91.905039	17.
^{64}Zn	64	63.929146	48.63(60)	^{94}Zr	94	93.906314	17.
^{66}Zn	66	65.926036	27.90(27)	^{96}Zr	96	95.908275	2.
^{67}Zn	67	66.927131	4.10(13)	^{93}Nb	93	92.906376	~
^{68}Zn	68	67.924847	18.75(51)	^{92}Mo	92	91.906810	14.
^{70}Zn	70	69.925325	0.62(3)	^{94}Mo	94	93.905087	9.2
^{69}Ga	69	68.925581	60.108(9)	^{95}Mo	95	94.905841	15.
^{71}Ga	71	70.924707	39.892(9)	^{96}Mo	96	95.904678	16.
^{70}Ge	70	69.924250	20.84(87)	^{97}Mo	97	96.906020	9.
^{72}Ge	72	71.922076	27.54(34)	^{98}Mo	98	97.905407	24.
^{73}Ge	73	72.923460	7.73(5)	^{100}Mo	100	99.90748	9.6
^{74}Ge	74	73.921178	36.28(73)	^{96}Ru	96	95.90760	5.5
^{76}Ge	76	75.921403	7.61(38)	^{98}Ru	98	97.90529	1.
^{75}As	75	74.921597	~100	^{99}Ru	99	98.905939	12.
^{74}Se	74	73.922477	0.89(4)	^{100}Ru	100	99.904219	12.
^{76}Se	76	75.919214	9.37(29)	^{101}Ru	101	100.905582	17.
^{77}Se	77	76.919915	7.63(16)	^{102}Ru	102	101.904349	31.
^{78}Se	78	77.917310	23.77(28)	^{104}Ru	104	103.905430	18.
^{80}Se	80	79.916522	49.61(41)	^{103}Rh	103	102.905504	~
^{82}Se	82	81.916700	8.73(22)	^{102}Pd	102	101.905607	1.
^{79}Br	79	78.918338	50.69(7)	^{104}Pd	104	103.904034	11.
^{81}Br	81	80.916291	49.31(7)	^{105}Pd	105	104.905083	22
^{78}Kr	78	77.92039	0.35(1)	^{106}Pd	106	105.903484	27.
^{80}Kr	80	79.916379	2.28(6)	^{108}Pd	108	107.903895	26.
^{82}Kr	82	81.913485	11.58(14)	^{110}Pd	110	109.905153	11.
^{83}Kr	83	82.914137	11.49(6)	^{107}Ag	107	106.905093	51.
^{84}Kr	84	83.911508	57.00(4)	^{109}Ag	109	108.904756	48.
^{86}Kr	86	85.910615	17.30(22)	^{106}Cd	106	105.90646	1.
^{85}Rb	85	84.911792	72.17(2)	^{108}Cd	108	107.90418	0.
^{87}Rb	87	86.909186	27.83(2)	^{110}Cd	110	109.903006	12.4
^{84}Sr	84	83.913426	0.56(1)	^{111}Cd	111	110.904182	12.
^{86}Sr	86	85.909265	9.86(1)	^{112}Cd	112	111.902758	24.

Isotope	*Nominal mass*	*Mass*	*Relative abundance*	*Isotope*	*Nominal mass*	*Mass*	*Relati abundar*
^{113}Cd	113	112.904401	12.22(12)	^{134}Ba	134	133.904504	2.417(18
^{114}Cd	114	113.903359	28.73(42)	^{135}Ba	135	134.905684	6.592(12
^{116}Cd	116	115.904756	7.49(18)	^{136}Ba	136	135.904571	7.854(24
^{113}In	113	112.904062	4.29(5)	^{137}Ba	137	136.905822	11.232(2
^{115}In	115	114.903879	95.71(5)	^{138}Ba	138	137.905242	71.698(4
^{112}Sn	112	111.904822	0.97(1)	^{138}La	138	137.907107	0.090(1
^{114}Sn	114	113.902783	0.65(1)	^{139}La	139	138.906349	99.910(
^{115}Sn	115	114.903347	0.34(1)	^{136}Ce	136	135.90714	0.19(1)
^{116}Sn	116	115.901745	14.45(9)	^{138}Ce	138	137.90599	0.25(1)
^{117}Sn	117	116.902955	7.68(7)	^{140}Ce	140	139.905435	88.48(1
^{118}Sn	118	117.901608	24.22(9)	^{142}Ce	142	141.909241	11.08(1
^{119}Sn	119	118.903311	8.59(4)	^{141}Pr	141	140.907648	~100
^{120}Sn	120	119.902199	32.59(9)	^{142}Nd	142	141.907719	27.13(12
^{122}Sn	122	121.903441	4.63(3)	^{143}Nd	143	142.909810	12.18(6
^{124}Sn	124	124.905275	5.79(5)	^{144}Nd	144	143.910083	23.80(12
^{121}Sb	121	120.903822	57.21(5)	^{145}Nd	145	144.912569	8.30(6)
^{123}Sb	123	122.904216	42.79(5)	^{146}Nd	146	145.913113	17.19(9
^{120}Te	120	119.90403	009(1)	^{148}Nd	148	147.916889	5.76(3)
^{122}Te	122	121.903056	2.55(12)	^{150}Nd	150	149.920887	5.64(3)
^{123}Te	123	122.904271	0.89(3)	^{144}Sm	144	143.911996	3.1(1)
^{124}Te	124	123.902819	4.74(14)	^{147}Sm	147	146.914894	15.0(2)
^{125}Te	125	124.904424	7.07(15)	^{148}Sm	148	147.914818	11.3(1)
^{126}Te	126	125.903305	18.84(25)	^{149}Sm	149	148.917180	13.8(1)
^{128}Te	128	127.904462	31.74(8)	^{150}Sm	150	149.917272	7.4(1)
^{130}Te	130	129.906223	34.08(62)	^{152}Sm	152	151.919729	26.7(2)
^{127}I	127	126.904468	~100	^{154}Sm	154	153.922206	22.7(2)
^{124}Xe	124	123.905895	0.09(1)	^{151}Eu	151	150.919846	47.8(1.5
^{126}Xe	126	125.90427	0.09(1)	^{153}Eu	153	152.921227	52.2(15
^{128}Xe	128	127.903531	1.92(3)	^{152}Gd	152	151.919789	0.20(1)
^{129}Xe	129	128.904780	26.44(24)	^{154}Gd	154	153.920862	2.18(3)
^{130}Xe	130	129.903509	4.08(2)	^{155}Gd	155	154.922619	14.80(5
^{131}Xe	131	130.905083	21.18(3)	^{156}Gd	156	155.922120	20.47(4
^{132}Xe	132	131.904155	26.89(6)	^{157}Gd	157	156.923957	15.65(3
^{134}Xe	134	133.905395	10.44(10)	^{158}Gd	158	157.924101	24.84(1
^{136}Xe	136	135.90722	8.87(16)	^{160}Gd	160	159.927051	21.86(4
^{133}Cs	133	132.905447	~100	^{159}Td	159	158.925343	~100
^{130}Ba	130	129.90631	0.106(1)	^{156}Dy	156	155.92428	0.06(1)
^{132}Ba	132	131.905056	0.101(1)	^{158}Dy	158	157.924405	0.10(1)

(Con

Isotope	Nominal mass	Mass	Relative abundance
^{160}Dy	160	159.925194	2.34(6)
^{161}Dy	161	160.926930	18.9(2)
^{162}Dy	162	161.926795	25.5(2)
^{163}Dy	163	162.928728	24.9(2)
^{164}Dy	164	163.929171	28.2(2)
^{165}Ho	165	164.930319	100
^{162}Er	162	161.928775	0.14(1)
^{164}Er	164	163.929197	1.61(2)
^{166}Er	166	165.930290	33.6(2)
^{167}Er	167	166.932046	22.95(15)
^{168}Er	168	167.932368	26.8(2)
^{170}Er	170	169.935461	14.9(2)
^{169}Tm	169	168.934211	~100
^{168}Yb	168	167.933895	0.13(1)
^{170}Yb	170	169.934759	3.05(6)
^{171}Yb	171	170.936323	14.3(2)
^{172}Yb	172	171.936378	21.9(3)
^{173}Yb	173	172.938207	16.12(21)
^{174}Yb	174	173.938858	31.8(4)
^{176}Yb	176	175.942569	12.7(2)
^{175}Lu	175	174.940768	97.41(2)
^{176}Lu	176	175.942683	2.59(2)
^{174}Hf	174	173.940042	0.162(3)
^{176}Hf	176	175.941403	5.206(5)
^{177}Hf	177	176.943220	18.606(4)
^{178}Hf	178	177.943698	27.297(4)
^{179}Hf	179	178.945815	13.629(6)
^{180}Hf	180	179.946549	35.100(7)
^{180}Ta	180	179.947466	0.012(2)
^{181}Ta	181	180.947996	99.988(2)
^{180}W	180	179.946706	0.120(1)
^{182}W	182	181.948205	26.498(29)
^{183}W	183	182.950224	14.314(4)
^{184}W	184	183.950932	30.642(8)
^{186}W	186	185.954362	28.426(37)
^{185}Re	185	184.952955	37.40(2)
^{187}Re	187	186.955751	62.60(2)
^{184}Os	184	183.952491	0.020(3)
^{186}Os	186	185.953838	1.58(10)
^{187}Os	187	186.955748	1.6(1)
^{188}Os	188	187.955836	13.3(2)
^{189}Os	189	188.958145	16.1(3)
^{190}Os	190	189.958445	26.4(4)
^{192}Os	192	191.961479	41.03(3)
^{191}Ir	191	190.960591	37.3(5)
^{193}Ir	193	192.962923	62.7(5)
^{190}Pt	190	189.95993	0.01(1)
^{192}Pt	192	191.961035	0.79(6)
^{194}Pt	194	193.962663	32.9(6)
^{195}Pt	195	194.964774	33.8(6)
^{196}Pt	196	195.964934	25.3(6)
^{198}Pt	198	197.967875	7.2(2)
^{197}Au	197	196.966551	~100
^{196}Hg	196	195.965814	0.15(1)
^{198}Hg	198	197.966752	9.97(8)
^{199}Hg	199	198.968262	16.87(10)
^{200}Hg	200	199.968309	23.10(16)
^{201}Hg	201	200.970285	13.18(8)
^{202}Hg	202	201.970625	29.86(20)
^{204}Hg	204	203.973475	6.87(4)
^{203}Tl	203	202.972329	29.524(14)
^{205}Tl	205	204.974412	70.476(14)
^{204}Pb	204	203.973028	1.4(1)
^{206}Pb	206	205.974449	24.1(1)
^{207}Pb	207	206.975880	22.1(1)
^{208}Pb	208	207.976636	52.4(1)
^{209}Bi	209	208.980384	~100
^{232}Th	232	232.038050	~100
^{234}U	234	234.040945	0.0055(5)
^{235}U	235	235.043922	0.720(1)
^{238}U	238	238.050784	99.2745(15)

Appendix 3

INTENSITIES OF MOLECULAR IONS FOR COMPOUNDS CONTAINING COMBINATIONS OF BROMINE AND CHLORINE

		Relative intensity		
Halogen	M	M + 2	M + 4	M + 6
Br	1.0	0.98	–	–
Br_2	1.0	1.95	0.95	–
Br_3	1.0	2.93	2.86	0.93
Cl	1.0	0.33	–	–
Cl_2	1.0	0.65	0.1	–
Cl_3	1.0	0.98	0.32	0.03
BrCl	1.0	1.30	0.32	–
Br_2Cl	1.0	2.28	1.59	0.32
$BrCl_2$	1.0	1.63	0.74	0.010

Appendix 4

MASS-TO-CHARGE RATIOS OF MCLAFFERTY REARRANGEMENT IONS FOR COMMON CARBONYL COMPOUNDS

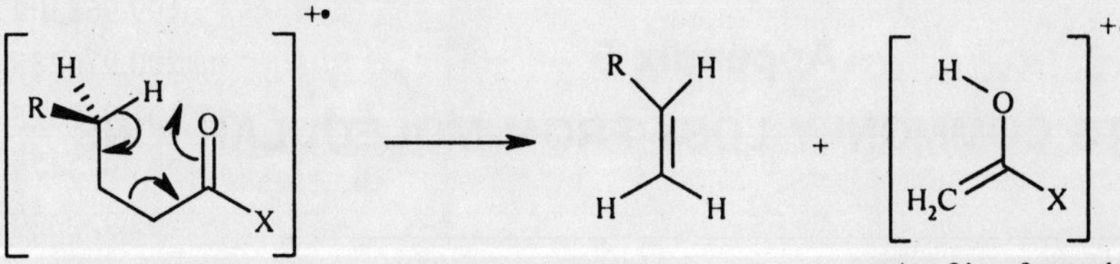

m/e of ion formed

Functional group	X	m/e
Aldehyde	–H	44
Methyl Ketone	$-CH_3$	58
Amide	$-NH_2$	59
Carboxylic acid	–OH	60
Ethyl ketone	$-CH_2CH_3$	72
Methyl ester	$-OCH_3$	74
Ethyl ester	$-OCH_2CH_3$	88

Appendix 5

PRIMARY FRAGMENTATIONS ASSOCIATED WITH SOME COMMON FUNCTIONAL GROUPS.

nctional group	Fragmentation
mine	$[R_1(CH_2)_n N(R_2)-CH_2R_3]^{+\bullet} \longrightarrow R_1(CH_2)_n \overset{+}{N}(R_2)=CH_2 + R_3^{\bullet} \longrightarrow H\overset{+}{N}(R_2)=CH_2 + \text{alkene}$
dehydes (R_2 = H) d Ketones	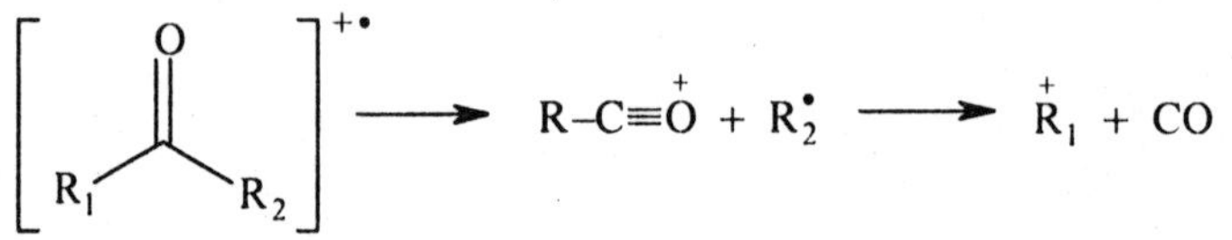
alides	$[R-X]^{+\bullet} \longrightarrow R^{+} + X\bullet$
cyl Compounds	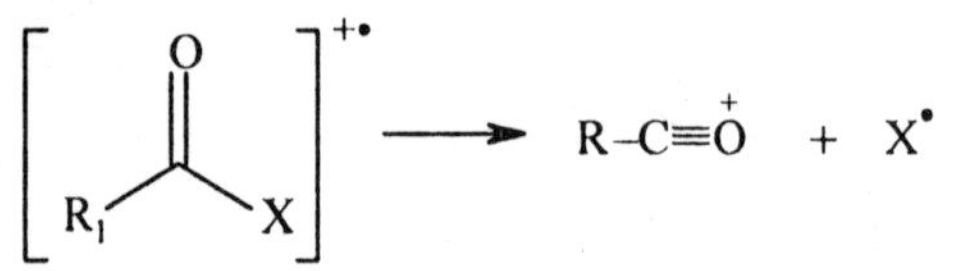
cohols and Thiols	$[R_1CH(R_2)-XH]^{+\bullet} \longrightarrow R_1CH_2=\overset{+}{X}H + R_2^{\bullet}$

Appendix 6

FRAGMENTS COMMONLY LOST FROM MOLECULAR IONS

Mass	*Group*	*Mass*	*Group*
15	CH_3	32	CH_3OH
16	NH_2	44	C_3H_5
17	OH	42	CH_2CO
18	H_2O	42	C_3H_6
19	F	43	C_3H_7
20	HF	43	CH_3CO
26	C_2H_2	44	CO_2
29	CHO	44	C_3H_8
29	CH_2CH_3	45	CO_2H
30	CH_2O	45	OCH_2CH_3
31	OCH_3	46	CH_3CH_2OH

Appendix 7

SES AND POSSIBLE STRUCTURES OF COMMON FRAGMENT IONS

	Associated structures		
	$CHO^+, CH_3CH_2^+$		
	$H_2C{=}NH_2^+$		
	$H_2C{=}OH^+$		
	$H_2C{=}CH{-}CH_2^+$		
	$H_2C{=}CH{-}CH_3^{+\bullet}$		
	$CH_3C\equiv O^+, CH_3^+CHCH_3$		
	$CH_3CHNH_2^+, CO_2^{+\bullet}, O{=}C{=}NH_2^{+\bullet}, C_3H_3^{+\bullet}, H_2C=CHOH^{+\bullet}$		
	$H_2C{=}\overset{+}{O}CH_3, CH_3CH{=}OH^+$		
	$H_2C{=}CH{-}CH{=}CH_2^{+\bullet}$		
	$C_4H_9^+, CH_3CH_2C\equiv O^+$		
	$CH_3CH_2NH^+{=}CH_2, H_2C{=}C(OH)CH_2^{+\bullet}, CH_2CH_2CH{=}NH_2^+$		
	$CH_3CH_2CH{=}OH^+, H_2C{=}C(OH)NH_2^{+\bullet}, H_2C{=}O^+{-}CH_2CH_3, CH_3O{-}C\equiv O^+$		
	$H_2C{=}C(OH)OH^{+\bullet}$		
	$C_5H_5^+$, H– 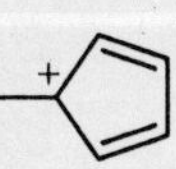		
	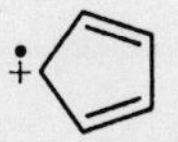	67	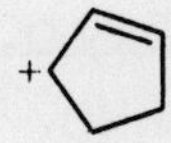
	$CH_3CH_2CH_2C\equiv O^+$ (and isomers)		
	$H_2C{=}C(OH)CH_2CH_3^{+\bullet}$		
	$^+O\equiv C{-}OCH_2CH_3$	74	$H_2C{=}C(OH)OCH_3^{+\bullet}$
	$C_6H_4^{+\bullet}$	77	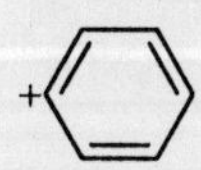
	$C_6H_5^{+\bullet}$	79 and 81	$Br^{+\bullet}$
d 82	$HBr^{+\bullet}$	85	$C_4H_9C\equiv O^+$
	$H_2C{=}C(OH)OCH_2CH_3^{+\bullet}$		
	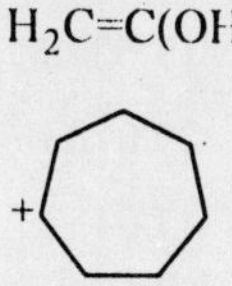 (and isomers)		
	$^+O\equiv C$– 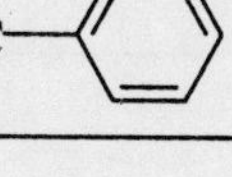, CH_3– 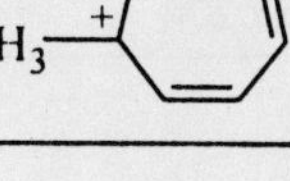 (and isomers)		

Appendix 8

AMINO ACID RESIDUE MASSES AND MODIFYING GROUPS

Residue	*Code*	*Elemental compostion*	*Monoisotopic mass*	*Average mass*
Alanine	A	C_3H_5NO	71.03711	71.0788
Cysteine	C	C_3H_5NOS	103.00919	103.1448
Aspartic acid	D	$C_4H_5NO_3$	115.02694	115.0886
Glutamic acid	E	$C_5H_7NO_3$	129.04259	129.1155
Phenylalanine	F	C_9H_9NO	147.06841	147.1766
Glycine	G	C_2H_3NO	57.02146	57.0520
Histidine	H	$C_6H_7N_3O$	137.05891	137.1412
Isoleucine	I	$C_6H_{11}NO$	113.08406	113.1595
Lysine	K	$C_6H_{12}N_2O$	128.09496	128.1742
Leucine	L	$C_6H_{11}NO$	113.08406	113.1595
Methionine	M	C_5H_9NOS	131.04049	131.1986
Asparagine	N	$C_4H_6N_2O_2$	114.04293	114.1039
Proline	P	C_5H_7NO	97.05276	97.1167
Glutamine	Q	$C_5H_8N_2O_2$	128.05858	128.1742
Arginine	R	$C_6H_{12}N_4O$	156.10111	156.1876
Serine	S	$C_3H_5NO_2$	87.03203	87.0782
Threonine	T	$C_4H_7NO_2$	101.04768	101.1051
Valine	V	C_5H_9NO	99.06841	99.1326
Tryptophan	W	$C_{11}H_{10}N_2O$	186.07931	186.2133
Tyrosine	Y	$C_9H_9NO_2$	163.06333	163.1760

Modifying group	*Elemental composition*	*Monoisotopic mass*	*Average mass*
Hydrogen	H	1.00782	1.0079
Methyl	CH_3	15.02347	15.0348
Formyl	CHO	29.00274	29.0183
Acetyl	C_2H_3O	43.01839	43.0452
t-Butyl	C_4H_9	57.07042	57.1154
Hydroxyl	HO	17.00274	17.0073

Appendix 9

MONOSACCHARIDE RESIDUE MASSES

Residue	*Abbreviation*	*Monoisotopic mass*	*Average mass*
Pentoses	Ara Rib Xyl	132.04226	132.1161
Deoxyhexoses	Fuc Rha	146.05791	146.1430
Hexosamines	GalN GlcN	161.06881	161.1577
Hexoses	Fru Gal Glc Man	162.05282	162.1424
Glucuronic acid	HexA	176.0321	176.1259
N-Acetylhexosamines	GalNAc GlcNAc	203.07937	203.1950
N-Acetylneuraminic Acid	NeuAc	291.09542	291.2579
N-Glycolylneuram-inic Acid	NeuGc	307.09033	307.2573

Appendix 10

ISOTOPIC ABUNDANCES (IN %) FOR VARIOUS ELEMENTAL COMPOSITIONS (C, H, O, N) (M = 100%)

		M + 1	M + 2
2	C	1.11	0.00
3	CH	1.13	0.00
4	N	0.37	0.00
	CH_2	1.14	0.00
5	HN	0.39	0.00
	CH_3	1.16	0.00
6	O	0.04	0.20
	H_2N	0.40	0.00
	CH_4	1.17	0.00
7	HO	0.06	0.20
	H_3N	0.42	0.00
8	H_2O	0.07	0.20
4	C_2	2.22	0.01
5	C_2H	2.24	0.01
6	CN	1.48	0.00
	C_2H_2	2.25	0.01
7	CHN	1.50	0.00
	C_2H_3	2.27	0.01
8	N_2	0.74	0.00
	CO	1.15	0.20
	CH_2N	1.51	0.00
	C_2H_4	2.28	0.01
9	HN_2	0.76	0.00
	CHO	1.17	0.20
	CH_3N	1.53	0.00
	C_2H_5	2.30	0.01
[illegible]	NO	0.41	0.20
	H_2N_2	0.77	0.00
	CH_2O	1.18	0.20
	CH_4N	1.54	0.01
	C_2H_6	2.31	0.01
[illegible]	HNO	0.43	0.20
	H_3N_2	0.79	0.00
	CH_3O	1.20	0.20
	CH_5N	1.56	0.01
32	O_2	0.08	0.40
	H_2NO	0.44	0.20
	H_4N_2	0.80	0.00
	CH_4O	1.21	0.20
33	HO_2	0.10	0.40
	H_3NO	0.46	0.20
34	H_2O_2	0.11	0.40
36	C_3	3.33	0.04
37	C_3H	3.35	0.04
38	C_2N	2.59	0.02
	C_3H_2	3.36	0.04
39	C_2HN	2.61	0.02
	C_3H_3	3.38	0.04
40	CN_2	1.85	0.01
	C_2O	2.26	0.21
	C_2H_2N	2.62	0.02
	C_3H_4	3.39	0.04
41	CHN_2	1.87	0.01
	C_2HO	2.28	0.21
	C_2H_3N	2.64	0.02
	C_3H_5	3.41	0.04
42	N_3	1.11	0.00
	CNO	1.52	0.21
	CH_2N_2	1.88	0.01
	C_2H_2O	2.29	0.21
	C_2H_4N	2.65	0.02
	C_3H_6	3.42	0.04
43	HN_3	1.13	0.00
	CHNO	1.54	0.21
	CH_3N_2	1.90	0.01
	C_2H_3O	2.31	0.21
	C_2H_5N	2.67	0.02
	C_3H_7	3.44	0.04
44	N_2O	0.78	0.20
	H_2N_3	1.14	0.00

(Contd.)

		M + 1	M + 2
	CO_2	1.19	0.40
	CH_2NO	1.55	0.21
	CH_4N_2	1.91	0.01
	C_2H_4O	2.32	0.21
	C_2H_6N	2.68	0.02
	C_3H_8	3.45	0.04
	HN_2O	0.80	0.20
	H_3N_3	1.16	0.00
	CHO_2	1.21	0.40
	CH_3NO	1.57	0.21
	CH_5N_2	1.93	0.01
	C_2H_5O	2.34	0.21
	C_2H_7N	2.70	0.02
	NO_2	0.45	0.40
	H_2N_2O	0.81	0.20
	H_4N_3	1.17	0.01
	CH_2O_2	1.22	0.40
	CH_4NO	1.58	0.21
	CH_6N_2	1.94	0.01
	C_2H_6O	2.35	0.22
	HNO_2	0.47	0.40
	H_3N_2O	0.83	0.20
	H_5N_3	1.19	0.01
	CH_3O_2	1.24	0.40
	CH_5NO	1.60	0.21
	O_3	0.12	0.60
	H_2NO_2	0.48	0.40
	H_4N_2O	0.84	0.20
	CH_4O_2	1.25	0.40
	C_4	4.44	0.07
	HO_3	0.14	0.60
	H_3NO_2	0.50	0.40
	C_4H	4.46	0.07
	H_2O_3	0.15	0.60
	C_3N	3.70	0.05
	C_4H_2	4.47	0.07
	C_3HN	3.72	0.05
	C_4H_3	4.49	0.08
	C_2N_2	2.96	0.03
	C_3O	3.37	0.24
	C_3H_2N	3.73	0.05
	C_4H_4	4.50	0.08
53	C_2HN_2	2.98	0.03
	C_3HO	3.39	0.24
	C_3H_3N	3.75	0.05
	C_4H_5	4.52	0.08
54	CN_3	2.22	0.02
	C_2NO	2.63	0.22
	$C_2H_2N_2$	2.98	0.03
	C_3H_2O	3.40	0.24
	C_3H_4N	3.76	0.05
	C_4H_6	4.53	0.08
55	CHN_3	2.24	0.02
	C_2HNO	2.65	0.22
	$C_2H_3N_2$	3.01	0.03
	C_3H_3O	3.42	0.24
	C_3H_5N	3.78	0.05
	C_4H_7	4.55	0.08
56	N_4	1.48	0.01
	CN_2O	1.89	0.21
	CH_2N_3	2.25	0.02
	C_2O_2	2.30	0.41
	C_2H_2NO	2.66	0.22
	$C_2H_4N_2$	3.02	0.03
	C_3H_4O	3.43	0.24
	C_3H_6N	3.79	0.05
	C_4H_8	4.56	0.08
57	HN_4	1.50	0.01
	CHN_2O	1.91	0.21
	CH_3N_3	2.27	0.02
	C_2HO_2	2.32	0.41
	C_2H_3NO	2.68	0.22
	$C_2H_5N_2$	3.04	0.03
	C_3H_5O	3.45	0.24
	C_3H_7N	3.81	0.05
	C_4H_9	4.59	0.08
58	N_3O	1.15	0.20
	H_2N_4	1.51	0.01
	CNO_2	1.56	0.41
	CH_2N_2O	1.92	0.21

(Contd.)

		M + 1	M + 2			M + 1	M + 2
	CH_4N_3	2.28	0.02		$H_2N_2O_2$	0.85	0.40
	$C_2H_2O_2$	2.33	0.42		H_4N_3O	1.21	0.42
	C_2H_4NO	2.69	0.22		H_6N_4	1.57	0.01
	$C_2H_6N_2$	3.05	0.03		CH_2O_3	1.26	0.60
	C_3H_6O	3.46	0.24		CH_4NO_2	1.62	0.41
	C_3H_8N	3.82	0.05		CH_6N_2O	1.98	0.21
	C_4H_{10}	4.59	0.08		$C_2H_6O_2$	2.39	0.42
59	HN_3O	1.17	0.20		C_4N	4.81	0.09
	H_3N_4	1.53	0.01		C_5H_2	5.58	0.12
	$CHNO_2$	1.58	0.41	63	HNO_3	0.51	0.60
	CH_3N_2O	1.94	0.21		$H_3N_2O_2$	0.87	0.40
	CH_5N_3	2.30	0.02		H_5N_3O	1.23	0.21
	$C_2H_3O_2$	2.35	0.42		CH_3O_3	1.28	0.60
	C_2H_5NO	2.71	0.22		CH_5NO_2	1.64	0.41
	$C_2H_7N_2$	3.07	0.03		C_4HN	4.83	0.09
	C_3H_7O	3.48	0.24		C_5H_3	5.60	0.12
	C_3H_9N	3.84	0.05	64	O_4	0.16	0.80
60	N_2O_2	0.82	0.40		H_2NO_3	0.52	0.60
	H_2N_3O	1.18	0.20		$H_4N_2O_2$	0.88	0.40
	H_4N_4	1.54	0.01		CH_4O_3	1.29	0.60
	CO_3	1.23	0.60		C_3N_2	4.07	0.06
	CH_2NO_2	1.59	0.41		C_4O	4.48	0.27
	CH_4N_2O	1.95	0.21		C_4H_2N	4.84	0.09
	CH_6N_3	2.31	0.02		C_5H_4	5.61	0.12
	$C_2H_4O_2$	2.36	0.42	65	HO_4	0.18	0.80
	C_2H_6NO	2.72	0.22		H_3NO_3	0.54	0.60
	$C_2H_8N_2$	3.08	0.03		C_3HN_2	4.09	0.06
	C_3H_8O	3.49	0.24		C_4HO	4.50	0.27
	C_5	5.55	0.12		C_4H_3N	4.86	0.09
61	HN_2O_2	0.84	0.40		C_5H_5	5.63	0.12
	H_3N_3O	1.20	0.21	66	H_2O_4	0.19	0.80
	H_5N_4	1.56	0.01		C_2N_3	3.33	0.04
	CHO_3	1.25	0.60		C_3NO	3.74	0.25
	CH_3NO_2	1.61	0.41		$C_3H_2N_2$	4.10	0.06
	CH_5N_2O	1.97	0.21		C_4H_4N	4.87	0.09
	CH_7N_3	2.33	0.02		C_5H_6	5.64	0.12
	$C_2H_5O_2$	2.38	0.42	67	C_2HN_3	3.35	0.04
	C_2H_7NO	2.74	0.22		C_3HNO	3.76	0.25
	C_5H	5.57	0.12		$C_3H_3N_2$	4.12	0.06
62	NO_3	0.49	0.60		C_4H_3O	4.53	0.27

(Contd.)

		M + 1	M + 2
	C_4H_5N	4.89	0.09
	C_5H_7	5.66	0.12
68	CN_4	2.59	0.02
	C_2N_2O	3.00	0.23
	$C_2H_2N_3$	3.36	0.04
	C_3O_2	3.41	0.44
	C_3H_2NO	3.77	0.25
	$C_3H_4N_2$	4.13	0.06
	C_4H_4O	4.54	0.28
	C_4H_6N	4.90	0.09
	C_5H_8	5.67	0.13
69	CHN_4	2.61	0.03
	C_2HN_2O	3.02	0.23
	$C_2H_3N_3$	3.38	0.04
	C_3HO_2	3.43	0.44
	C_3H_3NO	3.79	0.25
	$C_3H_5N_2$	4.15	0.06
	C_4H_5O	4.56	0.28
	C_4H_7N	4.92	0.09
	C_5H_5	5.63	0.12
	C_5H_9	5.69	0.13
70	CN_3O	2.26	0.22
	CH_2N_4	2.62	0.03
	C_2NO_2	2.67	0.42
	$C_2H_2N_2O$	3.03	0.23
	$C_2H_4N_3$	3.39	0.04
	$C_3H_2O_2$	3.44	0.44
	C_3H_4NO	3.80	0.25
	$C_3H_6N_2$	4.16	0.07
	C_4H_6O	4.57	0.28
	C_4H_8N	4.93	0.09
	C_5H_{10}	5.70	0.13
71	CHN_3O	2.28	0.22
	CH_3N_4	2.64	0.03
	C_2HNO_2	2.69	0.42
	$C_2H_3N_2O$	3.05	0.23
	$C_2H_5N_3$	3.41	0.04
	$C_3H_3O_2$	3.46	0.44
	C_3H_5NO	3.82	0.25
	$C_3H_7N_2$	4.18	0.07
	C_4H_7O	4.59	0.28
	C_4H_9N	4.95	0.10
	C_5H_{11}	5.72	0.13
72	N_4O	1.52	0.21
	CN_2O_2	1.93	0.41
	CH_2N_3O	2.29	0.22
	CH_4N_4	2.65	0.03
	C_2O_3	2.34	0.62
	$C_2H_2NO_2$	2.70	0.42
	$C_2H_4N_2O$	3.06	0.23
	$C_2H_6N_3$	3.42	0.04
	$C_3H_4O_2$	3.47	0.44
	C_3H_6NO	3.83	0.25
	$C_3H_8N_2$	4.19	0.07
	C_4H_8O	4.60	0.28
	$C_4H_{10}N$	4.96	0.09
	C_5H_{12}	5.73	0.13
	C_6	6.66	0.18
73	HN_4O	1.54	0.21
	CHN_2O_2	1.95	0.41
	CH_3N_3O	2.31	0.22
	CH_5N_4	2.67	0.03
	C_2HO_3	2.36	0.62
	$C_2H_3NO_2$	2.72	0.42
	$C_2H_5N_2O$	3.08	0.23
	$C_2H_7N_3$	3.44	0.04
	$C_3H_5O_2$	3.49	0.44
	C_3H_7NO	3.85	0.25
	$C_3H_9N_2$	4.21	0.07
	C_4H_9O	4.62	0.28
	$C_4H_{11}N$	4.98	0.09
	C_6H	6.68	0.18
74	N_3O_2	1.19	0.41
	H_2N_2O	1.55	0.21
	CNO_3	1.60	0.61
	$CH_2N_2O_2$	1.96	0.41
	CH_4N_3O	2.32	0.22
	CH_6N_4	2.68	0.03
	$C_2H_2O_3$	2.37	0.62
	$C_2H_4NO_2$	2.73	0.42

(Contd.)

		M + 1	M + 2
	$C_2H_6N_2O$	3.09	0.23
	$C_2H_8N_3$	3.45	0.05
	$C_3H_6O_2$	3.50	0.44
	C_3H_8NO	3.86	0.25
	$C_3H_{10}N_2$	4.22	0.07
	$C_4H_{10}O$	4.63	0.28
	C_5N	5.92	0.14
	C_6H_2	6.69	0.18
75	HN_3O_2	1.21	0.41
	H_3N_4O	1.57	0.21
	$CHNO_3$	1.62	0.61
	$CH_3N_2O_2$	1.98	0.41
	CH_5N_3O	2.34	0.22
	CH_7N_4	2.70	0.03
	$C_2H_3O_3$	2.39	0.62
	$C_2H_5NO_2$	2.75	0.43
	$C_2H_7N_2O$	3.11	0.23
	$C_2H_9N_3$	3.47	0.05
	$C_3H_7O_2$	3.52	0.44
	C_3H_9NO	3.88	0.25
	C_5HN	5.94	0.14
	C_6H_3	6.71	0.18
76	N_2O_3	0.86	0.60
	$H_2N_3O_2$	1.22	0.41
	H_4N_4O	1.58	0.21
	CO_4	1.27	0.80
	CH_2NO_3	1.63	0.61
	$CH_4N_2O_2$	1.99	0.41
	CH_6N_3O	2.35	0.22
	CH_8N_4	2.71	0.03
	$C_2H_4O_3$	2.40	0.62
	$C_2H_6NO_2$	2.76	0.43
	$C_2H_8N_2O$	3.12	0.24
	$C_3H_8O_2$	3.53	0.44
	C_4N_2	5.18	0.10
	C_5O	5.59	0.32
	C_5H_2N	5.95	0.14
	C_6H_4	6.72	0.19
77	HN_2O_3	0.88	0.60
	$H_3N_3O_2$	1.24	0.41

		M + 1
	H_5N_4O	1.60
	CHO_4	1.29
	CH_3NO_3	1.65
	$CH_5N_2O_2$	2.01
	CH_7N_3O	2.37
	$C_2H_5O_3$	2.42
	$C_2H_7NO_2$	2.78
	C_4HN_2	5.20
	C_5HO	5.61
	C_5H_3N	5.97
	C_6H_5	6.74
78	NO_4	0.53
	$H_2N_2O_3$	0.89
	$H_4N_3O_2$	1.25
	H_6N_4O	1.61
	CH_2O_4	1.30
	CH_4NO_3	1.66
	$CH_6N_2O_2$	2.02
	$C_2H_6O_3$	2.43
	C_3N_3	4.44
	C_4NO	4.85
	$C_4H_2N_2$	5.21
	C_5H_2O	5.62
	C_5H_4N	5.98
	C_6H_6	6.75
79	HNO_4	0.55
	$H_3N_2O_3$	0.91
	$H_5N_3O_2$	1.27
	CH_3O_4	1.32
	CH_5NO_3	1.68
	C_3HN_3	4.46
	C_4HNO	4.87
	$C_4H_3N_2$	5.23
	C_5H_3O	5.64
	C_5H_5N	6.00
	C_6H_7	6.77
80	H_2NO_4	0.56
	$H_4N_2O_3$	0.92
	CH_4O_4	1.33
	C_2N_4	3.70

(C

		M + 1	M + 2
	C_3N_2O	4.11	0.26
	$C_3H_2N_3$	4.47	0.08
	C_4O_2	4.52	0.47
	C_4H_2NO	4.88	0.29
	$C_4H_4N_2$	5.24	0.11
	C_5H_4O	5.65	0.32
	C_5H_6N	6.01	0.14
	C_6H_8	6.78	0.19
81	H_3NO_4	0.58	0.80
	C_2NH_4	3.72	0.05
	C_3HN_2O	4.13	0.26
	$C_3H_3N_3$	4.49	0.08
	C_4HO_2	4.54	0.48
	C_4H_3NO	4.90	0.29
	$C_4H_5N_2$	6.26	0.11
	C_5H_5O	5.67	0.32
	C_5H_7N	6.02	0.14
	C_6H_9	6.80	0.19
82	C_2N_3O	3.37	0.24
	$C_2H_2N_4$	3.73	0.05
	C_3NO_2	3.78	0.45
	$C_3H_2N_2O$	4.14	0.26
	$C_3H_4N_3$	4.50	0.08
	$C_4H_2O_2$	4.55	0.48
	C_4H_4NO	4.91	0.29
	$C_4H_6N_2$	5.27	0.11
	C_5H_6O	5.68	0.32
	C_5H_8N	6.04	0.14
	C_6H_{10}	6.81	0.19
83	C_2HN_3O	3.39	0.24
	$C_2H_3N_4$	3.75	0.06
	C_3HNO_2	3.80	0.45
	$C_3H_3N_2O$	4.16	0.27
	$C_3H_5N_3$	4.52	0.08
	$C_4H_3O_2$	4.57	0.48
	C_4H_5NO	4.93	0.29
	$C_4H_7N_2$	5.29	0.11
	C_5H_7O	5.70	0.33
	C_5H_9N	6.06	0.15
	C_6H_{11}	6.83	0.19
84	CN_4O	2.63	0.23
	$C_2H_2N_3O$	3.40	0.24
	$C_2N_2O_2$	3.04	0.43
	$C_2H_4N_4$	3.76	0.06
	C_3O_3	3.45	0.64
	$C_3H_2NO_2$	3.81	0.45
	$C_3H_4N_2O$	4.17	0.27
	$C_3H_6N_3$	4.53	0.08
	$C_4H_4O_2$	4.58	0.48
	C_4H_6NO	4.94	0.29
	$C_4H_8N_2$	5.30	0.11
	C_5H_8O	5.71	0.33
	$C_5H_{10}N$	6.07	0.15
	C_6H_{12}	6.84	0.19
	C_7	7.77	0.26
85	CHN_4O	2.65	0.23
	$C_2HN_2O_2$	3.06	0.43
	$C_2H_3N_3O$	3.42	0.24
	$C_2H_5N_4$	3.78	0.06
	C_3HO_3	3.47	0.64
	$C_3H_3NO_2$	3.83	0.45
	$C_3H_5N_2O$	4.19	0.27
	$C_3H_7N_3$	4.55	0.08
	$C_4H_5O_2$	4.60	0.48
	C_4H_7NO	4.96	0.29
	$C_4H_9N_2$	5.32	0.11
	C_5H_9O	5.73	0.33
	$C_5H_{11}N$	6.09	0.16
	C_6H_{13}	6.86	0.20
	C_7H	7.79	0.26
86	CN_3O_2	2.30	0.41
	CH_2N_4O	2.66	0.21
	C_2NO_3	2.71	0.62
	$C_2H_2N_2O_2$	3.07	0.43
	$C_2H_4N_3O$	3.43	0.24
	$C_2H_6N_4$	3.79	0.06
	$C_3H_2O_3$	3.48	0.64
	$C_3H_4NO_2$	3.84	0.45
	$C_3H_6N_2O$	4.20	0.27
	$C_3H_8N_3$	4.56	0.08

(Con

		M + 1	M + 2
	$C_4H_6O_2$	4.61	0.48
	C_4H_8NO	4.97	0.30
	$C_4H_{10}N_2$	5.33	0.11
	$C_5H_{10}O$	5.74	0.33
	$C_5H_{12}N$	6.10	0.16
	C_6H_{14}	6.87	0.21
	C_6N	7.03	0.21
	C_7H_2	7.80	0.26
87	CHN_3O_2	2.32	0.42
	CH_3N_4O	2.68	0.23
	C_2HNO_3	2.73	0.62
	$C_2H_3N_2O_2$	3.09	0.43
	$C_2H_5N_3O$	3.45	0.25
	$C_2H_7N_4$	3.81	0.06
	$C_3H_3O_3$	3.50	0.64
	$C_3H_5NO_2$	3.86	0.45
	$C_3H_7N_2O$	4.22	0.27
	$C_3H_9N_3$	4.58	0.08
	$C_4H_7O_2$	4.63	0.48
	C_4H_9NO	4.99	0.30
	$C_4H_{11}N_2$	5.35	0.11
	$C_5H_{11}O$	5.76	0.33
	$C_5H_{13}N$	6.12	0.15
	C_6HN	7.05	0.21
	C_7H_3	7.82	0.26
88	N_4O_2	1.56	0.41
	CN_2O_3	1.97	0.61
	$CH_2N_3O_2$	2.33	0.42
	CH_4N_4O	2.69	0.23
	C_2O_4	2.38	0.82
	$C_2H_2NO_3$	2.74	0.63
	$C_2H_4N_2O_2$	3.10	0.43
	$C_2H_6N_3O$	3.46	0.25
	$C_2H_8N_4$	3.82	0.06
	$C_3H_4O_3$	3.51	0.64
	$C_3H_6NO_2$	3.87	0.45
	$C_3H_8N_2O$	4.23	0.27
	$C_3H_{10}N_5$	4.59	0.08
	$C_4H_8O_2$	4.64	0.48
	$C_4H_{10}NO$	5.00	0.30
	$C_4H_{12}N_2$	5.36	0.11
	$C_5H_{12}O$	5.77	0.33
	C_5N_2	6.29	0.16
	C_6O	6.70	0.38
	C_6H_2N	7.06	0.21
	C_7H_4	7.83	0.26
89	HN_4O_2	1.58	0.41
	CHN_2O_3	1.99	0.61
	$CH_3N_3O_2$	2.35	0.42
	CH_5N_4O	2.71	0.23
	C_2HO_4	2.40	0.82
	$C_2H_3NO_3$	2.76	0.63
	$C_2H_5N_2O_2$	3.12	0.44
	$C_2H_7N_3O$	3.48	0.25
	$C_2H_9N_4$	3.84	0.06
	$C_3H_5O_3$	3.53	0.64
	$C_3H_7NO_2$	3.89	0.46
	$C_3H_9N_2O$	4.25	0.27
	$C_3H_{11}N_3$	4.61	0.08
	$C_4H_9O_2$	4.66	0.48
	$C_4H_{11}NO$	5.02	0.30
	C_5HN_2	6.31	0.16
	C_6HO	6.72	0.38
	C_6H_3N	7.08	0.21
	C_7H_5	7.85	0.26
90	N_3O_3	1.23	0.60
	$H_2N_4O_2$	1.59	0.40
	CNO_4	1.64	0.80
	$CH_2N_2O_3$	2.00	0.61
	$CH_4N_3O_2$	2.36	0.42
	CH_6N_4O	2.72	0.23
	$C_2H_2O_4$	2.41	0.82
	$C_2H_4NO_3$	2.77	0.63
	$C_2H_6N_2O_2$	3.13	0.44
	$C_2H_8N_3O$	3.49	0.25
	$C_2H_{10}N_4$	3.85	0.06
	$C_3H_6O_3$	3.54	0.64
	$C_3H_8NO_2$	3.90	0.46
	$C_3H_{10}N_2O$	4.26	0.27
	$C_4H_{10}O_2$	4.67	0.48

(Contd.)

		M + 1	M + 2			M + 1	M + 2
	C_4N_3	5.55	0.13		$C_5H_4N_2$	6.35	0.17
	C_5NO	5.96	0.34		C_6H_4O	5.76	0.38
	$C_5H_2N_2$	6.32	0.17		C_6H_6N	7.12	0.21
	C_6H_2O	6.73	0.38		C_7H_8	7.89	0.27
	C_6H_4N	7.09	0.21	93	HN_2O_4	0.92	0.80
	C_7H_6	7.86	0.26		$H_3N_3O_3$	1.28	0.60
91	HN_3O_3	1.25	0.60		$H_5N_4O_2$	1.64	0.41
	$H_3N_4O_2$	1.61	0.41		CH_3NO_4	1.69	0.81
	$CHNO_4$	1.66	0.81		$CH_5N_2O_3$	2.05	0.61
	$CH_3N_2O_3$	2.02	0.61		$CH_7N_3O_2$	2.41	0.42
	$CH_5N_3O_2$	2.38	0.42		$C_2H_5O_4$	2.46	0.82
	CH_7N_4O	2.74	0.23		$C_2H_7NO_3$	2.82	0.63
	$C_2H_3O_4$	2.43	0.82		C_3HN_4	4.83	0.09
	$C_2H_5NO_3$	2.79	0.63		C_4HN_2O	5.24	0.31
	$C_2H_7N_2O_2$	3.15	0.44		$C_4H_3N_3$	5.60	0.13
	$C_2H_9N_3O$	3.51	0.25		C_5HO_2	5.65	0.52
	$C_3H_7O_3$	3.56	0.64		C_5H_3NO	6.01	0.35
	$C_3H_9NO_2$	3.92	0.46		$C_5H_5N_2$	6.37	0.17
	C_4HN_3	5.57	0.13		C_6H_5O	6.78	0.38
	C_5HNO	5.98	0.34		C_6H_7N	7.14	0.22
	$C_5H_3N_2$	6.34	0.17		C_7H_9	7.91	0.27
	C_6H_3O	6.75	0.38	94	$H_2N_2O_4$	0.93	0.80
	C_6H_5N	7.22	0.21		$H_4N_3O_3$	1.29	0.61
	C_7H_7	7.88	0.26		$H_6N_4O_2$	1.65	0.41
92	N_2O_4	0.90	0.80		CH_4NO_4	1.70	0.81
	$H_2N_3O_3$	1.26	0.60		$CH_6N_2O_3$	2.06	0.62
	$H_4N_4O_2$	1.62	0.41		$C_2H_6O_4$	2.47	0.82
	CH_2NO_4	1.67	0.81		C_3N_3O	4.48	0.28
	$CH_4N_2O_3$	2.03	0.61		$C_3H_2N_4$	4.84	0.09
	$CH_6N_3O_2$	2.39	0.42		C_4NO_2	4.89	0.49
	CH_8N_4O	2.75	0.23		$C_4H_2N_2O$	5.25	0.31
	$C_2H_4O_4$	2.44	0.82		$C_4H_4N_3$	5.61	0.13
	$C_2H_6NO_3$	2.80	0.63		$C_5H_2O_2$	5.66	0.52
	$C_2H_8N_2O_2$	3.16	0.44		C_5H_4NO	6.02	0.35
	$C_3H_8O_3$	3.57	0.64		$C_5H_6N_2$	6.38	0.17
	C_3N_4	4.81	0.09		C_6H_6O	6.79	0.38
	C_4N_2O	5.22	0.31		C_6H_8N	7.15	0.22
	$C_4H_2N_3$	5.58	0.13		C_7H_{10}	7.92	0.27
	C_5O_2	5.63	0.52	95	$H_3N_2O_4$	0.95	0.80
	C_5H_2NO	5.99	0.34		$H_5N_3O_3$	1.31	0.60

(Contd.)

		M + 1	M + 2
	CH_5NO_4	1.72	0.81
	C_3HN_3O	4.50	0.28
	$C_3H_3N_4$	4.86	0.10
	C_4HNO_2	4.91	0.49
	$C_4H_3N_2O$	5.27	0.31
	$C_4H_5N_3$	5.63	0.13
	$C_5H_3O_2$	5.68	0.52
	C_5H_5NO	6.04	0.35
	$C_5H_7N_2$	6.40	0.17
	C_6H_7O	6.81	0.39
	C_6H_9N	7.17	0.22
	C_7H_{11}	7.94	0.27
96	$H_4N_2O_4$	0.96	0.80
	C_2N_4O	3.74	0.26
	$C_3N_2O_2$	4.15	0.47
	$C_3H_2N_3O$	4.51	0.28
	$C_3H_4N_4$	4.87	0.10
	C_4O_3	4.56	0.67
	$C_4H_2NO_2$	4.92	0.49
	$C_4H_4N_2O$	5.28	0.31
	$C_4H_6N_3$	5.64	0.13
	$C_5H_4O_2$	5.69	0.53
	C_5H_6NO	6.05	0.35
	$C_5H_8N_2$	6.41	0.17
	C_6H_8O	6.82	0.39
	$C_6H_{10}N$	7.18	0.22
	C_7H_{12}	7.95	0.27
	C_8	8.88	0.34
97	C_2HN_4O	3.76	0.26
	$C_3HN_2O_2$	4.17	0.47
	$C_3H_3N_3O$	4.53	0.28
	$C_3H_5N_4$	4.89	0.10
	C_4HO_3	4.58	0.68
	$C_4H_3NO_2$	4.94	0.49
	$C_4H_5N_2O$	5.30	0.31
	$C_4H_7N_3$	5.66	0.13
	$C_5H_5O_2$	5.71	0.53
	C_5H_7NO	6.07	0.35
	$C_5H_9N_2$	6.43	0.17
	C_6H_9O	6.84	0.39
	$C_6H_{11}N$	7.20	0.22
	C_7H_{13}	7.97	0.27
	C_8H	8.90	0.34
98	$C_2N_3O_2$	3.41	0.44
	$C_2H_2N_4O$	3.77	0.26
	C_3NO_3	3.82	0.65
	$C_3H_2N_2O_2$	4.18	0.47
	$C_3H_4N_3O$	4.54	0.28
	$C_3H_6N_4$	4.90	0.10
	$C_4H_2O_3$	4.59	0.68
	$C_4H_4NO_2$	4.95	0.49
	$C_4H_6N_2O$	5.31	0.31
	$C_4H_8N_3$	5.67	0.13
	$C_5H_6O_2$	5.72	0.53
	C_5H_8NO	6.08	0.35
	$C_5H_{10}N_2$	6.44	0.17
	$C_6H_{10}O$	6.85	0.39
	$C_6H_{12}N$	7.21	0.21
	C_7H_{14}	7.98	0.26
	C_7N	8.14	0.27
	C_8H_2	8.91	0.33
99	$C_2HN_3O_2$	3.43	0.44
	$C_2H_3N_4O$	3.79	0.25
	C_3HNO_3	3.84	0.65
	$C_3H_3N_2O_2$	4.20	0.47
	$C_3H_5N_3O$	4.56	0.28
	$C_3H_7N_4$	4.92	0.10
	$C_4H_3O_3$	4.61	0.68
	$C_4H_5NO_2$	4.97	0.49
	$C_4H_7H_2O$	5.33	0.31
	$C_4H_9N_3$	5.69	0.13
	$C_5H_7O_2$	5.74	0.53
	C_5H_9NO	6.11	0.35
	$C_5H_{11}N_2$	6.46	0.17
	$C_6H_{11}O$	6.86	0.39
	$C_6H_{13}N$	7.23	0.22
	C_7H_{15}	8.00	0.27
	C_7HN	8.16	0.29
	C_8H_3	8.93	0.35
100	CN_4O_2	2.67	0.43

(Contd.)

		M + 1	M + 2
	$C_2N_2O_3$	3.08	0.63
	$C_2H_2N_3O_2$	3.44	0.45
	$C_2H_4N_4O$	3.80	0.26
	C_3O_4	3.45	0.84
	$C_3H_2NO_3$	3.85	0.65
	$C_3H_4N_2O_2$	4.21	0.47
	$C_3H_6N_3O$	4.57	0.28
	$C_3H_8N_4$	4.94	0.10
	$C_4H_4O_3$	4.62	0.68
	$C_4H_6NO_2$	4.98	0.49
	$C_4H_8N_2O$	5.34	0.31
	$C_4H_{10}N_3$	5.70	0.13
	$C_5H_8O_2$	5.76	0.53
	$C_5H_{10}NO$	6.11	0.35
	$C_5H_{12}N_2$	6.47	0.18
	$C_6H_{12}O$	6.88	0.39
	$C_6H_{14}N$	7.24	0.22
	C_6N_2	7.40	0.23
	C_7H_{16}	8.01	0.28
	C_7O	7.81	0.46
	C_7H_2N	8.17	0.29
	C_8H_4	8.94	0.35
101	CHN_4O_2	2.701	0.428
	$C_2HN_2O_3$	3.057	0.635
	$C_2H_3N_3O_2$	3.432	0.446
	$C_2H_5N_4O$	3.806	0.258
	C_3HO_4	3.414	0.842
	$C_3H_3NO_3$	3.789	0.654
	$C_3H_5N_2O_2$	4.163	0.468
	$C_3H_7N_3O$	4.537	0.283
	$C_3H_9N_4$	4.912	0.100
	$C_4H_5O_3$	4.520	0.680
	$C_4H_7NO_2$	4.894	0.496
	$C_4H_9N_2O$	5.268	0.314
	$C_4H_{11}N_3$	5.643	0.137
	$C_5H_9O_2$	5.625	0.529
	$C_5H_{11}NO$	6.000	0.350
	$C_5H_{13}N_2$	6.374	0.172
	C_6HN_2	7.263	0.227
	$C_6H_{13}O$	6.731	0.391
	$C_6H_{15}N$	7.105	0.216
	C_7HO	7.619	0.449
	C_7H_3N	7.994	0.277
	C_8H_5	8.725	0.333
102	$CH_2N_4O_2$	2.717	0.429
	$C_2H_2N_2O_3$	3.073	0.635
	$C_2H_4N_3O_2$	3.448	0.446
	$C_2H_6N_4O$	3.822	0.258
	$C_3H_2O_4$	3.430	0.843
	$C_3H_4NO_3$	3.805	0.655
	$C_3H_6N_2O_2$	4.179	0.470
	$C_3H_8N_3O$	4.553	0.284
	$C_3H_{10}N_4$	4.928	0.101
	$C_4H_6O_3$	4.536	0.681
	$C_4H_8NO_2$	4.910	0.497
	$C_4H_{10}N_2O$	5.284	0.315
	$C_4H_{12}N_3$	5.659	0.135
	$C_5H_{10}O_2$	5.641	0.531
	$C_5H_{12}NO$	6.016	0.351
	$C_5H_{14}N_2$	6.390	0.173
	$C_6H_2N_2$	7.279	0.228
	$C_6H_{14}O$	6.747	0.393
	C_7H_2O	7.635	0.451
	C_7H_4N	8.010	0.279
	C_8H_6	8.741	0.333
103	CHN_3O_3	2.358	0.621
	$CH_3N_4O_2$	2.733	0.429
	C_2HNO_4	2.715	0.826
	$C_2H_3N_2O_3$	3.089	0.636
	$C_2H_5N_3O_2$	3.464	0.447
	$C_2H_7N_4O$	3.838	0.260
	$C_3H_3O_4$	3.446	0.844
	$C_3H_3NO_3$	3.821	0.656
	$C_3H_7N_2O_2$	4.195	0.470
	$C_3H_9N_3O$	4.569	0.285
	$C_3H_{11}N_4$	4.944	0.102
	$C_4H_7O_3$	4.552	0.681
	$C_4H_9NO_2$	4.926	0.498
	$C_4H_{11}N_2O$	5.300	0.316
	$C_4H_{13}N_3$	5.675	0.135

(Contd.)

		M + 1	M + 2
	C_5HN_3	6.563	0.184
	$C_5H_{11}O_2$	5.657	0.531
	$C_5H_{13}NO$	6.032	0.352
	C_6HNO	6.920	0.404
	$C_6H_3N_2$	7.295	0.229
	C_7H_3O	7.651	0.452
	C_7H_5N	8.026	0.280
	C_8H_7	8.757	0.336
104	$CH_2N_3O_3$	2.374	0.621
	$CH_4N_4O_2$	2.749	0.430
	$C_2H_2NO_4$	2.731	0.826
	$C_2H_4N_2O_3$	3.105	0.636
	$C_2H_6N_3O_2$	3.480	0.447
	$C_2H_8N_4O$	3.854	0.260
	$C_3H_4O_4$	3.462	0.844
	$C_3H_6NO_3$	3.837	0.656
	$C_3H_8N_2O_2$	4.211	0.470
	$C_3H_{10}N_3O$	4.585	0.285
	$C_3H_{12}N_4$	4.960	0.102
	$C_4H_8O_3$	4.568	0.682
	$C_4H_{10}NO_2$	4.942	0.499
	$C_4H_{12}N_2O$	5.316	0.317
	$C_5H_2N_3$	6.579	0.185
	$C_5H_{12}O_2$	5.673	0.532
	C_6H_2NO	6.936	0.405
	$C_6H_4N_2$	7.311	0.230
	C_7H_4O	7.667	0.453
	C_7H_6N	8.042	0.281
	C_8H_8	8.773	0.338
105	CHN_2O_4	2.016	0.814
	$CH_3N_3O_3$	2.390	0.622
	$CH_5N_4O_2$	2.765	0.430
	$C_2H_3NO_4$	2.747	0.827
	$C_2H_5N_2O_3$	3.121	0.637
	$C_2H_7N_3O_2$	3.496	0.448
	$C_2H_9N_4O$	3.870	0.260
	$C_3H_5O_4$	3.478	0.844
	$C_3H_7NO_3$	3.853	0.657
	$C_3H_9N_2O_2$	4.227	0.471
	$C_3H_{11}N_3O$	4.601	0.286
	C_4HN_4	5.864	0.145
	$C_4H_9O_3$	4.584	0.683
	$C_4H_{11}NO_2$	4.958	0.499
	C_5HN_2O	6.221	0.363
	$C_5H_3N_3$	6.595	0.186
	C_6HO_2	6.578	0.582
	C_6H_3NO	6.952	0.406
	$C_6H_5N_2$	7.327	0.231
	C_7H_5O	7.683	0.454
	C_7H_7N	8.058	0.283
	C_8H_9	8.789	0.339
106	$CH_2N_2O_4$	2.032	0.815
	$CH_4N_3O_3$	2.406	0.622
	$CH_6N_4O_2$	2.781	0.431
	$C_2H_4NO_4$	2.763	0.828
	$C_2H_6N_2O_3$	3.137	0.638
	$C_2H_8N_3O_2$	3.512	0.449
	$C_2H_{10}N_4O$	3.886	0.261
	$C_3H_6O_4$	3.494	0.845
	$C_3H_8NO_3$	3.869	0.658
	$C_3H_{10}N_2O_2$	4.243	0.472
	$C_4H_2N_4$	5.880	0.146
	$C_4H_{10}O_3$	4.600	0.683
	$C_5H_2N_2O$	6.237	0.364
	$C_5H_4N_3$	6.611	0.187
	$C_6H_2O_2$	6.594	0.583
	C_6H_4NO	6.968	0.407
	$C_6H_6N_2$	7.343	0.233
	C_7H_6O	7.699	0.456
	C_7H_8N	8.074	0.284
	C_8H_{10}	8.805	0.341
107	$CH_3N_2O_4$	2.048	0.816
	$CH_5N_3O_3$	2.422	0.623
	$CH_7N_4O_2$	2.797	0.431
	$C_2H_5NO_4$	2.779	0.828
	$C_2H_7N_2O_3$	3.153	0.638
	$C_2H_9N_3O_2$	3.528	0.449
	$C_3H_7O_4$	3.510	0.846
	$C_3H_9NO_3$	3.885	0.659
	C_4HN_3O	5.522	0.327

(Contd.)

		M + 1	M + 2
	$C_4H_3N_4$	5.896	0.148
	C_5HNO_2	5.879	0.544
	$C_5H_3N_2O$	6.253	0.365
	$C_5H_5N_3$	6.627	0.188
	$C_6H_3O_2$	6.610	0.584
	C_6H_5NO	6.984	0.409
	$C_6H_7N_2$	7.359	0.234
	C_7H_7O	7.715	0.457
	C_7H_9N	8.090	0.286
	C_8H_{11}	8.821	0.342
108	$CH_4N_2O_4$	2.064	0.815
	$CH_6N_3O_3$	2.438	0.623
	$CH_8N_4O_2$	2.813	0.432
	$C_2H_6NO_4$	2.795	0.828
	$C_2H_8N_2O_3$	3.169	0.638
	$C_3H_8O_4$	3.526	0.846
	$C_4H_2N_3O$	5.538	0.328
	$C_4H_4N_4$	5.912	0.148
	$C_5H_2NO_2$	5.895	0.544
	$C_5H_4N_2O$	6.269	0.366
	C_5H_6Na	6.643	0.189
	$C_6H_4O_2$	6.626	0.585
	C_6H_6NO	7.000	0.409
	$C_6H_8N_2$	7.375	0.235
	C_7H_8O	7.731	0.458
	$C_7H_{10}N$	8.106	0.286
	C_8H_{12}	8.837	0.343
109	$CH_5N_2O_4$	2.080	0.816
	$CH_7N_3O_3$	2.454	0.624
	$C_2H_7NO_4$	2.811	0.829
	C_3HN_4O	4.823	0.296
	$C_4HN_2O_2$	5.179	0.510
	$C_3H_3N_3O$	5.554	0.329
	$C_4H_5N_4$	5.928	0.149
	C_5HO_3	5.536	0.725
	$C_5H_3NO_2$	5.911	0.545
	$C_5H_5N_2O$	6.285	0.367
	$C_5H_7N_3$	6.659	0.190
	$C_6H_5O_2$	6.642	0.587
	C_6H_7NO	7.016	0.411
	$C_6H_9N_2$	7.391	0.237
	C_7H_9O	7.747	0.460
	$C_7H_{11}N$	8.122	0.288
	C_8H_{13}	8.853	0.345
	C_9H	9.741	0.421
110	$CH_6N_2O_4$	2.096	0.816
	$C_3H_2N_4O$	4.839	0.297
	$C_4H_2N_2O_2$	5.196	0.511
	$C_4H_4N_3O$	5.570	0.330
	$C_4H_6N_4$	5.944	0.150
	$C_5H_2O_3$	5.552	0.726
	$C_5H_4NO_2$	5.927	0.546
	$C_5H_6N_2O$	6.301	0.368
	$C_5H_8N_3$	6.675	0.191
	$C_6H_6O_2$	6.658	0.587
	C_6H_8NO	7.032	0.412
	$C_6H_{10}N_2$	7.407	0.237
	$C_7H_{10}O$	7.763	0.460
	$C_7H_{12}N$	8.138	0.289
	C_8H_{14}	8.869	0.346
	C_9H_2	9.757	0.423
111	$C_3HN_3O_2$	4.480	0.481
	$C_3H_3N_4O$	4.855	0.297
	C_4HNO_3	4.837	0.694
	$C_4H_3N_2O_2$	5.212	0.511
	$C_4H_5N_3O$	5.586	0.330
	$C_4H_7N_4$	5.960	0.151
	$C_5H_3O_3$	5.568	0.727
	$C_5H_5NO_2$	5.943	0.547
	$C_5H_7N_2O$	6.317	0.369
	$C_5H_9N_3$	6.691	0.192
	$C_6H_7O_2$	6.674	0.588
	C_6H_9NO	7.048	0.413
	$C_6H_{11}N_2$	7.423	0.239
	$C_7H_{11}O$	7.779	0.462
	$C_7H_{13}N$	8.154	0.291
	C_8HN	9.042	0.361
	C_8H_{15}	8.885	0.348
	C_9H_3	9.773	0.425
112	$C_3H_2N_3O_2$	4.496	0.482

(Contd.)

		M + 1	M + 2
	$C_3H_4N_4O$	4.871	0.298
	$C_4H_2NO_3$	4.853	0.695
	$C_4H_4N_2O_2$	5.228	0.512
	$C_4H_6N_3O$	5.602	0.331
	$C_4H_8N_4$	5.976	0.152
	$C_5H_4O_3$	5.584	0.728
	$C_5H_6NO_2$	5.959	0.548
	$C_5H_8N_2O$	6.333	0.370
	$C_5H_{10}N_3$	6.707	0.193
	$C_6H_8O_2$	6.690	0.589
	$C_6H_{10}NO$	7.064	0.414
	$C_6H_{12}N_2$	7.439	0.240
	$C_7H_{12}O$	7.795	0.463
	$C_7H_{14}N$	8.170	0.292
	C_8H_2N	9.058	0.362
	C_8H_{16}	8.901	0.349
	C_9H_4	9.789	0.426
113	$C_2HN_4O_2$	3.781	0.458
	$C_3HN_2O_3$	4.138	0.668
	$C_3H_3N_3O_2$	4.512	0.483
	$C_3H_5N_4O$	4.887	0.299
	C_4HO_4	4.495	0.880
	$C_4H_3NO_3$	4.869	0.696
	$C_4H_5N_2O_2$	5.244	0.514
	$C_4H_7N_3O$	5.618	0.333
	$C_4H_9N_4$	5.992	0.153
	$C_5H_5O_3$	5.600	0.729
	$C_5H_7NO_2$	5.975	0.550
	$C_5H_9N_2O$	6.349	0.371
	$C_5H_{11}N_3$	6.723	0.194
	$C_6H_9O_2$	6.706	0.590
	$C_6H_{11}NO$	7.080	0.415
	$C_6H_{13}N_2$	7.455	0.241
	C_7HN_2	8.343	0.305
	$C_7H_{13}O$	7.811	0.464
	$C_7H_{15}N$	8.186	0.293
	C_8HO	8.700	0.532
	C_8H_3N	9.074	0.364
	C_8H_{17}	8.917	0.350
	C_9H_5	9.805	0.428
114	$C_2H_2N_4O_2$	3.797	0.458
	$C_3H_2N_2O_3$	4.154	0.668
	$C_3H_4N_3O_2$	4.528	0.483
	$C_3H_6N_4O$	4.903	0.300
	$C_4H_2O_4$	4.511	0.880
	$C_4H_4NO_3$	4.885	0.696
	$C_4H_6N_2O_2$	5.260	0.514
	$C_4H_8N_3O$	5.634	0.336
	$C_4H_{10}N_4$	6.008	0.154
	$C_5H_6O_3$	5.616	0.729
	$C_5H_8NO_2$	5.991	0.550
	$C_5H_{10}N_2O$	6.365	0.372
	$C_5H_{12}N_3$	6.739	0.195
	$C_6H_{10}O_2$	6.722	0.591
	$C_6H_{12}NO$	7.096	0.416
	$C_6H_{14}N_2$	7.471	0.242
	$C_7H_2N_2$	8.359	0.307
	$C_7H_{14}O$	7.827	0.465
	$C_7H_{16}N$	8.202	0.294
	C_8H_2O	8.716	0.533
	C_8H_4N	9.090	0.365
	C_8H_{18}	8.933	0.352
	C_9H_6	9.821	0.429
115	$C_2HN_3O_3$	3.439	0.647
	$C_2H_3N_4O_2$	3.813	0.459
	C_3HNO_4	3.796	0.856
	$C_3H_3N_2O_3$	4.170	0.669
	$C_3H_5N_3O_2$	4.544	0.485
	$C_3H_7N_4O$	4.919	0.301
	$C_4H_3O_4$	4.527	0.881
	$C_4H_5NO_3$	4.901	0.697
	$C_4H_7N_2O_2$	5.276	0.515
	$C_4H_9N_3O$	5.650	0.335
	$C_4H_{11}N_4$	6.024	0.155
	$C_5H_7O_3$	5.632	0.731
	$C_5H_9NO_2$	6.007	0.551
	$C_5H_{11}N_2O$	6.381	0.373
	$C_5H_{13}N_3$	6.755	0.197
	C_6HN_3	7.644	0.255
	$C_6H_{11}O_2$	6.738	0.593

(Contd.)

		M + 1	M + 2			M + 1	M + 2
	$C_6H_{13}NO$	7.112	0.418		$C_3H_9N_4O$	4.951	0.303
	$C_6H_{15}N_2$	7.487	0.244		$C_4H_5O_4$	4.560	0.882
	C_7HNO	8.001	0.479		$C_4H_7NO_3$	4.933	0.699
	$C_7H_3N_2$	8.375	0.308		$C_4H_9N_2O_2$	5.308	0.517
	$C_7H_{15}O$	7.843	0.467		$C_4H_{11}N_3O$	5.682	0.336
	$C_7H_{17}N$	8.218	0.296		$C_4H_{13}N_4$	6.056	0.157
	C_8H_3O	8.732	0.535		C_5HN_4	6.945	0.209
	C_8H_5N	9.106	0.367		$C_5H_9O_3$	5.664	0.733
	C_9H_7	9.837	0.431		$C_5H_{11}NO_2$	6.039	0.553
116	$C_2H_2N_3O_3$	3.455	0.647		$C_5H_{13}N_2O$	6.413	0.375
	$C_2H_4N_4O_2$	3.829	0.460		$C_5H_{15}N_3$	6.787	0.199
	$C_3H_2NO_4$	3.812	0.856		C_6HN_2O	7.302	0.431
	$C_3H_4N_2O_3$	4.186	0.670		$C_6H_3N_3$	7.676	0.257
	$C_3H_6N_3O_2$	4.560	0.485		$C_6H_{13}O_2$	6.770	0.595
	$C_3H_8N_4O$	4.935	0.301		$C_6H_{15}NO$	7.144	0.420
	$C_4H_4O_4$	4.543	0.881		C_7HO_2	7.658	0.653
	$C_4H_6NO_3$	4.917	0.698		C_7H_3NO	8.033	0.482
	$C_4H_8N_2O_2$	5.292	0.516		$C_7H_5N_2$	8.407	0.311
	$C_4H_{10}N_3O$	5.666	0.335		C_8H_5O	8.764	0.538
	$C_4H_{12}N_4$	6.040	0.156		C_8H_7N	9.138	0.370
	$C_5H_8O_3$	5.648	0.731		C_9H_9	9.869	0.435
	$C_5H_{10}NO_2$	6.023	0.552	118	$C_2H_2N_2O_4$	3.113	0.837
	$C_5H_{12}N_2O$	6.397	0.374		$C_2H_4N_3O_3$	3.487	0.648
	$C_5H_{14}N_3$	6.771	0.197		$C_2H_6N_4O_2$	3.861	0.461
	$C_6H_2N_3$	7.660	6.256		$C_3H_4NO_4$	3.844	0.858
	$C_6H_{12}O_2$	6.754	0.594		$C_3H_6N_2O_3$	4.218	0.671
	$C_6H_{14}NO$	7.128	0.418		$C_3H_8N_3O_2$	4.592	0.487
	$C_6H_{16}N_2$	7.503	0.244		$C_3H_{10}N_4O$	4.967	0.303
	C_7H_2NO	8.017	0.480		$C_4H_6O_4$	4.575	0.883
	$C_7H_4N_2$	8.391	0.309		$C_4H_8NO_3$	4.949	0.700
	$C_7H_{16}O$	7.859	0.468		$C_4H_{10}N_2O_2$	5.324	0.518
	C_8H_4O	8.748	0.536		$C_4H_{12}N_3O$	5.698	0.337
	C_8H_6N	9.122	0.368		$C_4H_{14}N_4$	6.072	0.158
	C_9H_8	9.853	0.432		$C_5H_2N_4$	6.961	0.210
117	$C_2HN_2O_4$	3.097	0.837		$C_5H_{10}O_3$	5.680	0.734
	$C_2H_3N_3O_3$	3.471	0.648		$C_5H_{12}NO_2$	6.055	0.554
	$C_2H_5N_4O_2$	3.845	0.460		$C_5H_{14}N_2O$	6.429	0.376
	$C_3H_3NO_4$	3.828	0.857		$C_6H_2N_2O$	7.318	0.431
	$C_3H_5N_2O_3$	4.202	0.671		$C_6H_4N_3$	7.692	0.259
	$C_3H_7N_3O_2$	4.576	0.486		$C_6H_{14}O_2$	6.786	0.596

(Contd.)

		M + 1	M + 2
	$C_7H_2O_2$	7.674	0.655
	C_7H_4NO	8.049	0.483
	$C_7H_6N_2$	8.423	0.312
	C_8H_6O	8.780	0.539
	C_8H_8N	9.154	0.372
	C_9H_{10}	9.885	0.436
119	$C_2H_3N_2O_4$	3.129	0.838
	$C_2H_5N_3O_3$	3.503	0.649
	$C_2H_7N_4O_2$	3.877	0.462
	$C_3H_5NO_4$	3.860	0.858
	$C_3H_7N_2O_3$	4.234	0.672
	$C_3H_9N_3O_2$	4.608	0.487
	$C_3H_{11}N_4O$	4.983	0.304
	$C_4H_7O_4$	4.591	0.884
	$C_4H_9NO_3$	4.965	0.701
	$C_4H_{11}N_2O_2$	5.340	0.519
	$C_4H_{13}N_3O$	5.714	0.338
	C_5HN_3O	6.602	0.387
	$C_5H_3N_4$	6.977	0.211
	$C_5H_{11}O_3$	5.696	0.735
	$C_5H_{13}NO_2$	6.071	0.555
	C_6HNO_2	6.959	0.607
	$C_6H_3N_2O$	7.334	0.433
	$C_6H_5N_3$	7.708	0.260
	$C_7H_3O_2$	7.690	0.656
	C_7H_5NO	8.065	0.484
	$C_7H_7N_2$	8.439	0.314
	C_8H_7O	8.796	0.541
	C_8H_9N	9.170	0.373
	C_9H_{11}	9.901	0.438
120	$C_2H_4N_2O_4$	3.145	0.838
	$C_2H_6N_3O_3$	3.519	0.650
	$C_2H_8N_4O_2$	3.893	0.462
	$C_3H_6NO_4$	3.876	0.859
	$C_3H_8N_2O_3$	4.250	0.673
	$C_3H_{10}N_3O_2$	4.624	0.488
	$C_3H_{12}N_4O$	4.999	0.305
	$C_4H_8O_4$	4.607	0.885
	$C_4H_{10}NO_3$	4.981	0.701
	$C_4H_{12}N_2O_2$	5.356	0.520
	$C_5H_2N_3O$	6.618	0.388
	$C_5H_4N_4$	6.993	0.212
	$C_5H_{12}O_3$	5.712	0.735
	$C_6H_2NO_2$	6.975	0.608
	$C_6H_4N_2O$	7.350	0.434
	$C_6H_6N_3$	7.724	0.261
	$C_7H_4O_2$	7.706	0.657
	C_7H_6NO	8.081	0.485
	$C_7H_8N_2$	8.455	0.315
	C_8H_8O	8.812	0.542
	$C_8H_{10}N$	9.186	0.374
	C_9H_{12}	9.917	0.439
121	$C_2H_5N_2O_4$	3.161	0.839
	$C_2H_7N_3O_3$	3.535	0.650
	$C_2H_9N_4O_2$	3.909	0.463
	$C_3H_7NO_4$	3.892	0.859
	$C_3H_9N_2O_3$	4.266	0.673
	$C_3H_{11}N_3O_2$	4.640	0.489
	C_4HN_4O	5.903	0.349
	$C_4H_9O_4$	4.623	0.885
	$C_4H_{11}NO_3$	4.997	0.702
	$C_5HN_2O_2$	6.260	0.566
	$C_5H_3N_3O$	6.635	0.389
	$C_5H_5N_4$	7.009	0.214
	C_6HO_3	6.617	0.785
	$C_6H_3NO_2$	6.991	0.610
	$C_6H_5N_2O$	7.366	0.435
	$C_6H_7N_3$	7.740	0.262
	$C_7H_5O_2$	7.722	0.658
	C_7H_7NO	8.097	0.487
	$C_7H_9N_2$	8.471	0.317
	C_8H_9O	8.828	0.543
	$C_8H_{11}N$	9.202	0.376
	C_9H_{13}	9.933	0.441
	$C_{10}H$	10.822	0.527
122	$C_2H_6N_2O_4$	3.177	0.839
	$C_2H_8N_3O_3$	3.551	0.651
	$C_2H_{10}N_4O_2$	3.925	0.463
	$C_3H_8NO_4$	3.908	0.860
	$C_3H_{10}N_2O_3$	4.282	0.674

(Contd.)

		M + 1	M + 2
	$C_4H_2N_4O$	5.919	0.349
	$C_4H_{10}O_4$	4.639	0.886
	$C_5H_2N_2O_2$	6.276	0.567
	$C_5H_4N_3O$	6.651	0.390
	$C_5H_6N_4$	7.025	0.215
	$C_6H_2O_3$	6.633	0.786
	$C_6H_4NO_2$	7.00	0.611
	$C_6H_6N_2O$	7.382	0.436
	$C_6H_8N_3$	7.756	0.264
	$C_7H_6O_2$	7.738	0.660
	C_7H_8NO	8.113	0.488
	$C_7H_{10}N_2$	8.487	0.318
	$C_8H_{10}O$	8.844	0.545
	$C_8H_{12}N$	9.218	0.377
	C_9H_{14}	9.949	0.442
	$C_{10}H_2$	10.838	0.529
123	$C_2H_7N_2O_4$	3.193	0.840
	$C_2H_9N_3O_3$	3.567	0.651
	$C_3H_9NO_4$	3.924	0.861
	$C_4HN_3O_2$	5.561	0.530
	$C_4H_3N_4O$	5.935	0.350
	C_5HNO_3	5.918	0.747
	$C_5H_3N_2O_2$	6.292	0.568
	$C_5H_5N_3O$	6.667	0.391
	$C_5H_7N_4$	7.041	0.216
	$C_6H_3O_3$	6.649	0.787
	$C_6H_5NO_2$	7.023	0.612
	$C_6H_7N_2O$	7.398	0.438
	$C_6H_9N_3$	7.772	0.265
	$C_7H_7O_2$	7.754	0.661
	C_7H_9NO	8.129	0.489
	$C_7H_{11}N_2$	8.503	0.319
	$C_8H_{11}O$	8.860	0.546
	$C_8H_{13}N$	9.234	0.379
	C_9HN	10.123	0.459
	C_9H_{15}	9.965	0.444
	$C_{10}H_3$	10.854	0.531
124	$C_2H_8N_2O_4$	3.209	0.840
	$C_4H_2N_3O_2$	5.577	0.531
	$C_4H_4N_4O$	5.951	0.351
	$C_5H_2NO_3$	5.934	0.748
	$C_5H_4N_2O_2$	6.308	0.569
	$C_5H_6N_3O$	6.683	0.392
	$C_5H_8N_4$	7.057	0.217
	$C_6H_4O_3$	6.665	0.789
	$C_6H_6NO_2$	7.039	0.613
	$C_6H_8N_2O$	7.414	0.439
	$C_6H_{10}N_3$	7.788	0.266
	$C_7H_8O_2$	7.770	0.662
	$C_7H_{10}NO$	8.145	0.491
	$C_7H_{12}N_2$	8.519	0.321
	$C_8H_{12}O$	8.876	0.548
	$C_8H_{14}N$	9.250	0.380
	C_9H_2N	10.139	0.461
	C_9H_{16}	9.981	0.446
	$C_{10}H_4$	10.870	0.532
125	$C_3HN_4O_2$	4.862	0.499
	$C_4HN_2O_3$	5.219	0.713
	$C_4H_3N_3O_2$	5.593	0.532
	$C_4H_5N_4O$	5.967	0.352
	C_5HO_4	5.575	0.928
	$C_5H_3NO_3$	5.950	0.749
	$C_5H_5N_2O_2$	6.324	0.570
	$C_5H_7N_3O$	6.699	0.393
	$C_5H_9N_4$	7.073	0.218
	$C_6H_5O_3$	6.681	0.790
	$C_6H_7NO_2$	7.055	0.614
	$C_6H_9N_2O$	7.430	0.440
	$C_6H_{11}N_3$	7.804	0.267
	$C_7H_9O_2$	7.786	0.663
	$C_7H_{11}NO$	8.161	0.492
	$C_7H_{13}N_2$	8.535	0.322
	C_8HN_2	9.424	0.396
	$C_8H_{13}O$	8.892	0.549
	$C_8H_{15}N$	9.266	0.382
	C_9HO	9.781	0.626
	C_9H_3N	10.155	0.462
	C_9H_{17}	9.998	0.447
	$C_{10}H_5$	10.886	0.534
126	$C_3H_2N_4O_2$	4.878	0.500

(Contd.)

		M + 1	M + 2
	$C_4H_2N_2O_3$	5.235	0.714
	$C_4H_4N_3O_2$	5.609	0.533
	$C_4H_6N_4O$	5.983	0.353
	$C_5H_2O_4$	5.591	0.929
	$C_5H_4NO_3$	5.966	0.749
	$C_5H_6N_2O_2$	6.340	0.571
	$C_5H_8N_3O$	6.715	0.350
	$C_5H_{10}N_4$	7.089	0.219
	$C_6H_6O_3$	6.697	0.791
	$C_6H_8NO_2$	7.071	0.615
	$C_6H_{10}N_2O$	7.446	0.441
	$C_6H_{12}N_3$	7.820	0.268
	$C_7H_{10}O_2$	7.802	0.664
	$C_7H_{12}NO$	8.177	0.493
	$C_7H_{14}N_2$	8.551	0.323
	$C_8H_2N_2$	9.440	0.397
	$C_8H_{14}O$	8.908	0.550
	$C_8H_{16}N$	9.282	0.383
	C_9H_2O	9.797	0.628
	C_9H_4N	10.171	0.464
	C_9H_{18}	10.013	0.448
	$C_{10}H_6$	10.902	0.535
127	$C_3HN_3O_3$	4.519	0.684
	$C_3H_3N_4O_2$	4.894	0.500
	C_4HNO_4	4.876	0.897
	$C_4H_3N_2O_3$	5.251	0.715
	$C_4H_5N_3O_2$	5.625	0.534
	$C_4H_7N_4O$	5.999	0.354
	$C_5H_3O_4$	5.607	0.930
	$C_5H_5NO_3$	5.982	0.750
	$C_5H_7N_2O_2$	6.356	0.572
	$C_5H_9N_3O$	6.731	0.396
	$C_5H_{11}N_4$	7.105	0.220
	$C_6H_7O_3$	6.713	0.792
	$C_6H_9NO_2$	7.087	0.616
	$C_6H_{11}N_2O$	7.462	0.442
	$C_6H_{13}N_3$	7.836	0.270
	C_7HN_3	8.725	0.338
	$C_7H_{11}O_2$	7.818	0.666
	$C_7H_{13}NO$	8.193	0.495

		M + 1	M + 2
	$C_7H_{15}N_2$	8.567	0.325
	C_8HNO	9.081	0.565
	$C_8H_3N_2$	9.456	0.399
	$C_8H_{15}O$	8.924	0.552
	$C_8H_{17}N$	9.298	0.385
	C_9H_3O	9.813	0.629
	C_9H_5N	10.187	0.466
	C_9H_{19}	10.030	0.450
	$C_{10}H_7$	10.918	0.548
128	$C_3H_2N_3O_3$	4.535	0.685
	$C_3H_4N_4O_2$	5.910	0.501
	$C_4H_2NO_4$	4.892	0.898
	$C_4H_4N_2O_3$	5.267	0.715
	$C_4H_6N_3O_2$	5.641	0.535
	$C_4H_8N_4O$	6.015	0.355
	$C_5H_4O_4$	5.623	0.931
	$C_5H_6NO_3$	5.998	0.751
	$C_5H_8N_2O_2$	6.372	0.573
	$C_5H_{10}N_3O$	6.747	0.397
	$C_5H_{12}N_4$	7.121	0.221
	$C_6H_8O_3$	6.729	0.793
	$C_6H_{10}NO_2$	7.103	0.618
	$C_6H_{12}N_2O$	7.478	0.444
	$C_6H_{14}N_3$	7.852	0.271
	$C_7H_2N_3$	8.741	0.339
	$C_7H_{12}O_2$	7.834	0.667
	$C_7H_{14}NO$	8.209	0.496
	$C_7H_{16}N_2$	8.583	0.326
	C_8H_2NO	9.097	0.567
	$C_8H_4N_2$	9.472	0.400
	$C_8H_{16}O$	8.940	0.553
	$C_8H_{18}N$	9.314	0.386
	C_9H_4O	9.829	0.631
	C_9H_6N	10.203	0.467
	C_9H_{20}	10.045	0.452
	$C_{10}H_8$	10.935	0.539
129	$C_3HN_2O_4$	4.177	0.870
	$C_3H_3N_3O_3$	4.551	0.685
	$C_3H_5N_4O_2$	4.926	0.502
	$C_4H_3NO_4$	4.908	0.898

(Contd.)

		M + 1	M + 2			M + 1	M + 2
	$C_4H_5N_2O_3$	5.283	0.716		$C_6H_{12}NO_2$	7.135	0.620
	$C_4H_7N_3O_2$	5.657	0.535		$C_6H_{14}N_2O$	7.510	0.446
	$C_4H_9N_4O$	6.031	0.356		$C_6H_{16}N_3$	7.884	0.274
	$C_5H_5O_4$	5.639	0.932		$C_7H_2N_2O$	8.398	0.511
	$C_5H_7NO_3$	6.014	0.752		$C_7H_4N_3$	8.773	0.342
	$C_5H_9N_2O_2$	6.388	0.574		$C_7H_{14}O_2$	7.866	0.670
	$C_5H_{11}N_3O$	6.763	0.398		$C_7H_{16}NO$	8.241	0.498
	$C_5H_{13}N_4$	7.137	0.223		$C_7H_{18}N_2$	8.615	0.329
	C_6HN_4	8.025	0.284		$C_8H_2O_2$	8.755	0.738
	$C_6H_9O_3$	6.745	0.794		C_8H_4NO	9.129	0.570
	$C_6H_{11}NO_2$	7.119	0.619		$C_8H_6N_2$	9.504	0.403
	$C_6H_{13}N_2O$	7.494	0.445		$C_8H_{18}O$	8.972	0.556
	$C_6H_{15}N_3$	7.868	0.272		C_9H_6O	9.861	0.634
	C_7HN_2O	8.382	0.510		C_9H_8N	10.235	0.471
	$C_7H_3N_3$	8.757	0.340		$C_{10}H_{10}$	10.966	0.543
	$C_7H_{13}O_2$	7.850	0.668	131	$C_3H_3N_2O_4$	4.209	0.972
	$C_7H_{15}NO$	8.225	0.497		$C_3H_5N_3O_3$	4.583	0.687
	$C_7H_{17}N_2$	8.599	0.327		$C_3H_7N_4O_2$	4.958	0.503
	C_8HO_2	8.739	0.736		$C_4H_5NO_4$	4.940	0.900
	C_8H_3NO	9.113	0.568		$C_4H_7N_2O_2$	5.315	0.717
	$C_8H_5N_2$	9.488	0.402		$C_4H_9N_3O_2$	5.689	0.537
	$C_8H_{17}O$	8.956	0.555		$C_4H_{11}N_4O$	6.063	0.358
	$C_8H_{19}N$	9.330	0.388		$C_5H_7O_4$	5.671	0.933
	C_9H_5O	9.845	0.633		$C_5H_9NO_3$	6.046	0.754
	C_9H_7N	10.219	4.688		$C_5H_{11}N_2O_2$	6.420	0.576
	$C_{10}H_9$	10.950	0.541		$C_5H_{13}N_3O$	6.795	0.399
130	$C_3H_2N_2O_4$	4.193	0.871		$C_5H_{15}N_4$	7.169	0.224
	$C_3H_4N_3O_3$	4.567	0.686		C_6HN_3O	7.683	0.458
	$C_3H_6N_4O_2$	4.942	0.503		$C_6H_3N_4$	8.057	0.286
	$C_4H_4NO_4$	4.924	0.899		$C_6H_{11}O_3$	6.777	0.796
	$C_4H_6N_2O_3$	5.299	0.717		$C_6H_{13}NO_2$	7.151	0.621
	$C_4H_8N_3O_2$	5.673	0.536		$C_6H_{15}N_2O$	7.526	0.447
	$C_4H_{10}N_4O$	6.047	0.357		$C_6H_{17}N_3$	7.900	0.274
	$C_5H_6O_4$	5.655	0.933		C_7HNO_2	8.040	0.682
	$C_5H_8NO_3$	6.030	0.753		$C_7H_3N_2O$	8.414	0.512
	$C_5H_{10}N_2O_2$	6.404	0.575		$C_7H_5N_3$	8.789	0.343
	$C_5H_{12}N_3O$	6.779	0.399		$C_{17}H_{15}O_2$	7.882	0.670
	$C_5H_{14}N_4$	7.153	0.224		$C_7H_{17}NO$	8.257	0.499
	$C_6H_2N_4$	8.041	0.285		$C_8H_3O_2$	8.771	0.738
	$C_6H_{10}O_3$	6.761	0.795		C_8H_5NO	9.145	0.571

(Contd.)

		M + 1	M + 2
	$C_8H_7N_2$	9.520	0.405
	C_9H_7O	9.877	0.635
	C_9H_9N	10.251	0.472
	$C_{10}H_{11}$	10.982	0.544
132	$C_3H_4N_2O_4$	4.225	0.872
	$C_3H_6N_3O_3$	4.599	0.688
	$C_3H_8N_4O_2$	4.974	0.504
	$C_4H_6NO_4$	4.956	0.900
	$C_4H_8N_2O_3$	5.331	0.718
	$C_4H_{10}N_3O_2$	5.705	0.538
	$C_4H_{12}N_4O$	6.079	0.359
	$C_5H_8O_4$	5.687	6.934
	$C_5H_{10}NO_3$	6.062	0.755
	$C_5H_{12}N_2O_2$	6.436	0.577
	$C_5H_{14}N_3O$	6.811	0.401
	$C_5H_{16}N_4$	7.185	0.226
	$C_6H_2N_3O$	7.699	0.460
	$C_6H_4N_4$	8.073	0.288
	$C_6H_{12}O_3$	6.793	0.797
	$C_6H_{14}NO_2$	7.167	0.622
	$C_6H_{16}N_2O$	7.542	0.448
	$C_7H_2NO_2$	8.056	0.683
	$C_7H_4N_2O$	8.430	0.514
	$C_7H_6N_3$	8.805	0.345
	$C_7H_{16}O_2$	7.898	0.672
	$C_8H_4O_2$	8.787	0.740
	C_8H_6NO	9.161	0.573
	$C_8H_8N_2$	9.536	0.407
	C_9H_8O	9.893	0.637
	$C_9H_{10}N$	10.267	0.474
	$C_{10}H_{12}$	10.998	0.546
133	$C_3H_5N_2O_4$	4.241	0.8729
	$C_3H_7N_3O_3$	4.616	0.688
	$C_3H_9N_4O_2$	4.990	0.505
	$C_4H_7NO_4$	4.972	0.901
	$C_4H_9N_2O_3$	5.347	0.720
	$C_4H_{11}N_3O_2$	5.721	0.539
	$C_4H_{13}N_4O$	6.095	0.360
	C_5HN_4O	6.984	0.412
	$C_5H_9O_4$	5.703	0.935
	$C_5H_{11}NO_3$	6.078	0.756
	$C_5H_{13}N_2O_2$	6.452	5.784
	$C_5H_{15}N_3O$	6.827	0.402
	$C_6HN_2O_2$	7.341	0.634
	$C_6H_3N_3O$	7.715	0.461
	$C_6H_5N_4$	8.089	0.289
	$C_6H_{13}O_3$	6.809	0.798
	$C_6H_{15}NO_2$	7.183	0.623
	C_7HO_3	7.698	0.857
	$C_7H_3NO_2$	8.072	0.685
	$C_7H_5N_2O$	8.446	0.515
	$C_7H_7N_3$	8.821	0.346
	$C_8H_5O_2$	8.803	0.742
	C_8H_7NO	9.177	0.574
	$C_8H_9N_2$	9.552	0.408
	C_9H_9O	9.909	0.638
	$C_9H_{11}N$	10.283	0.475
	$C_{10}H_{13}$	11.014	0.548
	$C_{11}H$	11.903	0.644
134	$C_3H_6N_2O_4$	4.257	0.874
	$C_3H_8N_3O_3$	4.632	0.689
	$C_3H_{10}N_4O_2$	5.006	0.506
	$C_4H_8NO_4$	4.988	0.902
	$C_4H_{10}N_2O_3$	5.363	0.720
	$C_4H_{12}N_3O_2$	5.737	0.540
	$C_4H_{14}N_4O$	6.111	0.361
	$C_5H_2N_4O$	7.000	0.413
	$C_5H_{10}O_4$	5.719	0.936
	$C_5H_{12}NO_3$	6.094	0.757
	$C_5H_{14}N_2O_2$	6.468	0.580
	$C_6H_2N_2O_2$	7.357	0.635
	$C_6H_4N_3O$	7.731	0.462
	$C_6H_6N_4$	8.105	0.291
	$C_6H_{14}O_3$	6.825	0.799
	$C_7H_2O_3$	7.714	0.858
	$C_7H_4NO_2$	8.088	0.686
	$C_7H_6N_2O$	8.462	0.516
	$C_7H_8N_3$	8.837	0.347
	$C_8H_6O_2$	8.819	0.743
	C_8H_8NO	9.193	0.576

(Contd.)

		M + 1	M + 2
	$C_8H_{10}N_2$	9.568	0.410
	$C_9H_{10}O$	9.925	0.640
	$C_9H_{12}N$	10.299	0.477
	$C_{10}H_{14}$	11.030	0.550
	$C_{11}H_2$	11.919	0.646
135	$C_3H_7N_2O_4$	4.273	0.874
	$C_3H_9N_3O_3$	4.648	0.690
	$C_3H_{11}N_4O_2$	5.022	0.507
	$C_4H_9NO_4$	5.004	0.903
	$C_4H_{11}N_2O_2$	5.379	0.721
	$C_4H_{13}N_3O_2$	5.753	0.541
	$C_5HN_3O_2$	6.642	0.590
	$C_5H_3N_4O$	7.016	0.415
	$C_5H_{11}O_4$	5.735	0.937
	$C_5H_{13}NO_3$	6.110	0.758
	C_6HNO_3	6.998	0.810
	$C_6H_3N_2O_2$	7.373	0.636
	$C_6H_5N_3O$	7.747	0.463
	$C_6H_7N_4$	8.121	0.291
	$C_7H_3O_3$	7.730	0.859
	$C_7H_5NO_2$	8.104	0.687
	$C_7H_7N_2O$	8.478	0.517
	$C_7H_9N_3$	8.853	0.348
	$C_8H_7O_2$	8.835	0.744
	C_8H_9NO	9.209	0.577
	$C_8H_{11}N_2$	9.584	0.411
	$C_9H_{11}O$	9.941	0.642
	$C_9H_{13}N$	10.315	0.478
	$C_{10}HN$	11.203	0.569
	$C_{10}H_{15}$	11.046	0.552
	$C_{11}H_3$	11.935	0.648
136	$C_3H_8N_2O_4$	4.289	0.875
	$C_3H_{10}N_3O_3$	4.664	0.691
	$C_3H_{12}N_4O_2$	5.038	0.507
	$C_4H_{10}NO_4$	5.020	0.904
	$C_4H_{12}N_2O_3$	5.395	0.722
	$C_5H_2N_3O_2$	6.658	0.591
	$C_5H_4N_4O$	7.032	0.416
	$C_5H_{12}O_4$	5.751	0.938
	$C_6H_2NO_3$	7.014	0.812
	$C_6H_4N_2O_2$	7.389	0.637
	$C_6H_6N_3O$	7.763	0.465
	$C_6H_8N_4$	8.137	0.293
	$C_7H_4O_3$	7.746	0.861
	$C_7H_6NO_2$	8.120	0.689
	$C_7H_8N_2O$	8.494	0.519
	$C_7H_{10}N_3$	8.869	0.350
	$C_8H_8O_2$	8.851	0.746
	$C_8H_{10}NO$	9.225	0.579
	$C_8H_{12}N_2$	9.600	0.413
	$C_9H_{12}O$	9.957	0.644
	$C_9H_{14}N$	10.331	0.480
	$C_{10}H_2N$	11.219	0.570
	$C_{10}H_{16}$	11.062	0.553
	$C_{11}H_4$	11.951	0.650
137	$C_3H_9N_2O_4$	4.305	0.876
	$C_3H_{11}N_3O_3$	4.680	0.691
	$C_4HN_4O_2$	5.942	0.551
	$C_4H_{11}NO_4$	5.036	0.905
	$C_5HN_2O_3$	6.299	0.769
	$C_5H_3N_3O_2$	6.674	0.592
	$C_5H_5N_4O$	7.048	0.417
	C_6HO_4	6.656	0.988
	$C_6H_3NO_3$	7.030	0.813
	$C_6H_5N_2O_2$	7.405	0.639
	$C_6H_7N_3O$	7.779	0.466
	$C_6H_9N_4$	8.153	0.294
	$C_7H_5O_3$	7.762	0.862
	$C_7H_7NO_2$	8.136	0.690
	$C_7H_9N_2O$	8.510	0.520
	$C_7H_{11}N_3$	8.885	0.352
	$C_8H_9O_2$	8.867	0.747
	$C_8H_{11}NO$	9.241	0.580
	$C_8H_{13}N_2$	9.616	0.414
	C_9HN_2	10.504	0.498
	$C_9H_{13}O$	9.973	0.645
	$C_9H_{15}N$	10.347	0.482
	$C_{10}HO$	10.861	0.732
	$C_{10}H_3N$	11.235	0.572
	$C_{10}H_{17}$	11.078	0.555

(Contd.)

		M + 1	M + 2
	$C_{11}H_5$	11.967	0.652
138	$C_3H_{10}N_2O_4$	4.321	0.876
	$C_4H_2N_4O_2$	5.958	0.552
	$C_5H_2N_2O_3$	6.315	0.770
	$C_5H_4N_3O_2$	6.690	0.593
	$C_5H_6N_4O$	7.064	0.418
	$C_6H_2O_4$	6.672	0.989
	$C_6H_4NO_3$	7.046	0.814
	$C_6H_6N_2O_2$	7.421	0.639
	$C_6H_8N_3O$	7.795	0.467
	$C_6H_{10}N_4$	8.169	0.295
	$C_7H_6O_3$	7.778	0.863
	$C_7H_8NO_2$	8.152	0.691
	$C_7H_{10}N_2O$	8.526	0.521
	$C_7H_{12}N_3$	8.901	0.353
	$C_8H_{10}O_2$	8.883	0.748
	$C_8H_{12}NO$	9.257	0.581
	$C_8H_{14}N_2$	9.632	0.415
	$C_9H_2N_2$	10.520	0.499
	$C_9H_{14}O$	9.989	0.646
	$C_9H_{16}N$	10.363	0.483
	$C_{10}H_2O$	10.877	0.733
	$C_{10}H_4N$	11.251	0.573
	$C_{10}H_{18}$	11.094	0.557
	$C_{11}H_6$	11.983	0.653
139	$C_4H_3N_3O_3$	5.600	0.733
	$C_4H_3N_4O_2$	5.974	0.553
	C_5HNO_4	5.957	0.949
	$C_5H_3N_2O_3$	6.331	0.771
	$C_5H_5N_3O_2$	6.706	0.594
	$C_5H_7N_4O$	7.080	0.419
	$C_6H_3O_4$	6.688	0.991
	$C_6H_5NO_3$	7.062	0.815
	$C_6H_7N_2O_2$	7.437	0.641
	$C_6H_9N_3O$	7.811	0.468
	$C_6H_{11}N_4$	8.185	0.297
	$C_7H_7O_3$	7.794	0.864
	$C_7H_9NO_2$	8.168	0.692
	$C_7H_{11}N_2O$	8.542	0.523
	$C_7H_{13}N_3$	8.917	0.354
	C_8HN_3	9.805	0.431
	$C_8H_{11}O_2$	8.899	0.750
	$C_8H_{13}NO$	9.273	0.583
	$C_8H_{15}N_2$	9.648	0.417
	C_9HNO	10.162	0.663
	$C_9H_3N_2$	10.536	0.501
	$C_9H_{15}O$	10.005	0.648
	$C_9H_{17}N$	10.379	0.485
	$C_{10}H_3O$	10.893	0.735
	$C_{10}H_5N$	11.267	0.575
	$C_{10}H_{19}$	11.110	0.558
	$C_{11}H_7$	11.999	0.655
140	$C_4H_2N_3O_3$	5.616	0.734
	$C_4H_4N_4O_2$	5.990	0.554
	$C_5H_2NO_4$	5.973	0.950
	$C_5H_4N_2O_3$	6.347	0.772
	$C_5H_6N_3O_2$	6.722	0.596
	$C_5H_8N_4O$	7.096	0.420
	$C_6H_4O_4$	6.704	0.992
	$C_6H_6NO_3$	7.078	0.816
	$C_6H_8N_2O_2$	7.453	0.642
	$C_6H_{10}N_3O$	7.827	0.470
	$C_6H_{12}N_4$	8.201	9.298
	$C_7H_8O_3$	7.810	0.866
	$C_7H_{10}NO_2$	8.184	0.694
	$C_7H_{12}N_2O$	8.558	0.524
	$C_7H_{14}N_3$	8.933	0.356
	$C_8H_2N_3$	9.821	0.433
	$C_8H_{12}O_2$	8.915	0.751
	$C_8H_{14}NO$	9.289	0.584
	$C_8H_{16}N_2$	9.664	0.418
	C_9H_2NO	10.178	0.665
	$C_9H_4N_2$	10.552	0.502
	$C_9H_{16}O$	10.021	0.650
	$C_9H_{18}N$	10.395	0.487
	$C_{10}H_4O$	10.909	0.737
	$C_{10}H_6N$	11.283	0.577
	$C_{10}H_{20}$	11.126	0.560
	$C_{11}H_8$	12.015	0.657
141	$C_4HN_2O_4$	5.258	0.915

(Contd.)

		M + 1	M + 2
	$C_4H_3N_3O_3$	5.632	0.735
	$C_4H_5N_4O_2$	6.006	0.555
	$C_5H_3NO_4$	5.989	0.951
	$C_5H_5N_2O_3$	6.363	0.773
	$C_5H_7N_3O_2$	6.738	0.597
	$C_5H_9N_4O$	7.112	0.421
	$C_6H_5O_4$	6.720	0.993
	$C_6H_7NO_3$	7.094	0.817
	$C_6H_9N_2O_2$	7.469	0.643
	$C_6H_{11}N_3O$	7.843	0.471
	$C_6H_{13}N_4$	8.217	0.300
	C_7HN_4	9.106	0.371
	$C_7H_9O_3$	7.826	0.867
	$C_7H_{11}NO_2$	8.200	0.696
	$C_7H_{13}N_2O$	8.574	0.526
	$C_7H_{15}N_3$	8.949	0.357
	C_8HN_2O	9.463	0.600
	$C_8H_3N_3$	9.837	0.435
	$C_8H_{13}O_2$	8.931	0.753
	$C_8H_{15}NO$	9.305	0.586
	$C_8H_{17}N_2$	9.680	0.420
	C_9HO_2	9.820	0.830
	C_9H_3NO	10.194	0.666
	$C_9H_5N_2$	10.568	0.504
	$C_9H_{17}O$	10.037	0.651
	$C_9H_{19}N$	10.411	0.488
	$C_{10}H_5O$	10.925	0.738
	$C_{10}H_7N$	11.299	0.579
	$C_{10}H_{21}$	11.142	0.562
	$C_{11}H_9$	12.031	0.659
142	$C_4H_2N_2O_4$	5.274	0.916
	$C_4H_4N_3O_3$	5.648	0.735
	$C_4H_6N_4O_2$	6.022	0.556
	$C_5H_4NO_4$	6.005	0.952
	$C_5H_6N_2O_3$	6.379	0.774
	$C_5H_8N_3O_2$	6.754	0.598
	$C_5H_{10}N_4O$	7.128	0.422
	$C_6H_6O_4$	6.736	0.994
	$C_6H_8NO_3$	7.110	0.818
	$C_6H_{10}N_2O_2$	7.485	0.645
	$C_6H_{12}N_3O$	7.859	0.472
	$C_6H_{14}N_4$	8.233	0.301
	$C_7H_2N_4$	9.122	0.372
	$C_7H_{10}O_3$	7.842	0.868
	$C_7H_{12}NO_2$	8.216	0.697
	$C_7H_{14}N_2O$	8.590	0.527
	$C_7H_{16}N_3$	8.965	0.359
	$C_8H_2N_2O$	9.479	0.602
	$C_8H_4N_3$	9.853	0.437
	$C_8H_{14}O_2$	8.947	0.755
	$C_8H_{16}NO$	9.321	0.588
	$C_8H_{18}N_2$	9.696	0.422
	$C_9H_2O_2$	9.836	0.832
	C_9H_4NO	10.210	0.668
	$C_9H_6N_2$	10.584	0.506
	$C_9H_{18}O$	10.053	0.653
	$C_9H_{20}N$	10.427	0.490
	$C_{10}H_6O$	10.941	0.741
	$C_{10}H_8N$	11.315	0.581
	$C_{10}H_{22}$	11.158	0.564
	$C_{11}H_{10}$	12.047	0.661
143	$C_4H_3N_2O_4$	5.290	0.917
	$C_4H_5N_3O_3$	5.664	0.736
	$C_4H_7N_4O_2$	6.038	0.557
	$C_5H_5NO_4$	6.021	0.953
	$C_5H_7N_2O_3$	6.395	0.775
	$C_5H_9N_3O_2$	6.770	0.599
	$C_5H_{11}N_4O$	7.144	0.424
	$C_6H_7O_4$	6.752	0.995
	$C_6H_9NO_3$	7.126	0.820
	$C_6H_{11}N_2O_2$	7.501	0.646
	$C_6H_{13}N_3O$	7.875	0.473
	$C_6H_{15}N_4$	8.249	0.302
	C_7HN_3O	8.764	0.541
	$C_7H_3N_4$	9.138	0.374
	$C_7H_{11}O_3$	7.858	0.869
	$C_7H_{13}NO_2$	8.232	0.698
	$C_7H_{15}N_2O$	8.606	0.529
	$C_7H_{17}N_3$	8.981	0.360
	C_8HNO_2	9.120	0.769

(Contd.)

		M + 1	M + 2
	$C_8H_3N_2O$	9.495	0.603
	$C_8H_5N_3$	9.869	0.438
	$C_8H_{15}O_2$	8.963	0.755
	$C_8H_{17}NO$	9.337	0.589
	$C_8H_{19}N_2$	9.712	0.423
	$C_9H_3O_2$	9.852	0.834
	C_9H_5NO	10.226	0.670
	$C_9H_7N_2$	10.600	0.508
	$C_9H_{19}O$	10.069	0.655
	$C_9H_{21}N$	10.443	0.492
	$C_{10}H_7O$	10.957	0.742
	$C_{10}H_9N$	11.331	0.582
	$C_{11}H_{11}$	12.063	0.663
144	$C_4H_9N_2O_4$	5.306	0.917
	$C_4H_6N_3O_3$	5.680	0.737
	$C_4H_8N_4O_2$	6.054	0.558
	$C_5H_6NO_4$	6.037	0.954
	$C_5H_8N_2O_2$	6.411	0.776
	$C_5H_{10}N_3O_2$	6.786	0.599
	$C_5H_{12}N_4O$	7.160	0.424
	$C_6H_8O_4$	6.768	0.995
	$C_7H_{10}NO_3$	7.142	0.820
	$C_6H_{12}N_2O_2$	7.517	0.647
	$C_6H_{14}N_3O$	7.891	0.474
	$C_6H_{16}N_4$	8.265	0.303
	$C_7H_2N_3O$	8.780	0.542
	$C_7H_4N_4$	9.154	0.375
	$C_7H_{12}O_3$	7.874	0.870
	$C_7H_{14}NO_2$	8.248	0.699
	$C_7H_{16}N_2O$	8.622	0.529
	$C_7H_{18}N_3$	8.997	0.361
	$C_8H_2NO_2$	9.136	0.770
	$C_8H_4N_2O$	9.511	0.604
	$C_8H_6N_3$	9.885	0.439
	$C_8H_{16}O_2$	8.979	0.757
	$C_8H_{18}NO$	9.353	0.590
	$C_8H_{20}N_2$	9.728	0.425
	$C_9H_4O_2$	9.868	0.835
	C_9H_6NO	10.242	0.671
	$C_9H_8N_2$	10.616	0.509
	$C_9H_{20}O$	10.085	0.656
	$C_{10}H_8O$	10.973	0.744
	$C_{10}H_{10}N$	11.347	0.584
	$C_{11}H_{12}$	12.079	0.665
145	$C_4H_5N_2O_4$	5.322	0.918
	$C_4H_7N_3O_3$	5.696	0.738
	$C_4H_9N_4O_2$	6.070	0.558
	$C_5H_7NO_4$	6.053	0.955
	$C_5H_9N_2O_3$	6.427	0.777
	$C_5H_{11}N_3O_2$	6.802	0.600
	$C_5H_{13}N_4O$	7.176	0.425
	C_6HN_4O	8.065	0.487
	$C_6H_9O_4$	6.784	0.997
	$C_6H_{11}NO_3$	7.158	0.821
	$C_6H_{13}N_2O_2$	7.533	0.648
	$C_6H_{15}N_3O$	7.907	0.475
	$C_6H_{17}N_4$	8.282	0.305
	$C_7HN_2O_2$	8.421	0.713
	$C_7H_3N_3O$	8.796	0.544
	$C_7H_5N_4$	9.170	0.376
	$C_7H_{13}O_3$	7.890	0.871
	$C_7H_{15}NO_2$	8.264	0.701
	$C_7H_{17}N_2O$	8.638	0.531
	$C_7H_{19}N_3$	9.013	0.363
	C_8HO_3	8.778	0.940
	$C_8H_3NO_2$	9.152	0.772
	$C_8H_5N_2O$	9.527	0.606
	$C_8H_7N_3$	9.901	0.441
	$C_8H_{17}O_2$	8.995	0.759
	$C_8H_{19}NO$	9.369	0.592
	$C_9H_5O_2$	9.884	0.837
	C_9H_7NO	10.258	0.673
	$C_9H_9N_2$	10.632	0.511
	$C_{10}H_9O$	10.989	0.746
	$C_{10}H_{11}N$	11.363	0.587
	$C_{11}H_{13}$	12.095	0.667
	$C_{12}H$	12.983	0.773
146	$C_4H_6N_2O_4$	5.338	9.195
	$C_4H_8N_3O_3$	5.712	0.739
	$C_4H_{10}N_4O_2$	6.086	0.559

(Contd.)

		M + 1	M + 2
	$C_5H_8NO_4$	6.069	0.956
	$C_5H_{10}N_2O_3$	6.443	0.778
	$C_5H_{12}N_3O_2$	6.818	0.602
	$C_5H_{14}N_4O$	7.192	0.427
	$C_6H_2N_4O$	8.081	0.489
	$C_6H_{10}O_4$	6.800	0.998
	$C_6H_{12}NO_3$	7.174	0.823
	$C_6H_{14}N_2O_2$	7.549	0.649
	$C_6H_{16}N_3O$	7.923	0.477
	$C_6H_{18}N_4$	8.298	0.306
	$C_7H_2N_2O_2$	8.437	0.715
	$C_7H_4N_3O$	8.812	0.546
	$C_7H_6N_4$	9.186	0.378
	$C_7H_{14}O_3$	7.906	0.873
	$C_7H_{16}NO_2$	8.280	0.702
	$C_7H_{18}N_2O$	8.654	0.533
	$C_8H_2O_3$	8.794	0.941
	$C_8H_4NO_2$	9.168	0.773
	$C_8H_6N_2O$	9.543	0.602
	$C_8H_8N_3$	9.917	0.443
	$C_8H_{18}O_2$	9.011	0.760
	$C_9H_6O_2$	9.900	0.838
	C_9H_8NO	10.274	0.675
	$C_9H_{10}N_2$	10.648	0.513
	$C_{10}H_{10}O$	11.005	0.748
	$C_{10}H_{12}N$	11.379	0.588
	$C_{11}H_{14}$	12.111	0.669
	$C_{12}H_2$	12.999	0.774
147	$C_4H_7N_2O_4$	5.354	0.920
	$C_4H_9N_3O_3$	5.728	0.740
	$C_4H_{11}N_4O_2$	6.102	0.561
	$C_5H_9NO_4$	6.085	0.957
	$C_5H_{11}N_2O_3$	6.459	0.779
	$C_5H_{13}N_3O_2$	6.834	0.603
	$C_5H_{15}N_4O$	7.208	0.428
	$C_6HN_3O_2$	7.722	0.662
	$C_6H_3N_4O$	8.097	0.490
	$C_6H_{11}O_4$	6.816	0.999
	$C_6H_{13}NO_3$	7.190	0.824
	$C_6H_{15}N_2O_2$	7.565	0.651
	$C_6H_{17}N_3O$	7.939	0.478
	C_7HNO_3	8.079	0.886
	$C_7H_3N_2O_2$	8.453	0.716
	$C_7H_5N_3O$	8.828	0.547
	$C_7H_7N_4$	9.202	0.380
	$C_7H_{15}O_3$	7.922	0.874
	$C_{17}H_{17}NO_2$	8.296	0.703
	$C_8H_3O_3$	8.810	0.943
	$C_8H_5NO_2$	9.185	0.775
	$C_8H_7N_2O$	9.559	0.609
	$C_8H_9N_3$	9.933	0.444
	$C_9H_7O_2$	9.916	0.840
	C_9H_9NO	10.290	6.766
	$C_9H_{11}N_2$	10.664	0.515
	$C_{10}H_{11}O$	11.021	0.749
	$C_{10}H_{13}N$	11.395	5.902
	$C_{11}HN$	12.284	0.690
	$C_{11}H_{15}$	12.127	0.671
	$C_{12}H_3$	13.015	7.769
148	$C_4H_8N_2O_4$	5.370	0.921
	$C_4H_{10}N_3O_3$	5.744	0.741
	$C_4H_{12}N_4O_2$	6.118	0.562
	$C_5H_{10}NO_4$	6.101	0.958
	$C_5H_{12}N_2O_3$	6.475	0.780
	$C_5H_{14}N_3O_2$	6.850	0.604
	$C_5H_{16}N_4O$	7.224	0.429
	$C_6H_2N_3O_2$	7.738	0.663
	$C_6H_4N_4O$	8.113	0.492
	$C_6H_{12}O_4$	6.832	1.000
	$C_6H_{14}NO_3$	7.206	0.825
	$C_6H_{16}N_2O_2$	7.581	0.652
	$C_7H_2NO_3$	8.095	0.888
	$C_7H_4N_2O_2$	8.469	0.717
	$C_7H_6N_3O$	8.844	0.549
	$C_7H_8N_4$	9.218	0.381
	$C_7H_{16}O_3$	7.938	0.876
	$C_8H_4O_3$	8.826	0.944
	$C_8H_6NO_2$	9.201	0.777
	$C_8H_8N_2O$	9.575	0.611
	$C_8H_{10}N_3$	9.949	0.446

(Contd.)

		M + 1	M + 2
	$C_9H_8O_2$	9.932	0.842
	$C_9H_{10}NO$	10.306	0.678
	$C_9H_{12}N_2$	10.680	0.516
	$C_{10}H_{12}O$	11.037	0.751
	$C_{10}H_{14}N$	11.411	0.592
	$C_{11}H_2N$	12.300	0.692
	$C_{11}H_{16}$	12.143	0.673
	$C_{12}H_4$	13.031	0.779
149	$C_4H_9N_2O_4$	5.386	0.922
	$C_4H_{11}N_3O_3$	5.760	0.742
	$C_4H_{13}N_4O_2$	6.134	0.563
	$C_5HN_4O_2$	7.023	0.616
	$C_5H_{11}NO_4$	6.117	0.959
	$C_5H_{13}N_2O_3$	6.491	0.781
	$C_5H_{15}N_3O_2$	6.866	0.605
	$C_6HN_2O_3$	7.380	0.837
	$C_6H_3N_3O_2$	7.754	0.664
	$C_6H_5N_4O$	8.129	0.493
	$C_6H_{13}O_4$	6.848	1.001
	$C_6H_{15}NO_3$	7.222	0.827
	C_7HO_4	7.737	1.060
	$C_7H_3NO_3$	8.111	0.889
	$C_7H_5N_2O_2$	8.485	0.719
	$C_7H_7N_3O$	8.860	0.550
	$C_7H_9N_4$	9.234	0.382
	$C_8H_5O_3$	8.842	0.945
	$C_8H_7NO_2$	9.217	0.778
	$C_8H_9N_2O$	9.591	0.612
	$C_8H_{11}N_3$	9.965	0.447
	$C_9H_9O_2$	9.948	0.843
	$C_9H_{11}NO$	10.322	0.679
	$C_9H_{13}N_2$	10.696	0.518
	$C_{10}HN_2$	11.585	0.611
	$C_{10}H_{13}O$	11.053	0.752
	$C_{10}H_{15}N$	11.427	0.593
	$C_{11}HO$	11.942	0.849
	$C_{11}H_3N$	12.316	0.693
	$C_{11}H_{17}$	12.159	0.674
	$C_{12}H_5$	13.047	0.781
150	$C_4H_{10}N_2O_4$	5.402	0.923
	$C_4H_{12}N_3O_3$	5.776	0.743
	$C_4H_{14}N_4O_2$	6.150	0.564
	$C_5H_2N_4O_2$	7.039	0.617
	$C_5H_{12}NO_4$	6.133	0.960
	$C_5H_{14}N_2O_3$	6.507	0.783
	$C_6H_2N_2O_3$	7.396	0.838
	$C_6H_4N_3O_2$	7.770	0.666
	$C_6H_6N_4O$	8.145	0.494
	$C_6H_{14}O_4$	6.864	1.002
	$C_7H_2O_4$	7.753	1.061
	$C_7H_4NO_3$	8.127	0.890
	$C_7H_6N_2O_2$	8.501	0.720
	$C_7H_8N_3O$	8.876	0.551
	$C_7H_{10}N_4$	9.250	0.384
	$C_8H_6O_3$	8.858	0.947
	$C_8H_8NO_2$	9.233	0.780
	$C_8H_{10}N_2O$	9.607	0.614
	$C_8H_{12}N_3$	9.981	0.449
	$C_9H_{10}O_2$	9.964	0.845
	$C_9H_{12}NO$	10.338	0.682
	$C_9H_{14}N_2$	10.712	0.520
	$C_{10}H_2N_2$	11.601	0.613
	$C_{10}H_{14}O$	11.069	0.755
	$C_{10}H_{16}N$	11.443	0.596
	$C_{11}H_2O$	11.958	0.851
	$C_{11}H_4N$	12.332	0.695
	$C_{11}H_{18}$	12.175	0.677
	$C_{12}H_6$	13.062	0.783
151	$C_4H_{11}N_2O_4$	5.418	0.924
	$C_4H_{13}N_3O_3$	5.792	0.744
	$C_5HN_3O_3$	6.681	0.793
	$C_5H_3N_4O_2$	7.055	0.618
	$C_5H_{13}NO_4$	6.149	0.961
	C_6HNO_3	7.037	1.013
	$C_6H_3N_2O_3$	7.412	0.840
	$C_6H_5N_3O_2$	7.786	0.667
	$C_6H_7N_4O$	8.161	0.496
	$C_7H_3O_4$	7.769	1.062
	$C_7H_5NO_3$	8.143	0.891
	$C_7H_7N_2O_2$	8.517	0.721

(Contd.)

		M + 1	M + 2
	$C_7H_9N_3O$	8.892	0.553
	$C_7H_{11}N_4$	9.266	0.386
	$C_8H_7O_3$	8.874	0.949
	$C_8H_9NO_2$	9.249	0.781
	$C_8H_{11}N_2O$	9.623	0.615
	$C_8H_{13}N_3$	9.997	0.451
	C_9HN_3	10.866	0.538
	$C_9H_{11}O_2$	9.980	0.846
	$C_9H_{13}NO$	10.356	0.683
	$C_9H_{15}N_2$	10.728	0.522
	$C_{10}HNO$	11.243	0.773
	$C_{10}H_3N_2$	11.617	0.615
	$C_{10}H_{15}O$	11.085	0.757
	$C_{10}H_{17}N$	11.460	0.598
	$C_{11}H_3O$	11.974	0.853
	$C_{11}H_5N$	12.348	0.697
	$C_{11}H_{19}$	12.191	0.679
	$C_{12}H_7$	13.079	0.785
152	$C_4H_{12}N_2O_4$	5.434	0.925
	$C_5H_2N_3O_3$	6.697	0.794
	$C_5H_4N_4O_2$	7.071	0.619
	$C_6H_2NO_4$	7.053	1.015
	$C_6H_4N_2O_3$	7.428	0.841
	$C_6H_6N_3O_2$	7.802	0.668
	$C_6H_8N_4O$	8.177	0.497
	$C_7H_4O_4$	7.785	1.064
	$C_7H_6NO_3$	8.159	0.893
	$C_7H_8N_2O_2$	8.533	0.723
	$C_7H_{10}N_3O$	8.908	0.554
	$C_7H_{12}N_4$	9.282	0.387
	$C_8H_8O_3$	8.890	0.950
	$C_8H_{10}NO_2$	9.265	0.783
	$C_8H_{12}N_2O$	9.639	0.617
	$C_8H_{14}N_3$	10.013	0.452
	$C_9H_2N_3$	10.902	0.540
	$C_9H_{12}O_2$	9.996	0.848
	$C_9H_{14}NO$	10.370	0.685
	$C_9H_{16}N_2$	10.744	0.523
	$C_{10}H_2NO$	11.259	0.775
	$C_{10}H_4N_2$	11.633	0.617
	$C_{10}H_{16}O$	11.101	0.758
	$C_{10}H_{18}N$	11.476	0.599
	$C_{11}H_4O$	11.990	0.855
	$C_{11}H_6N$	12.364	0.699
	$C_{11}H_{20}$	12.207	0.681
	$C_{12}H_8$	13.095	0.787
153	$C_5HN_2O_4$	6.338	0.972
	$C_5H_3N_3O_3$	6.713	0.795
	$C_5H_5N_4O_2$	7.087	0.620
	$C_6H_3NO_4$	7.069	1.016
	$C_6H_5N_2O_3$	7.444	0.842
	$C_6H_7N_3O_2$	7.818	0.669
	$C_6H_9N_4O$	8.193	0.498
	$C_7H_5O_4$	7.801	1.065
	$C_7H_7NO_3$	8.175	0.894
	$C_7H_9N_2O_2$	8.549	0.724
	$C_7H_{11}N_3O$	8.924	0.556
	$C_7H_{13}N_4$	9.298	0.389
	C_8HN_4	10.187	0.469
	$C_8H_9O_3$	8.906	0.951
	$C_8H_{11}NO_2$	9.281	0.784
	$C_8H_{13}N_2O$	9.655	0.618
	$C_8H_{15}N_3$	10.029	0.454
	C_9HN_2O	10.543	0.702
	$C_9H_3N_3$	10.918	0.541
	$C_9H_{13}O_2$	10.012	0.850
	$C_9H_{15}NO$	10.386	0.687
	$C_9H_{17}N_2$	10.760	0.525
	$C_{10}HO_2$	10.900	0.937
	$C_{10}H_3NO$	11.275	0.777
	$C_{10}H_5N_2$	11.649	0.619
	$C_{10}H_{17}O$	11.117	0.760
	$C_{10}H_{19}N$	11.492	0.601
	$C_{11}H_5O$	12.006	0.857
	$C_{11}H_7N$	12.380	0.701
	$C_{11}H_{21}$	12.223	0.682
	$C_{12}H_9$	13.111	0.790
154	$C_5H_2N_2O_4$	6.354	0.973
	$C_5H_4N_3O_3$	6.729	0.796
	$C_5H_6N_4O_2$	7.103	0.621

(Contd.)

		M + 1	M + 2
	$C_6H_4NO_4$	7.085	1.017
	$C_6H_6N_2O_3$	7.460	0.843
	$C_6H_8N_3O_2$	7.834	0.671
	$C_6H_{10}N_4O$	8.209	0.499
	$C_7H_6O_4$	7.817	1.067
	$C_7H_8NO_3$	8.191	0.895
	$C_7H_{10}N_2O_2$	8.565	0.725
	$C_7H_{12}N_3O$	8.940	0.557
	$C_7H_{14}N_4$	9.314	0.390
	$C_8H_2N_4$	10.203	0.471
	$C_8H_{10}O_3$	8.922	0.953
	$C_8H_{12}NO_2$	9.297	0.786
	$C_8H_{14}N_2O$	9.671	0.620
	$C_8H_{16}N_3$	10.045	0.456
	$C_9H_2N_2O$	10.559	7.040
	$C_9H_4N_3$	10.934	0.543
	$C_9H_{14}O_2$	10.028	0.851
	$C_9H_{16}NO$	10.402	0.688
	$C_9H_{18}N_2$	10.776	0.527
	$C_{10}H_2O_2$	10.916	0.938
	$C_{10}H_4NO$	11.291	0.779
	$C_{10}H_6N_2$	11.665	0.621
	$C_{10}H_{18}O$	11.133	0.762
	$C_{10}H_{20}N$	11.508	0.603
	$C_{11}H_6O$	12.022	0.859
	$C_{11}H_8N$	12.396	0.703
	$C_{11}H_{22}$	12.239	0.685
	$C_{12}H_{10}$	13.127	0.792
155	$C_5H_3N_2O_4$	6.370	0.974
	$C_5H_5N_3O_3$	6.745	0.798
	$C_5H_7N_4O_2$	7.119	0.622
	$C_6H_5NO_4$	7.101	1.018
	$C_6H_7N_2O_3$	7.476	0.844
	$C_6H_9N_3O_2$	7.850	0.672
	$C_6H_{11}N_4O$	8.225	0.501
	$C_7H_7O_4$	7.833	1.067
	$C_7H_9NO_3$	8.207	0.897
	$C_7H_{11}N_2O_2$	8.581	0.727
	$C_7H_{13}N_3O$	8.956	0.558
	$C_7H_{15}N_4$	9.330	0.392
	C_8HN_3O	9.844	0.636
	$C_8H_3N_4$	10.219	0.473
	$C_8H_{11}O_3$	8.938	0.954
	$C_8H_{13}NO_2$	9.313	0.787
	$C_8H_{15}N_2O$	9.687	0.622
	$C_8H_{17}N_3$	10.061	0.457
	C_9HNO_2	10.201	0.868
	$C_9H_3N_2O$	10.575	0.706
	$C_9H_5N_3$	10.950	0.545
	$C_9H_{15}O_2$	10.044	0.853
	$C_9H_{17}NO$	10.418	0.690
	$C_9H_{19}N_2$	10.792	0.528
	$C_{10}H_3O_2$	10.932	0.940
	$C_{10}H_5NO$	11.307	0.781
	$C_{10}H_7N_2$	11.681	0.622
	$C_{10}H_{19}O$	11.149	0.764
	$C_{10}H_{21}N$	11.524	0.605
	$C_{11}H_7O$	12.038	0.861
	$C_{11}H_9N$	12.412	0.705
	$C_{11}H_{23}$	12.255	0.687
	$C_{12}H_{11}$	13.143	0.794
156	$C_5H_4N_2O_4$	6.386	0.975
	$C_5H_6N_3O_3$	6.761	0.799
	$C_5H_8N_4O_2$	7.135	0.623
	$C_6H_6NO_4$	7.117	1.019
	$C_6H_8N_2O_3$	7.492	0.846
	$C_6H_{10}N_3O_2$	7.866	0.673
	$C_6H_{12}N_4O$	8.241	0.502
	$C_7H_8O_4$	7.849	1.069
	$C_7H_{10}NO_3$	8.223	0.898
	$C_7H_{12}N_2O_2$	8.597	0.728
	$C_7H_{14}N_3O$	8.972	0.560
	$C_7H_{16}N_4$	9.346	0.393
	$C_8H_2N_3O$	9.860	0.638
	$C_8H_4N_4$	10.235	0.474
	$C_8H_{12}O_3$	8.954	0.956
	$C_8H_{14}NO_2$	9.329	0.789
	$C_8H_{16}N_2O$	9.703	0.623
	$C_8H_{18}N_3$	10.077	0.459
	$C_9H_2NO_2$	10.217	0.870

(Contd.)

		M + 1	M + 2
	$C_9H_4N_2O$	10.591	0.707
	$C_9H_6N_3$	10.966	0.547
	$C_9H_{16}O_2$	10.060	0.854
	$C_9H_{18}NO$	10.434	0.692
	$C_9H_{20}N_2$	10.808	0.530
	$C_{10}H_4O_2$	10.948	0.942
	$C_{10}H_6NO$	11.323	0.782
	$C_{10}H_8N_2$	11.697	0.624
	$C_{10}H_{20}O$	11.165	0.765
	$C_{10}H_{22}N$	11.540	0.606
	$C_{11}H_8O$	12.054	0.862
	$C_{11}H_{10}N$	12.428	0.707
	$C_{11}H_{24}$	12.271	0.688
	$C_{12}H_{12}$	13.159	0.795
157	$C_5H_5N_2O_4$	6.402	0.976
	$C_5H_7N_3O_3$	6.777	0.800
	$C_5H_9N_4O_2$	7.151	0.625
	$C_6H_7NO_4$	7.133	1.021
	$C_6H_9N_2O_3$	7.508	0.847
	$C_6H_{11}N_3O_2$	7.882	0.674
	$C_6H_{13}N_4O$	8.257	0.503
	C_7HN_4O	9.145	0.575
	$C_7H_9O_4$	7.865	1.070
	$C_7H_{11}NO_3$	8.239	0.899
	$C_7H_{13}N_2O_2$	8.613	0.730
	$C_7H_{15}N_3O$	8.988	0.561
	$C_7H_{17}N_4$	9.362	0.394
	$C_8HN_2O_2$	9.502	0.804
	$C_8H_3N_3O$	9.876	0.639
	$C_8H_5N_4$	10.251	0.476
	$C_8H_{13}O_3$	8.970	0.957
	$C_8H_{15}NO_2$	9.345	0.790
	$C_8H_{17}N_2O$	9.719	0.625
	$C_8H_{19}N_3$	10.093	0.461
	C_9HO_3	9.859	1.035
	$C_9H_3NO_2$	10.233	0.871
	$C_9H_5N_2O$	10.607	0.709
	$C_9H_7N_3$	10.982	0.548
	$C_9H_{17}O_2$	10.076	0.856
	$C_9H_{19}NO$	10.450	0.693
	$C_9H_{21}N_2$	10.824	0.532
	$C_{10}H_5O_2$	10.964	0.944
	$C_{10}H_7NO$	11.339	0.784
	$C_{10}H_9N_2$	11.713	0.626
	$C_{10}H_{21}O$	11.181	0.767
	$C_{10}H_{23}N$	11.556	0.609
	$C_{11}H_9O$	12.070	0.865
	$C_{11}H_{11}N$	12.444	0.709
	$C_{12}H_{13}$	13.175	7.979
	$C_{13}H$	14.064	0.913
158	$C_5H_6N_2O_4$	6.418	0.977
	$C_5H_8N_3O_3$	6.793	0.801
	$C_5H_{10}N_4O_2$	7.167	0.626
	$C_6H_8NO_4$	7.149	1.022
	$C_6H_{10}N_2O_3$	7.524	0.848
	$C_6H_{12}N_3O_2$	7.898	0.676
	$C_6H_{14}N_4O$	8.273	0.505
	$C_7H_2N_4O$	9.161	0.576
	$C_7H_{10}O_4$	7.881	1.072
	$C_7H_{12}NO_3$	8.255	0.901
	$C_7H_{14}N_2O_2$	8.629	0.731
	$C_7H_{16}N_3O$	9.004	0.563
	$C_7H_{18}N_4$	9.378	0.396
	$C_8H_2N_2O_2$	9.518	0.806
	$C_8H_4N_3O$	9.892	0.641
	$C_8H_6N_4$	10.267	0.477
	$C_8H_{14}O_3$	8.986	0.958
	$C_8H_{16}NO_2$	9.361	0.792
	$C_8H_{18}N_2O$	9.735	0.626
	$C_8H_{20}N_3$	10.109	0.462
	$C_9H_2O_3$	9.875	1.036
	$C_9H_4NO_2$	10.249	0.873
	$C_9H_6N_2O$	10.623	0.711
	$C_9H_8N_3$	10.998	0.550
	$C_9H_{18}O_2$	10.092	0.858
	$C_9H_{20}NO$	10.466	0.695
	$C_9H_{22}N_2$	10.840	0.534
	$C_{10}H_6O_2$	10.980	0.945
	$C_{10}H_8NO$	11.355	0.786
	$C_{10}H_{10}N_2$	11.729	0.628

(Contd.)

		M + 1	M + 2			M + 1	M + 2
	$C_{10}H_{22}O$	11.197	0.769		$C_{13}H_3$	14.096	0.917
	$C_{11}H_{10}O$	12.086	0.867	160	$C_5H_8N_2O_4$	6.450	0.979
	$C_{11}H_{12}N$	12.460	0.711		$C_5H_{10}N_3O_3$	6.825	0.803
	$C_{12}H_{14}$	13.191	0.800		$C_5H_{12}N_4O_2$	7.199	0.628
	$C_{13}H_2$	14.080	0.915		$C_6H_{10}NO_4$	7.181	1.024
159	$C_5H_7N_2O_4$	6.434	0.978		$C_6H_{12}N_2O_3$	7.556	0.850
	$C_5H_9N_3O_3$	6.809	0.802		$C_6H_{14}N_3O_2$	7.930	0.678
	$C_5H_{11}N_4O_2$	7.183	0.627		$C_6H_{16}N_4O$	8.305	0.507
	$C_6H_9NO_4$	7.165	1.023		$C_7H_2N_3O_2$	8.819	0.747
	$C_6H_{11}N_2O_3$	7.540	0.849		$C_7H_4N_4O$	9.193	0.579
	$C_6H_{13}N_3O_2$	7.914	0.677		$C_7H_{12}O_4$	7.913	1.074
	$C_6H_{15}N_4O$	8.285	0.506		$C_7H_{14}NO_3$	8.287	0.903
	$C_7HN_3O_2$	8.803	0.745		$C_7H_{16}N_2O_2$	8.661	0.734
	$C_7H_3N_4O$	9.177	0.578		$C_7H_{18}N_3O$	9.036	0.566
	$C_7H_{11}O_4$	7.897	1.073		$C_7H_{20}N_4$	9.410	0.399
	$C_7H_{13}NO_3$	8.271	0.902		$C_8H_2NO_3$	9.176	0.974
	$C_7H_{15}N_2O_2$	8.645	0.732		$C_8H_4N_2O_2$	9.550	0.809
	$C_7H_{17}N_3O$	9.020	0.564		$C_8H_6N_3O$	9.924	0.644
	$C_7H_{19}N_4$	9.394	0.397		$C_8H_8N_4$	10.299	0.481
	C_8HNO_3	9.160	0.974		$C_8H_{16}O_3$	9.018	0.961
	$C_8H_3N_2O_2$	9.534	0.807		$C_8H_{18}NO_2$	9.393	0.795
	$C_8H_5N_3O$	9.908	0.642		$C_8H_{20}N_2O$	9.767	0.629
	$C_8H_7N_4$	10.283	0.479		$C_9H_4O_3$	9.907	1.040
	$C_8H_{15}O_3$	9.002	0.960		$C_9H_6NO_2$	10.281	0.876
	$C_8H_{17}NO_2$	9.377	0.793		$C_9H_8N_2O$	10.655	0.714
	$C_8H_{19}N_2O$	9.751	0.628		$C_9H_{10}N_3$	11.030	0.554
	$C_8H_{21}N_3$	10.125	0.464		$C_9H_{20}O_2$	10.124	0.861
	$C_9H_3O_3$	9.891	1.038		$C_{10}H_8O_2$	11.012	0.949
	$C_9H_5NO_2$	10.265	0.875		$C_{10}H_{10}NO$	11.387	0.790
	$C_9H_7N_2O$	10.639	0.713		$C_{10}H_{12}N_2$	11.761	0.632
	$C_9H_9N_3$	11.014	0.552		$C_{11}H_{12}O$	12.118	0.870
	$C_9H_{19}O_2$	10.108	0.859		$C_{11}H_{14}N$	12.492	0.715
	$C_9H_{21}NO$	10.482	0.697		$C_{12}H_2N$	13.381	0.824
	$C_{10}H_7O_2$	10.996	0.947		$C_{12}H_{16}$	13.223	0.804
	$C_{10}H_9NO$	11.371	0.788		$C_{13}H_4$	14.112	0.920
	$C_{10}H_{11}N_2$	11.745	0.630	161	$C_5H_9N_2O_4$	6.466	0.980
	$C_{11}H_{11}O$	12.102	0.869		$C_5H_{11}N_3O_3$	6.841	0.804
	$C_{11}H_{13}N$	12.476	0.713		$C_5H_{13}N_4O_2$	7.215	0.629
	$C_{12}HN$	13.365	0.822		$C_6HN_4O_2$	8.104	0.691
	$C_{12}H_{15}$	13.207	0.802		$C_6H_{11}NO_4$	7.197	1.025

(Contd.)

		M + 1	M + 2
	$C_6H_{13}N_2O_3$	7.572	0.852
	$C_6H_{15}N_3O_2$	7.946	0.679
	$C_6H_{17}N_4O$	8.321	0.509
	$C_7HN_2O_3$	8.460	0.917
	$C_7H_3N_3O_2$	8.835	0.748
	$C_7H_5N_4O$	9.209	0.581
	$C_7H_{13}O_4$	7.929	1.075
	$C_7H_{15}NO_3$	8.303	0.905
	$C_7H_{17}N_2O_2$	8.677	0.735
	$C_7H_{19}N_3O$	9.052	0.567
	C_8HO_4	8.817	1.144
	$C_8H_3NO_3$	9.192	0.976
	$C_8H_5N_2O_2$	9.566	0.810
	$C_8H_7N_3O$	9.940	0.646
	$C_8H_9N_4$	10.315	0.482
	$C_8H_{17}O_3$	9.034	0.963
	$C_8H_{19}NO_2$	9.409	0.796
	$C_9H_5O_3$	9.923	1.041
	$C_9H_7NO_2$	10.297	0.878
	$C_9H_9N_2O$	10.671	0.716
	$C_9H_{11}N_3$	11.046	0.555
	$C_{10}H_9O_2$	11.028	0.951
	$C_{10}H_{11}NO$	11.403	0.791
	$C_{10}H_{13}N_2$	11.777	0.634
	$C_{11}HN_2$	12.666	0.736
	$C_{11}H_{13}O$	12.134	0.872
	$C_{11}H_{15}N$	12.508	0.717
	$C_{12}HO$	13.022	0.978
	$C_{12}H_3N$	13.397	0.827
	$C_{12}H_{17}$	13.239	0.806
	$C_{13}H_5$	14.128	0.922
162	$C_5H_{10}N_2O_4$	6.482	0.981
	$C_5H_{12}N_3O_3$	6.857	0.805
	$C_5H_{14}N_4O_2$	7.231	0.630
	$C_6H_2N_4O_2$	8.120	0.692
	$C_6H_{12}NO_4$	7.213	1.026
	$C_6H_{14}N_2O_3$	7.588	0.853
	$C_6H_{16}N_3O_2$	7.962	0.681
	$C_6H_{18}N_4O$	8.337	0.510
	$C_7H_2N_2O_3$	8.476	0.918
	$C_7H_4N_3O_2$	8.851	0.750
	$C_7H_6N_4O$	9.225	0.582
	$C_7H_{14}O_4$	7.945	1.077
	$C_7H_{16}NO_3$	8.319	0.906
	$C_7H_{18}N_2O_2$	8.693	0.737
	C_8H_2O4	8.833	1.145
	$C_8H_4NO_3$	9.208	0.978
	$C_8H_6N_2O_2$	9.582	0.812
	$C_8H_8N_3O$	9.956	0.647
	$C_8H_{10}N_4$	10.331	0.484
	$C_8H_{18}O_3$	9.050	0.964
	$C_9H_6O_3$	9.939	1.043
	$C_9H_8NO_2$	10.313	0.880
	$C_9H_{10}N_2O$	10.687	0.718
	$C_9H_{12}N_3$	11.062	0.557
	$C_{10}H_{10}O_2$	11.044	0.952
	$C_{10}H_{12}NO$	11.419	0.793
	$C_{10}H_{14}N_2$	11.793	0.636
	$C_{11}H_2N_2$	12.682	0.738
	$C_{11}H_{14}O$	12.150	0.874
	$C_{11}H_{16}N$	12.524	0.719
	$C_{12}H_2O$	13.038	0.980
	$C_{12}H_4N$	13.413	0.829
	$C_{12}H_{18}$	13.255	0.808
	$C_{13}H_6$	14.144	0.924
163	$C_5H_{11}N_2O_4$	6.498	0.982
	$C_5H_{13}N_3O_3$	6.873	0.806
	$C_5H_{15}N_4O_2$	7.247	0.631
	$C_6HN_3O_3$	7.761	0.865
	$C_6H_3N_4O_2$	8.136	0.694
	$C_6H_{13}NO_4$	7.230	1.027
	$C_6H_{15}N_2O_3$	7.604	0.854
	$C_6H_{17}N_3O_2$	7.978	0.682
	C_7HNO_4	8.118	1.090
	$C_7H_3N_2O_3$	8.492	0.920
	$C_7H_5N_3O_2$	8.867	0.751
	$C_7H_7N_4O$	9.241	0.584
	$C_7H_{15}O_4$	7.961	1.078
	$C_7H_{17}NO_3$	8.335	0.907
	$C_8H_3O_4$	8.849	1.147

(Contd.)

		M + 1	M + 2
	$C_8H_5NO_3$	9.224	0.979
	$C_8H_7N_2O_2$	9.598	0.813
	$C_8H_9N_3O$	9.972	0.649
	$C_8H_{11}N_4$	10.347	0.486
	$C_9H_7O_3$	9.955	1.044
	$C_9H_9NO_2$	10.329	0.881
	$C_9H_{11}N_2O$	10.703	0.719
	$C_9H_{13}N_3$	11.078	0.559
	$C_{10}HN_3$	11.966	0.655
	$C_{10}H_{11}O_2$	11.060	0.954
	$C_{10}H_{13}NO$	11.435	0.795
	$C_{10}H_{15}N_2$	11.809	0.637
	$C_{11}HNO$	12.323	0.895
	$C_{11}H_3N_2$	12.698	0.741
	$C_{11}H_{15}O$	12.166	0.876
	$C_{11}H_{17}N$	12.540	0.721
	$C_{12}H_3O$	13.054	0.983
	$C_{12}H_5N$	13.429	0.831
	$C_{12}H_{19}$	13.271	0.811
	$C_{13}H_7$	14.160	0.927
164	$C_5H_{12}N_2O_4$	6.514	0.983
	$C_5H_{14}N_3O_3$	6.889	0.807
	$C_5H_{16}N_4O_2$	7.263	0.633
	$C_6H_2N_3O_3$	7.777	0.867
	$C_6H_4N_4O_2$	8.152	0.695
	$C_6H_{14}NO_4$	7.246	1.029
	$C_6H_{16}N_2O_3$	7.620	0.855
	$C_7H_2NO_4$	8.134	1.091
	$C_7H_4N_2O_3$	8.508	0.921
	$C_7H_6N_3O_2$	8.883	0.752
	$C_7H_8N_4O$	9.257	0.585
	$C_7H_{16}O_4$	7.977	1.079
	$C_8H_4O_4$	8.865	1.148
	$C_8H_6NO_3$	9.240	0.981
	$C_8H_8N_2O_2$	9.614	0.815
	$C_8H_{10}N_3O$	9.988	0.650
	$C_8H_{12}N_4$	10.363	0.487
	$C_9H_8O_3$	9.971	1.046
	$C_9H_{10}NO_2$	10.345	0.883
	$C_9H_{12}N_2O$	10.719	0.721
	$C_9H_{14}Na$	11.094	0.561
	$C_{10}H_2N_3$	11.982	0.657
	$C_{10}H_{12}O_2$	11.076	0.956
	$C_{10}H_{14}NO$	11.451	0.797
	$C_{10}H_{16}N_2$	11.825	0.639
	$C_{11}H_2NO$	12.339	0.897
	$C_{11}H_4N_2$	12.714	0.743
	$C_{11}H_{16}O$	12.182	0.878
	$C_{11}H_{18}N$	12.556	0.723
	$C_{12}H_4O$	13.070	0.985
	$C_{12}H_6N$	13.445	0.833
	$C_{12}H_{20}$	13.287	0.813
	$C_{13}H_8$	14.176	0.929
165	$C_5H_{13}N_2O_4$	6.530	0.985
	$C_5H_{15}N_3O_3$	6.905	0.808
	$C_6HN_2O_4$	7.419	1.041
	$C_6H_3N_3O_3$	7.793	0.868
	$C_6H_5N_4O_2$	8.168	0.697
	$C_6H_{15}NO_4$	7.262	1.030
	$C_7H_3NO_4$	8.150	1.092
	$C_7H_5N_2O_3$	8.524	0.922
	$C_7H_7N_3O_2$	8.899	0.754
	$C_7H_9N_4O$	9.273	0.587
	$C_8H_5O_4$	8.881	1.150
	$C_8H_7NO_3$	9.256	0.982
	$C_8H_9N_2O_2$	9.630	0.817
	$C_8H_{11}N_3O$	10.004	0.652
	$C_8H_{13}N_4$	10.379	0.489
	C_9HN_4	11.267	0.579
	$C_9H_9O_3$	9.987	1.048
	$C_9H_{11}NO_2$	10.361	0.884
	$C_9H_{13}N_2O$	10.735	0.723
	$C_9H_{15}N_3$	11.110	0.562
	$C_{10}HN_2O$	11.624	0.816
	$C_{10}H_3N_3$	11.998	0.659
	$C_{10}H_{13}O_2$	11.092	0.958
	$C_{10}H_{15}NO$	11.467	0.799
	$C_{10}H_{17}N_2$	11.841	0.641
	$C_{11}HO_2$	11.981	1.054
	$C_{11}H_3NO$	12.355	0.899

(Contd.)

		M + 1	M + 2
	$C_{11}H_5N_2$	12.730	0.745
	$C_{11}H_{17}O$	12.198	0.880
	$C_{11}H_{19}N$	12.572	0.725
	$C_{12}H_5O$	13.086	0.987
	$C_{12}H_7N$	13.461	0.835
	$C_{12}H_{21}$	13.303	0.815
	$C_{13}H_9$	14.192	0.931
166	$C_5H_{14}N_2O_4$	6.546	0.986
	$C_6H_2N_2O_4$	7.435	1.042
	$C_6H_4N_3O_3$	7.809	0.869
	$C_6H_6N_4O_2$	8.184	0.698
	$C_7H_4NO_4$	8.166	1.094
	$C_7H_6N_2O_3$	8.540	0.924
	$C_7H_8N_3O_2$	8.915	0.755
	$C_7H_{10}N_4O$	9.289	0.588
	$C_8H_6O_4$	8.897	1.151
	$C_8H_8NO_3$	9.272	0.984
	$C_8H_{10}N_2O_2$	9.646	0.818
	$C_8H_{12}N_3O$	10.020	0.654
	$C_8H_{14}N_4$	10.395	0.491
	$C_9H_2N_4$	11.283	0.581
	$C_9H_{10}O_3$	10.003	1.049
	$C_9H_{12}NO_2$	10.377	0.886
	$C_9H_{14}N_2O$	10.751	0.724
	$C_9H_{16}N_3$	11.126	0.564
	$C_{10}H_2N_2O$	11.640	0.818
	$C_{10}H_4N_3$	12.014	0.661
	$C_{10}H_{14}O_2$	11.108	0.959
	$C_{10}H_{16}NO$	11.483	0.800
	$C_{10}H_{18}N_2$	11.857	0.643
	$C_{11}H_2O_2$	11.997	1.056
	$C_{11}H_4NO$	12.371	0.901
	$C_{11}H_6N_2$	12.746	0.747
	$C_{11}H_{18}O$	12.214	0.882
	$C_{11}H_{20}N$	12.588	0.727
	$C_{12}H_6O$	13.102	0.989
	$C_{12}H_8N$	13.477	0.837
	$C_{12}H_{22}$	13.319	0.817
	$C_{13}H_{10}$	14.208	0.933
167	$C_6H_3N_2O_4$	7.451	1.043
	$C_6H_5N_3O_3$	7.825	0.870
	$C_6H_7N_4O_2$	8.200	0.699
	$C_7H_5NO_4$	8.182	1.095
	$C_7H_7N_2O_3$	8.556	0.925
	$C_7H_9N_3O_2$	8.931	0.757
	$C_7H_{11}N_4O$	9.305	0.590
	$C_8H_7O_4$	8.913	1.152
	$C_8H_9NO_3$	9.288	0.985
	$C_8H_{11}N_2O_2$	9.662	0.820
	$C_8H_{13}N_3O$	10.036	0.655
	$C_8H_{15}N_4$	10.411	0.492
	C_9HN_3O	10.925	0.743
	$C_9H_3N_4$	11.299	0.583
	$C_9H_{11}O_3$	10.019	1.051
	$C_9H_{13}NO_2$	10.393	0.888
	$C_9H_{15}N_2O$	10.767	0.726
	$C_9H_{17}N_3$	11.142	0.566
	$C_{10}HNO_2$	11.282	0.978
	$C_{10}H_3N_2O$	11.656	8.199
	$C_{10}H_5Na$	12.030	0.663
	$C_{10}H_{15}O_2$	11.124	0.961
	$C_{10}H_{17}NO$	11.499	0.802
	$C_{10}H_{19}N_2$	11.873	0.645
	$C_{11}H_3O_2$	12.013	1.058
	$C_{11}H_5NO$	12.387	0.903
	$C_{11}H_7N_2$	12.762	0.749
	$C_{11}H_{19}O$	12.230	0.884
	$C_{11}H_{21}N$	12.604	0.729
	$C_{12}H_7O$	13.118	0.991
	$C_{12}H_9N$	13.493	0.840
	$C_{12}H_{23}$	13.335	0.819
	$C_{13}H_{11}$	14.224	0.936
168	$C_6H_4N_2O_4$	7.467	1.044
	$C_6H_6N_3O_3$	7.841	0.872
	$C_8H_8N_4O_2$	8.216	0.700
	$C_7H_6NO_4$	8.198	1.096
	$C_7H_8N_2O_3$	8.572	0.927
	$C_7H_{10}N_3O_2$	8.947	0.758
	$C_7H_{12}N_4O$	9.321	0.591
	$C_8H_8O_4$	8.929	1.154

(Contd.)

		M + 1	M + 2
	$C_8H_{10}NO_3$	9.304	9.868
	$C_8H_{12}N_2O_2$	9.678	0.821
	$C_8H_{14}N_3O$	10.052	0.657
	$C_8H_{16}N_4$	10.427	0.494
	$C_9H_2N_3O$	10.941	0.744
	$C_9H_4N_4$	11.315	0.585
	$C_9H_{12}O_3$	10.035	1.052
	$C_9H_{14}NO_2$	10.409	0.889
	$C_9H_{16}N_2O$	10.783	0.728
	$C_9H_{18}N_3$	11.158	0.568
	$C_{10}H_2NO_2$	11.298	0.980
	$C_{10}H_4N_2O$	11.672	0.822
	$C_{10}H_6N_3$	12.046	0.665
	$C_{10}H_{16}O_2$	11.140	0.963
	$C_{10}H_{18}NO$	11.515	0.804
	$C_{10}H_{20}N_2$	11.889	0.647
	$C_{11}H_4O_2$	12.029	1.060
	$C_{11}H_6NO$	12.403	0.905
	$C_{11}H_8N_2$	12.778	0.751
	$C_{11}H_{20}O$	12.246	0.886
	$C_{11}H_{22}N$	12.620	0.731
	$C_{12}H_8O$	13.134	0.993
	$C_{12}H_{10}N$	13.509	0.842
	$C_{12}H_{24}$	13.351	0.821
	$C_{13}H_{12}$	14.240	0.938
169	$C_6H_5N_2O_4$	7.483	1.045
	$C_6H_7N_3O_3$	7.857	0.873
	$C_6H_9N_4O_2$	8.232	0.702
	$C_7H_7NO_4$	8.214	1.098
	$C_7H_9N_2O_3$	8.588	9.279
	$C_7H_{11}N_3O_2$	8.963	0.760
	$C_7H_{13}N_4O$	9.337	0.593
	C_8HN_4O	10.226	0.674
	$C_8H_9O_4$	8.945	1.155
	$C_8H_{11}NO_3$	9.320	0.988
	$C_8H_{13}N_2O_2$	9.694	0.823
	$C_8H_{15}N_3O$	10.068	0.658
	$C_8H_{17}N_4$	10.443	0.496
	$C_9HN_2O_2$	10.582	0.907
	$C_9H_3N_3O$	10.957	0.746
	$C_9H_5N_4$	11.331	0.587
	$C_9H_{13}O_3$	10.051	1.054
	$C_9H_{15}NO_2$	10.425	0.891
	$C_9H_{17}N_2O$	10.799	0.730
	$C_9H_{19}N_3$	11.174	0.570
	$C_{10}HO_3$	10.939	1.141
	$C_{10}H_3NO_2$	11.314	0.982
	$C_{10}H_5N_2O$	11.688	0.824
	$C_{10}H_7N_3$	12.062	0.667
	$C_{10}H_{17}O_2$	11.156	0.965
	$C_{10}H_{19}NO$	11.531	0.806
	$C_{10}H_{21}N_2$	11.905	0.649
	$C_{11}H_5O_2$	12.045	1.062
	$C_{11}H_7NO$	12.419	0.907
	$C_{11}H_9N_2$	12.794	0.753
	$C_{11}H_{21}O$	12.262	0.888
	$C_{11}H_{23}N$	12.636	0.733
	$C_{12}H_9O$	13.150	0.995
	$C_{12}H_{11}N$	13.525	0.844
	$C_{12}H_{25}$	13.367	0.823
	$C_{13}H_{13}$	14.256	0.940
	$C_{14}H$	15.144	1.065
170	$C_6H_6N_2O_4$	7.499	1.046
	$C_6H_8N_3O_3$	7.873	0.874
	$C_6H_{10}N_4O_2$	8.248	0.703
	$C_7H_8NO_4$	8.230	1.099
	$C_7H_{10}N_2O_3$	8.604	0.929
	$C_7H_{12}N_3O_2$	8.979	0.761
	$C_7H_{14}N_4O$	9.353	0.594
	$C_8H_2N_4O$	10.242	0.675
	$C_8H_{10}O_4$	8.961	1.157
	$C_8H_{12}NO_3$	9.336	0.990
	$C_8H_{14}N_2O_2$	9.710	0.824
	$C_8H_{16}N_3O$	10.084	0.660
	$C_8H_{18}N_4$	10.459	0.497
	$C_9H_2N_2O_2$	10.598	0.909
	$C_9H_4N_3O$	10.973	0.748
	$C_9H_6N_4$	11.347	0.588
	$C_9H_{14}O_3$	10.067	1.056
	$C_9H_{16}NO_2$	10.441	0.893

(Contd.)

		M + 1	M + 2			M + 1	M + 2
	$C_9H_{18}N_2O$	10.815	0.731		$C_9H_{21}N_3$	11.206	0.573
	$C_9H_{20}N_3$	11.190	0.571		$C_{10}H_3O_3$	10.971	1.145
	$C_{10}H_2O_3$	10.955	1.143		$C_{10}H_5NO_2$	11.346	9.855
	$C_{10}H_4NO_2$	11.330	0.984		$C_{10}H_7N_2O$	11.720	0.827
	$C_{10}H_6N_2O$	11.704	0.826		$C_{10}H_9N_3$	12.094	0.671
	$C_{10}H_8N_3$	12.078	0.669		$C_{10}H_{19}O_2$	11.188	0.968
	$C_{10}H_{18}O_2$	11.172	0.967		$C_{10}H_{21}NO$	11.563	0.810
	$C_{10}H_{20}NO$	11.547	0.808		$C_{10}H_{23}N_2$	11.937	0.653
	$C_{10}H_{22}N_2$	11.921	0.651		$C_{11}H_7O_2$	12.077	1.066
	$C_{11}H_6O_2$	12.061	1.064		$C_{11}H_9NO$	12.451	0.911
	$C_{11}H_8NO$	12.435	0.909		$C_{11}H_{11}N_2$	12.826	0.757
	$C_{11}H_{10}N_2$	12.810	0.755		$C_{11}H_{23}O$	12.294	0.892
	$C_{11}H_{22}O$	12.278	0.890		$C_{11}H_{25}N$	12.668	0.737
	$C_{11}H_{24}N$	12.652	0.735		$C_{12}H_{11}O$	13.182	1.000
	$C_{12}H_{10}O$	13.166	0.997		$C_{12}H_{13}N$	13.557	0.848
	$C_{12}H_{12}N$	13.541	0.846		$C_{13}HN$	14.445	0.967
	$C_{12}H_{26}$	13.383	0.826		$C_{13}H_{15}$	14.288	0.945
	$C_{13}H_{14}$	14.272	0.942		$C_{14}H_3$	15.176	1.070
	$C_{14}H_2$	15.160	1.068	172	$C_6H_8N_2O_4$	7.531	1.049
171	$C_6H_7N_2O_4$	7.515	1.048		$C_9H_{10}N_3O_3$	7.905	0.877
	$C_6H_9N_3O_3$	7.889	0.875		$C_6H_{12}N_4O_2$	8.280	0.706
	$C_6H_{11}N_4O_2$	8.264	0.704		$C_7H_{10}NO_4$	8.262	1.102
	$C_7H_9NO_4$	8.246	1.100		$C_7H_{12}N_2O_3$	8.636	0.932
	$C_7H_{11}N_2O_3$	8.620	0.931		$C_7H_{14}N_3O_2$	9.011	0.764
	$C_7H_{13}N_3O_2$	8.995	0.762		$C_7H_{16}N_4O$	9.385	5.971
	$C_7H_{15}N_4O$	9.369	0.596		$C_8H_2N_3O_2$	9.899	0.842
	$C_8HN_3O_2$	9.883	0.841		$C_8H_4N_4O$	10.274	0.679
	$C_8H_3N_4O$	10.258	0.677		$C_8H_{12}O_4$	8.993	1.160
	$C_8H_{11}O_4$	8.977	1.158		$C_8H_{14}NO_3$	9.368	0.993
	$C_8H_{13}NO_3$	9.352	0.991		$C_8H_{16}N_2O_2$	9.742	0.827
	$C_8H_{15}N_2O_2$	9.726	0.826		$C_8H_{18}N_3O$	10.116	6.633
	$C_8H_{17}N_3O$	10.100	0.662		$C_8H_{20}N_4$	10.491	0.501
	$C_8H_{19}N_4$	10.475	0.499		$C_9H_2NO_3$	10.256	1.074
	C_9HNO_3	10.240	1.072		$C_9H_4N_2O_2$	10.630	0.912
	$C_9H_3N_2O_2$	10.614	0.910		$C_9H_6N_3O$	11.005	0.751
	$C_9H_5N_3O$	10.989	0.750		$C_9H_8N_4$	11.379	0.592
	$C_9H_7N_4$	11.363	0.590		$C_9H_{16}O_3$	10.099	1.058
	$C_9H_{15}O_3$	10.083	1.057		$C_9H_{18}NO_2$	10.473	0.896
	$C_9H_{17}NO_2$	10.457	0.894		$C_9H_{20}N_2O$	10.847	0.734
	$C_9H_{19}N_2O$	10.831	0.733		$C_9H_{22}N_3$	11.222	0.575

(Contd.)

		M + 1	M + 2			M + 1	M + 2
	$C_{10}H_4O_3$	10.987	1.147		$C_9H_{23}N_3$	11.238	0.577
	$C_{10}H_6NO_2$	11.362	0.987		$C_{10}H_5O_3$	11.003	1.148
	$C_{10}H_8N_2O$	11.736	0.829		$C_{10}H_7NO_2$	11.378	0.989
	$C_{10}H_{10}N_3$	12.110	0.673		$C_{10}H_9N_2O$	11.752	0.831
	$C_{10}H_{20}O_2$	11.204	0.970		$C_{10}H_{11}N_3$	12.126	0.675
	$C_{10}H_{22}NO$	11.579	0.812		$C_{10}H_{21}O_2$	11.220	0.972
	$C_{10}H_{24}N_2$	11.953	0.655		$C_{10}H_{23}NO$	11.595	0.814
	$C_{11}H_8O_2$	12.093	1.068		$C_{11}H_9O_2$	12.109	1.070
	$C_{11}H_{10}NO$	12.467	0.913		$C_{11}H_{11}NO$	12.483	0.915
	$C_{11}H_{12}N_2$	12.842	0.759		$C_{11}H_{13}N_2$	12.858	0.761
	$C_{11}H_{24}O$	12.310	0.894		$C_{12}HN_2$	13.746	0.873
	$C_{12}H_{12}O$	13.198	1.001		$C_{12}H_{13}O$	13.214	1.000
	$C_{12}H_{14}N$	13.573	0.850		$C_{12}H_{15}N$	13.589	0.852
	$C_{13}H_2N$	14.461	0.969		$C_{13}HO$	14.103	1.119
	$C_{13}H_{16}$	14.304	0.947		$C_{13}H_3N$	14.477	0.971
	$C_{14}H_4$	15.192	1.072		$C_{13}H_{17}$	14.320	0.949
173	$C_6H_9N_2O_4$	7.547	1.050		$C_{14}H_5$	15.208	1.075
	$C_6H_{11}N_3O_3$	7.921	0.878	174	$C_6H_{10}N_2O_4$	7.563	1.051
	$C_6H_{13}N_4O_2$	8.296	0.707		$C_6H_{12}N_3O_3$	7.937	0.879
	$C_7HN_4O_2$	9.184	0.779		$C_6H_{14}N_4O_2$	8.312	0.708
	$C_7H_{11}NO_4$	8.278	1.103		$C_7H_2N_4O_2$	9.200	0.780
	$C_7H_{13}N_2O_3$	8.652	0.933		$C_7H_{12}NO_4$	8.294	1.104
	$C_7H_{15}N_3O_2$	9.027	0.765		$C_7H_{14}N_2O_3$	8.668	0.935
	$C_7H_{17}N_4O$	9.401	0.599		$C_7H_{16}N_3O_2$	9.043	0.767
	$C_8HN_2O_3$	9.541	1.008		$C_7H_{18}N_4O$	9.417	0.600
	$C_8H_3N_3O_2$	9.915	8.436		$C_8H_2N_2O_3$	9.557	1.010
	$C_8H_5N_4O$	10.290	0.680		$C_8H_4N_3O_2$	9.931	0.845
	$C_8H_{13}O_4$	9.009	1.161		$C_8H_6N_4O$	10.306	0.682
	$C_8H_{15}NO_3$	9.384	0.994		$C_8H_{14}O_4$	9.025	1.162
	$C_8H_{17}N_2O_2$	9.758	0.829		$C_8H_{16}NO_3$	9.400	9.957
	$C_8H_{19}N_3O$	10.132	0.665		$C_8H_{18}N_2O_2$	9.774	0.830
	$C_8H_{21}N_4$	10.507	0.502		$C_8H_{20}N_3O$	10.148	0.667
	C_9HO_4	9.898	1.239		$C_8H_{22}N_4$	10.523	0.504
	$C_9H_3NO_3$	10.272	1.076		$C_9H_2O_4$	9.914	1.241
	$C_9H_5N_2O_2$	10.647	0.914		$C_9H_4NO_3$	10.288	1.077
	$C_9H_7N_3O$	11.021	0.753		$C_9H_6N_2O_2$	10.663	0.915
	$C_9H_9N_4$	11.395	0.594		$C_9H_8N_3O$	11.037	0.755
	$C_9H_{17}O_3$	10.115	1.060		$C_9H_{10}N_4$	11.411	0.596
	$C_9H_{19}NO_2$	10.489	0.898		$C_9H_{18}O_3$	10.131	1.062
	$C_9H_{21}N_2O$	10.863	0.737		$C_9H_{20}NO_2$	10.505	0.899

(Contd.)

		M + 1	M + 2			M + 1	M + 2
	$C_9H_{22}N_2O$	10.879	0.738		$C_{10}H_7O_3$	11.035	1.151
	$C_{10}H_6O_3$	11.019	1.150		$C_{10}H_9NO_2$	11.410	0.993
	$C_{10}H_8NO_2$	11.394	0.991		$C_{10}H_{11}N_2O$	11.784	0.835
	$C_{10}H_{10}N_2O$	11.768	0.833		$C_{10}H_{13}N_3$	12.158	0.679
	$C_{10}H_{12}N_3$	12.142	0.677		$C_{11}HN_3$	13.047	0.785
	$C_{10}H_{22}O_2$	11.236	0.974		$C_{11}H_{11}O_2$	12.141	1.073
	$C_{11}H_{10}O_2$	12.125	1.072		$C_{11}H_{13}NO$	12.515	0.919
	$C_{11}H_{12}NO$	12.449	0.917		$C_{11}H_{15}N_2$	12.890	7.650
	$C_{11}H_{14}N_2$	12.874	0.763		$C_{12}HNO$	13.404	1.028
	$C_{12}H_2N_2$	13.762	0.876		$C_{12}H_3N_2$	13.778	0.878
	$C_{12}H_{14}O$	13.230	1.006		$C_{12}H_{15}O$	13.246	1.008
	$C_{12}H_{16}N$	13.605	0.855		$C_{12}H_{17}N$	13.621	0.857
	$C_{13}H_2O$	14.119	1.121		$C_{13}H_3O$	14.135	1.124
	$C_{13}H_4N$	14.493	0.974		$C_{13}H_5N$	14.509	0.976
	$C_{13}H_{18}$	14.336	0.952		$C_{13}H_{19}$	14.352	0.954
	$C_{14}H_6$	15.224	1.077		$C_{14}H_7$	15.240	1.080
175	$C_6H_{11}N_2O_4$	7.579	1.052	176	$C_6H_{12}N_2O_4$	7.595	1.054
	$C_6H_{13}N_3O_3$	7.953	0.881		$C_6H_{14}N_3O_3$	7.969	0.882
	$C_6H_{15}N_4O_2$	8.328	0.710		$C_6H_{16}N_4O_2$	8.344	0.711
	$C_7HN_3O_3$	8.842	0.949		$C_7H_2N_3O_3$	8.858	0.951
	$C_7H_3N_4O_2$	9.216	0.782		$C_7H_4N_4O_2$	9.232	0.783
	$C_7H_{13}NO_4$	8.310	1.106		$C_7H_{14}NO_4$	8.326	1.107
	$C_7H_{15}N_2O_3$	8.684	0.936		$C_7H_{16}N_2O_3$	8.700	0.938
	$C_7H_{17}N_3O_2$	9.059	0.768		$C_7H_{18}N_3O_2$	9.075	0.770
	$C_7H_{19}N_4O$	9.432	0.602		$C_7H_{20}N_4O$	9.449	0.603
	C_8HNO_4	9.199	1.178		$C_8H_2NO_4$	9.215	1.179
	$C_8H_3N_2O_3$	9.573	1.012		$C_8H_4N_2O_3$	9.589	1.013
	$C_8H_5N_3O_2$	9.947	0.847		$C_8H_6N_3O_2$	9.963	0.848
	$C_8H_7N_4O$	10.322	0.684		$C_8H_8N_4O$	10.338	0.685
	$C_8H_{17}NO_3$	9.416	0.997		$C_8H_{16}O_4$	9.057	1.165
	$C_8H_{19}N_2O_2$	9.790	0.832		$C_8H_{18}NO_3$	9.432	0.999
	$C_8H_{21}N_3O$	10.164	0.668		$C_8H_{20}N_2O_2$	9.806	0.834
	$C_8H_{15}O_4$	9.041	1.164		$C_9H_4O_4$	9.946	1.244
	$C_9H_3O_4$	9.930	1.242		$C_9H_6NO_3$	10.320	1.081
	$C_9H_5NO_3$	10.304	1.079		$C_9H_8N_2O_2$	10.695	0.919
	$C_9H_7N_2O_2$	10.679	0.917		$C_9H_{10}N_3O$	11.069	0.758
	$C_9H_9N_3O$	11.053	7.566		$C_9H_{12}N_4$	11.443	0.599
	$C_9H_{11}N_4$	11.427	0.597		$C_9H_{20}O_3$	10.163	1.065
	$C_9H_{19}O_3$	10.147	1.064		$C_{10}H_8O_3$	11.051	1.154
	$C_9H_{21}NO_2$	10.521	0.901		$C_{10}H_{10}NO_2$	11.426	0.995

(Contd.)

		M + 1	M + 2			M + 1	M + 2
	$C_{10}H_{12}N_2O$	11.800	0.837		$C_{11}H_3N_3$	13.079	0.789
	$C_{10}H_{14}N_3$	12.174	0.681		$C_{11}H_{13}O_2$	12.173	1.078
	$C_{11}H_2N_3$	13.063	0.787		$C_{11}H_{15}NO$	12.547	0.923
	$C_{11}H_{12}O_2$	12.157	1.076		$C_{11}H_{17}N_2$	12.922	0.769
	$C_{11}H_{14}NO$	12.531	0.921		$C_{12}HO_2$	13.061	1.184
	$C_{11}H_{16}N_2$	12.906	0.767		$C_{12}H_3NO$	13.436	1.032
	$C_{12}H_2NO$	13.420	1.030		$C_{12}H_5N_2$	13.810	0.882
	$C_{12}H_4N_2$	13.794	0.880		$C_{12}H_{17}O$	13.278	1.012
	$C_{12}H_{16}O$	13.262	1.010		$C_{12}H_{19}N$	13.653	0.861
	$C_{12}H_{18}N$	13.637	0.859		$C_{13}H_5O$	14.167	1.128
	$C_{18}H_4O$	14.151	1.126		$C_{13}H_7N$	14.541	0.981
	$C_{13}H_6N$	14.525	0.978		$C_{13}H_{21}$	14.384	0.959
	$C_{13}H_{20}$	14.368	0.956		$C_{14}H_9$	15.272	1.085
	$C_{14}H_8$	15.256	1.082	178	$C_6H_{14}N_2O_4$	7.627	1.056
177	$C_6H_{13}N_2O_4$	7.611	1.055		$C_6H_{16}N_3O_3$	8.001	0.884
	$C_6H_{15}N_3O_3$	7.985	0.883		$C_6H_{18}N_4O_2$	8.376	0.714
	$C_6H_{17}N_4O_2$	8.360	0.712		$C_7H_2N_2O_4$	8.516	1.122
	$C_7HN_2O_4$	8.500	1.121		$C_7H_4N_3O_3$	8.890	0.054
	$C_7H_3N_3O_3$	8.874	0.952		$C_7H_6N_4O_2$	9.264	0.786
	$C_7H_5N_4O_2$	9.248	0.785		$C_7H_{16}NO_4$	8.358	1.110
	$C_7H_{15}NO_4$	8.342	1.108		$C_7H_{18}N_2O_3$	8.732	0.940
	$C_7H_{17}N_2O_3$	8.716	0.939		$C_8H_4NO_4$	9.247	1.182
	$C_7H_{19}N_3O_2$	9.091	0.771		$C_8H_6N_2O_3$	9.621	1.016
	$C_8H_3NO_4$	9.231	1:181		$C_8H_8N_3O_2$	9.995	0.852
	$C_8H_5N_2O_3$	9.605	1.014		$C_8H_{10}N_4O$	10.370	0.689
	$C_8H_7N_3O_2$	9.979	0.850		$C_8H_{18}O_4$	9.089	1.168
	$C_8H_9N_4O$	10.354	0.687		$C_9H_6O_4$	9.978	1.247
	$C_8H_{17}O_4$	9.073	1.166		$C_9H_8NO_3$	10.352	1.084
	$C_8H_{19}NO_3$	9.448	1.000		$C_9H_{10}N_2O_2$	10.727	0.922
	$C_9H_5O_4$	9.962	1.246		$C_9H_{12}N_3O$	11.101	0.762
	$C_9H_7NO_3$	10.336	1.082		$C_9H_{14}N_4$	11.475	0.603
	$C_9H_9N_2O_2$	10.711	0.921		$C_{10}H_2N_4$	12.364	0.703
	$C_9H_{11}N_3O$	11.085	0.760		$C_{10}H_{10}O_3$	11.083	1.157
	$C_9H_{13}N_4$	11.459	0.601		$C_{10}H_{12}NO_2$	11.458	0.998
	$C_{10}HN_4$	12.348	0.701		$C_{10}H_{14}N_2O$	11.832	0.841
	$C_{10}H_9O_3$	11.067	1.155		$C_{10}H_{16}N_3$	12.206	0.684
	$C_{10}H_{11}NO_2$	11.442	0.996		$C_{11}H_2N_2O$	12.721	0.944
	$C_{10}H_{13}N_2O$	11.816	0.839		$C_{11}H_4N_3$	13.095	0.791
	$C_{10}H_{15}N_3$	12.190	0.682		$C_{11}H_{14}O_2$	12.189	1.080
	$C_{11}HN_2O$	12.705	0.942		$C_{11}H_{16}NO$	12.563	0.925

(Contd.)

		M + 1	M + 2			M + 1	M + 2
	$C_{11}H_{18}N_2$	12.938	0.771		$C_{12}H_{19}O$	13.310	1.016
	$C_{12}H_2O_2$	13.077	1.186		$C_{12}H_{21}N$	13.685	8.655
	$C_{12}H_4NO$	13.452	1.034		$C_{13}H_7O$	14.199	1.133
	$C_{12}H_6N_2$	13.826	0.884		$C_{13}H_9N$	14.573	0.985
	$C_{12}H_{18}O$	13.294	1.014		$C_{13}H_{23}$	14.416	0.963
	$C_{12}H_{20}N$	13.669	0.863		$C_{14}H_{11}$	15.304	1.089
	$C_{13}H_6O$	14.183	1.130	180	$C_6H_{16}N_2O_4$	7.659	1.059
	$C_{13}H_8N$	14.557	0.983		$C_7H_4N_2O_4$	8.548	1.125
	$C_{13}H_{22}$	14.400	0.961		$C_7H_6N_3O_3$	8.922	0.956
	$C_{14}H_{10}$	15.288	1.087		$C_7H_8N_4O_2$	9.296	0.789
179	$C_6H_{15}N_2O_4$	7.643	1.058		$C_8H_6NO_4$	9.279	1.185
	$C_6H_{17}N_3O_3$	8.017	0.886		$C_8H_8N_2O_3$	9.653	1.019
	$C_7H_3N_2O_4$	8.532	1.124		$C_8H_{10}N_3O_2$	10.027	0.855
	$C_7H_5N_3O_3$	8.906	0.955		$C_8H_{12}N_4O$	10.402	0.692
	$C_7H_7N_4O_2$	9.280	0.788		$C_9H_8O_4$	10.010	1.250
	$C_7H_{17}NO_4$	8.374	1.111		$C_9H_{10}NO_3$	10.384	1.087
	$C_8H_5NO_4$	9.263	1.183		$C_9H_{12}N_2O_2$	10.759	0.926
	$C_8H_7N_2O_3$	9.637	1.018		$C_9H_{14}N_3O$	11.133	0.765
	$C_8H_9N_3O_2$	10.011	0.853		$C_9H_{16}N_4$	11.507	0.607
	$C_8H_{11}N_4O$	10.386	0.690		$C_{10}H_2N_3O$	12.021	0.863
	$C_9H_7O_4$	9.994	1.249		$C_{10}H_4N_4$	12.396	0.707
	$C_9H_9NO_3$	10.368	1.086		$C_{10}H_{12}O_3$	11.115	1.161
	$C_9H_{11}N_2O_2$	10.743	0.924		$C_{10}H_{14}NO_2$	11.490	1.002
	$C_9H_{13}N_3O$	11.117	0.764		$C_{10}H_{16}N_2O$	11.864	0.844
	$C_9H_{15}N_4$	11.491	0.605		$C_{10}H_{18}N_3$	12.238	0.688
	$C_{10}HN_3O$	12.005	0.861		$C_{11}H_2NO_2$	12.378	1.102
	$C_{10}H_3N_4$	12.380	0.705		$C_{11}H_4N_2O$	12.753	0.948
	$C_{10}H_{11}O_3$	11.099	1.159		$C_{11}H_6N_3$	13.127	0.795
	$C_{10}H_{13}NO_2$	11.474	1.000		$C_{11}H_{16}O_2$	12.221	1.083
	$C_{10}H_{15}N_2O$	11.848	0.843		$C_{11}H_{18}NO$	12.595	0.929
	$C_{10}H_{17}N_3$	12.222	0.686		$C_{11}H_{20}N_2$	12.970	0.775
	$C_{11}HNO_2$	12.362	1.001		$C_{12}H_4O_2$	13.109	1.190
	$C_{11}H_3N_2O$	12.737	0.946		$C_{12}H_6NO$	13.484	1.039
	$C_{11}H_5N_3$	13.111	0.793		$C_{12}H_8N_2$	13.858	0.889
	$C_{11}H_{15}O_2$	12.205	1.082		$C_{12}H_{20}O$	13.326	1.018
	$C_{11}H_{17}NO$	12.579	0.927		$C_{12}H_{22}N$	13.701	0.868
	$C_{11}H_{19}N_2$	12.954	0.773		$C_{13}H_8O$	14.215	1.135
	$C_{12}H_3O_2$	13.093	1.188		$C_{13}H_{10}N$	14.589	0.988
	$C_{12}H_5NO$	13.468	1.036		$C_{13}H_{24}$	14.432	0.966
	$C_{12}H_7N_2$	13.842	0.887		$C_{14}H_{12}$	15.321	1.092

(Contd.)

		M + 1	M + 2			M + 1	M + 2
181	$C_7H_5N_2O_4$	8.564	1.126		$C_8H_8NO_4$	9.311	1.188
	$C_7H_7N_3O_3$	8.938	0.958		$C_8H_{10}N_2O_3$	9.685	1.022
	$C_7H_9N_4O_2$	9.312	0.791		$C_8H_{12}N_3O_2$	10.059	0.858
	$C_8H_7NO_4$	9.295	1.186		$C_8H_{14}N_4O$	10.434	0.695
	$C_8H_9N_2O_3$	9.669	1.021		$C_8H_2N_4O$	11.322	0.786
	$C_8H_{11}N_3O_2$	10.043	0.856		$C_9H_{10}O_4$	10.042	1.254
	$C_8H_{13}N_4O$	10.418	0.694		$C_9H_{12}NO_3$	10.416	1.091
	C_9HN_4O	11.306	0.784		$C_9H_{14}N_2O_2$	10.791	0.929
	$C_9H_9O_4$	10.026	1.252		$C_9H_{16}N_3O$	11.165	0.769
	$C_9H_{11}NO_3$	10.400	1.089		$C_9H_{18}N_4$	11.539	0.610
	$C_9H_{13}N_2O_2$	10.775	0.927		$C_{10}H_2N_2O_2$	11.679	1.023
	$C_9H_{15}N_3O$	11.149	0.767		$C_{10}H_4N_3O$	12.053	0.866
	$C_9H_{17}N_4$	11.523	0.609		$C_{10}H_6N_4$	12.428	0.711
	$C_{10}HN_2O_2$	11.663	1.021		$C_{10}H_{14}O_3$	11.147	1.164
	$C_{10}H_3N_3O$	12.037	0.864		$C_{10}H_{16}NO_2$	11.522	1.006
	$C_{10}H_5N_4$	12.412	0.709		$C_{10}H_{18}N_2O$	11.896	0.848
	$C_{10}H_{13}O_3$	11.131	1.163		$C_{10}H_{20}N_3$	12.270	0.692
	$C_{10}H_{15}NO_2$	11.506	1.004		$C_{11}H_2O_3$	12.036	1.262
	$C_{10}H_{17}N_2O$	11.880	0.846		$C_{11}H_4NO_2$	12.410	1.106
	$C_{10}H_{19}N_3$	12.254	0.690		$C_{11}H_6N_2O$	12.785	0.952
	$C_{11}HO_3$	12.020	1.260		$C_{11}H_8N_3$	13.159	0.799
	$C_{11}H_3NO_2$	12.394	1.104		$C_{11}H_{18}O_2$	12.253	1.087
	$C_{11}H_5N_2O$	12.769	0.950		$C_{11}H_{20}NO$	12.627	0.933
	$C_{11}H_7N_3$	13.143	0.797		$C_{11}H_{22}N_2$	13.002	0.780
	$C_{11}H_{17}O_2$	12.237	1.085		$C_{12}H_6O_2$	13.141	1.194
	$C_{11}H_{19}NO$	12.611	0.931		$C_{12}H_8NO$	13.516	1.043
	$C_{11}H_{21}N_2$	12.986	0.777		$C_{12}H_{10}N_2$	13.890	0.893
	$C_{12}H_5O_2$	13.125	1.192		$C_{12}H_{22}O$	13.358	1.023
	$C_{12}H_7NO$	13.500	1.041		$C_{12}H_{24}N$	13.733	0.872
	$C_{12}H_9N_2$	13.874	0.891		$C_{13}H_{10}O$	14.247	1.139
	$C_{12}H_{21}O$	13.342	1.021		$C_{13}H_{18}N$	14.621	0.992
	$C_{12}H_{23}N$	13.717	0.870		$C_{13}H_{26}$	14.464	0.970
	$C_{13}H_9O$	14.231	1.137		$C_{14}H_{14}$	15.353	1.097
	$C_{13}H_{11}N$	14.605	0.990		$C_{15}H_2$	16.241	1.213
	$C_{13}H_{25}$	14.448	0.968	183	$C_7H_7N_2O_4$	8.596	1.129
	$C_{14}H_{13}$	15.337	1.094		$C_7H_8N_3O_3$	8.970	0.961
	$C_{15}H$	16.225	1.229		$C_7H_{11}N_4O_2$	9.344	0.794
182	$C_7H_6N_2O_4$	8.580	1.127		$C_8H_9NO_4$	9.327	1.189
	$C_7H_8N_3O_3$	8.954	0.959		$C_8H_{11}N_2O_3$	9.701	1.024
	$C_7H_{10}N_4O_2$	9.328	0.792		$C_8H_{13}N_3O_2$	10.075	0.860

(Contd.)

		M + 1	M + 2			M + 1	M + 2
	$C_8H_{15}N_4O$	10.450	0.697		$C_8H_{16}N_4O$	10.466	0.699
	$C_9HN_3O_2$	10.964	0.947		$C_9H_2N_3O_2$	10.980	0.949
	$C_9H_3N_4O$	11.338	0.788		$C_9H_4N_4O$	11.354	0.790
	$C_9H_{11}O_4$	10.058	1.255		$C_9H_{12}O_4$	10.074	1.257
	$C_9H_{13}NO_3$	10.432	1.092		$C_9H_{14}NO_3$	10.448	1.094
	$C_9H_{15}N_2O_2$	10.807	0.931		$C_9H_{16}N_2O_2$	10.823	0.933
	$C_9H_{17}N_3O$	11.181	0.771		$C_9H_{18}N_3O$	11.197	0.773
	$C_9H_{19}N_4$	11.555	0.612		$C_9H_{20}N_4$	11.571	0.614
	$C_{10}HNO_3$	11.321	1.183		$C_{10}H_2NO_3$	11.337	1.184
	$C_{10}H_3N_2O_2$	11.695	1.025		$C_{10}H_4N_2O_2$	11.711	1.027
	$C_{10}H_5N_3O$	12.069	0.868		$C_{10}H_6N_3O$	12.085	0.870
	$C_{10}H_7N_4$	12.444	0.713		$C_{10}H_8N_4$	12.460	0.715
	$C_{10}H_{15}O_3$	11.163	1.166		$C_{10}H_{16}O_3$	11.179	1.168
	$C_{10}H_{17}NO_2$	11.538	1.007		$C_{10}H_{18}NO_2$	11.554	1.009
	$C_{10}H_{19}N_2O$	11.912	0.850		$C_{10}H_{20}N_2O$	11.928	0.852
	$C_{10}H_{21}N_3$	12.286	0.694		$C_{10}H_{22}N_3$	12.302	0.696
	$C_{11}H_3O_3$	12.052	1.263		$C_{11}H_4O_3$	12.068	1.265
	$C_{11}H_5NO_2$	12.426	1.108		$C_{11}H_6NO_2$	12.442	1.110
	$C_{11}H_7N_2O$	12.801	0.954		$C_{11}H_8N_2O$	12.817	0.956
	$C_{11}H_9N_3$	13.175	0.802		$C_{11}H_{10}N_3$	13.191	0.804
	$C_{11}H_{19}O_2$	12.269	1.089		$C_{11}H_{20}O_2$	12.285	1.091
	$C_{11}H_{21}NO$	12.643	0.935		$C_{11}H_{22}NO$	12.659	0.937
	$C_{11}H_{23}N_2$	13.018	0.782		$C_{11}H_{24}N_2$	13.034	0.784
	$C_{12}H_7O_2$	13.157	1.197		$C_{12}H_8O_2$	13.173	1.199
	$C_{12}H_9NO$	13.532	1.045		$C_{12}H_{10}NO$	13.548	1.047
	$C_{12}H_{11}N_2$	13.906	0.895		$C_{12}H_{12}N_2$	13.922	0.898
	$C_{12}H_{23}O$	13.374	1.025		$C_{12}H_{24}O$	13.390	1.027
	$C_{12}H_{25}N$	13.749	0.874		$C_{12}H_{26}N$	13.765	0.877
	$C_{13}H_{11}O$	14.263	1.142		$C_{13}H_{12}O$	14.279	1.144
	$C_{13}H_{13}N$	14.637	0.995		$C_{13}H_{14}N$	14.653	0.997
	$C_{13}H_{27}$	14.480	0.972		$C_{13}H_{28}$	14.496	0.975
	$C_{14}HN$	15.526	1.123		$C_{14}H_2N$	15.542	1.125
	$C_{14}H_{15}$	15.369	1.099		$C_{14}H_{16}$	15.384	1.102
	$C_{15}H_3$	16.257	1.234		$C_{15}H_4$	16.273	1.237
184	$C_7H_8N_2O_4$	8.612	1.130	185	$C_7H_9N_2O_4$	8.628	1.132
	$C_7H_{10}N_3O_3$	8.986	0.962		$C_7H_{11}N_3O_3$	9.002	0.964
	$C_7H_{12}N_4O_2$	9.360	0.795		$C_7H_{13}N_4O_2$	9.376	0.797
	$C_8H_{10}NO_4$	9.343	1.191		$C_8HN_4O_2$	10.265	0.878
	$C_8H_{12}N_2O_3$	9.717	1.025		$C_8H_{11}NO_4$	9.359	1.192
	$C_8H_{14}N_3O_2$	10.091	0.861		$C_8H_{13}N_2O_3$	9.733	1.027

(Contd.)

		M + 1	M + 2
	$C_8H_{15}N_3O_2$	10.107	0.863
	$C_8H_{17}N_4O$	10.482	0.700
	$C_9HN_2O_3$	10.622	1.112
	$C_9H_3N_3O_2$	10.996	0.951
	$C_9H_5N_4O$	11.370	0.791
	$C_9H_{13}O_4$	10.090	1.258
	$C_9H_{15}NO_3$	10.464	1.096
	$C_9H_{17}N_2O_2$	10.839	0.934
	$C_9H_{19}N_3O$	11.213	0.774
	$C_9H_{21}N_4$	11.587	0.616
	$C_{10}HO_4$	10.978	1.346
	$C_{10}H_3NO_3$	11.353	1.187
	$C_{10}H_5N_2O_2$	11.727	1.029
	$C_{10}H_7N_3O$	12.101	0.872
	$C_{10}H_9N_4$	12.476	0.717
	$C_{10}H_{17}O_3$	11.195	1.170
	$C_{10}H_{19}NO_2$	11.570	1.011
	$C_{10}H_{21}N_2O$	11.944	0.854
	$C_{10}H_{23}N_3$	12.318	0.698
	$C_{11}H_5O_3$	12.084	1.267
	$C_{11}H_7NO_2$	12.458	1.112
	$C_{11}H_9N_2O$	12.833	0.958
	$C_{11}H_{11}N_3$	13.207	0.806
	$C_{11}H_{21}O_2$	12.301	1.093
	$C_{11}H_{23}NO$	1.268	0.939
	$C_{11}H_{25}N_2$	13.050	0.786
	$C_{12}H_9O_2$	13.189	1.201
	$C_{12}H_{11}NO$	13.564	1.050
	$C_{12}H_{13}N_2$	13.938	0.900
	$C_{12}H_{25}O$	13.406	1.029
	$C_{12}H_{27}N$	13.781	0.879
	$C_{13}HN_2$	14.827	1.022
	$C_{13}H_{13}O$	14.295	1.146
	$C_{13}H_{15}N$	14.669	0.999
	$C_{14}HO$	15.183	1.271
	$C_{14}H_3N$	15.558	1.128
	$C_{14}H_{17}$	15.400	1.104
	$C_{15}H_5$	16.289	1.239
186	$C_7H_{10}N_2O_4$	8.644	1.133
	$C_7H_{12}N_3O_3$	9.018	0.965

	M + 1	M + 2
$C_7H_{14}N_4O_2$	9.392	0.798
$C_8H_2N_4O_2$	10.281	0.880
$C_8H_{12}NO_4$	9.375	1.194
$C_8H_{14}N_2O_3$	9.749	1.029
$C_8H_{16}N_3O_2$	10.123	0.865
$C_8H_{18}N_4O$	10.498	0.702
$C_9H_2N_2O_3$	10.638	1.113
$C_9H_4N_3O_2$	11.012	0.953
$C_9H_6N_4O$	11.386	0.793
$C_9H_{14}O_4$	10.106	1.260
$C_9H_{16}NO_3$	10.480	1.097
$C_9H_{18}N_2O_2$	10.855	0.936
$C_9H_{20}N_3O$	11.229	0.776
$C_9H_{22}N_4$	11.603	0.618
$C_{10}H_2O_4$	10.994	1.347
$C_{10}H_4NO_3$	11.369	1.189
$C_{10}H_6N_2O_2$	11.743	1.031
$C_9H_{20}N_3O$	11.229	0.776
$C_9H_{22}N_4$	11.603	0.618
$C_{10}H_4NO_3$	11.369	1.189
$C_{10}H_6N_2O_2$	11.743	1.031
$C_{10}H_8N_3O$	12.117	0.874
$C_{10}H_{10}N_4$	12.492	0.719
$C_{10}H_{18}O_3$	11.211	1.172
$C_{10}H_{20}NO_2$	11.586	1.013
$C_{10}H_{22}N_2O$	11.960	0.856
$C_{10}H_{24}N_3$	12.334	0.700
$C_{11}H_6O_3$	12.100	1.269
$C_{11}H_8NO_2$	12.474	1.114
$C_{11}H_{10}N_2O$	12.849	0.960
$C_{11}H_{12}N_3$	13.223	0.808
$C_{11}H_{22}O_2$	12.317	1.095
$C_{11}H_{24}NO$	1.269	0.941
$C_{11}H_{26}N_2$	13.066	0.788
$C_{12}H_{10}O_2$	13.205	1.203
$C_{12}H_{12}NO$	13.580	1.052
$C_{12}H_{14}N_2$	13.954	0.902
$C_{12}H_{26}O$	13.422	1.031
$C_{13}H_2N_2$	14.843	1.024
$C_{13}H_{14}O$	14.311	1.149

(Contd.)

		M + 1	M + 2			M + 1	M + 2
	$C_{13}H_{16}N$	14.685	1.002		$C_{12}H_{13}NO$	13.596	1.054
	$C_{14}H_2O$	15.199	1.274		$C_{12}H_{15}N_2$	13.970	0.904
	$C_{14}H_4N$	15.574	1.130		$C_{13}HNO$	14.484	1.173
	$C_{14}H_{18}$	15.416	1.107		$C_{13}H_3N_2$	14.859	1.027
	$C_{15}H_6$	16.305	1.242		$C_{13}H_{15}O$	14.327	1.151
187	$C_7H_{11}N_2O_4$	8.660	1.135		$C_{13}H_{17}N$	14.701	1.004
	$C_7H_{13}N_3O_3$	9.034	0.966		$C_{14}H_3O$	15.216	1.276
	$C_7H_{15}N_4O_2$	9.408	0.800		$C_{14}H_5N$	15.590	1.133
	$C_8HN_3O_3$	9.922	1.045		$C_{14}H_{19}$	15.432	1.109
	$C_8H_3N_4O_2$	10.297	0.881		$C_{15}H_7$	16.321	1.244
	$C_8H_{13}NO_4$	9.391	1.195	188	$C_7H_{12}N_2O_4$	8.676	1.136
	$C_8H_{15}N_2O_3$	9.765	1.030		$C_7H_{14}N_3O_3$	9.050	0.968
	$C_8H_{17}N_3O_2$	10.139	0.866		$C_{17}H_{16}N_4O_2$	9.424	0.801
	$C_8H_{19}N_4O$	10.514	0.704		$C_8H_2N_3O_3$	9.938	1.046
	C_9HNO_4	10.279	1.277		$C_8H_4N_4O_2$	10.313	0.883
	$C_9H_3N_2O_3$	10.654	1.115		$C_8H_{14}NO_4$	9.407	1.197
	$C_9H_5N_3O_2$	11.028	0.954		$C_8H_{16}N_2O_3$	9.781	1.032
	$C_9H_7N_4O$	11.402	0.795		$C_8H_{18}N_3O_2$	10.155	0.868
	$C_9H_{15}O_4$	10.122	1.262		$C_8H_{20}N_4O$	10.530	0.705
	$C_9H_{17}NO_3$	10.496	1.099		$C_9H_2NO_4$	10.295	1.279
	$C_9H_{19}N_2O_2$	10.871	0.938		$C_9H_4N_2O_3$	10.670	1.117
	$C_9H_{21}N_3O$	11.245	0.778		$C_9H_6N_3O_2$	11.044	0.956
	$C_9H_{23}N_4$	11.619	0.620		$C_9H_8N_4O$	11.418	0.797
	$C_{10}H_3O_4$	11.010	1.349		$C_9H_{16}O_4$	10.138	1.263
	$C_{10}H_5NO_3$	11.385	1.190		$C_9H_{18}NO_3$	10.512	1.101
	$C_{10}H_7N_2O_2$	11.759	1.033		$C_9H_{20}N_2O_2$	10.887	0.940
	$C_{10}H_9N_3O$	12.133	0.876		$C_9H_{22}N_3O$	11.261	0.780
	$C_{10}H_{11}N_4$	12.508	0.721		$C_9H_{24}N_4$	11.636	0.621
	$C_{10}H_{19}O_3$	11.227	1.173		$C_{10}H_4O_4$	11.026	1.351
	$C_{10}H_{21}NO_2$	11.602	1.015		$C_{10}H_6NO_3$	11.401	1,192
	$C_{10}H_{23}N_2O$	11.976	0.858		$C_{10}H_8N_2O_2$	11.775	1.034
	$C_{10}H_{25}N_3$	12.350	0.702		$C_{10}H_{10}N_3O$	12.149	0.978
	$C_{11}H_7O_3$	12.116	1.271		$C_{10}H_{12}N_4$	12.524	0.723
	$C_{11}H_9NO_2$	12.490	1.116		$C_{10}H_{20}O_3$	11.243	1.175
	$C_{11}H_{11}N_2O$	12.865	0.962		$C_{10}H_{22}NO_2$	11.618	1.017
	$C_{11}H_{13}N_3$	13.239	0.801		$C_{10}H_{24}N_2O$	11.992	0.860
	$C_{11}H_{25}O_2$	12.333	10.972		$C_{11}H_8O_3$	12.132	1.273
	$C_{11}H_{25}NO$	12.707	0.943		$C_{11}H_{10}NO_2$	12.506	1.118
	$C_{12}HN_3$	14.128	0.926		$C_{11}H_{12}N_2O$	12.881	0.964
	$C_{12}H_{11}O_2$	13.221	1.205		$C_{11}H_{14}N_3$	13.255	0.812

(Contd.)

		M + 1	M + 2
	$C_{11}H_{24}O_2$	12.349	1.099
	$C_{12}H_2N_3$	14.144	0.928
	$C_{12}H_{12}O_2$	13.237	1.207
	$C_{12}H_{14}NO$	13.612	1.056
	$C_{12}H_{16}N_2$	13.986	0.907
	$C_{13}H_2NO$	14.500	1.175
	$C_{13}H_4N_2$	14.875	1.029
	$C_{13}H_{16}O$	14.343	1.153
	$C_{13}H_{18}N$	14.717	1.006
	$C_{14}H_4O$	15.232	1.279
	$C_{14}H_6N$	15.606	1.135
	$C_{14}H_{20}$	15.448	1.112
	$C_{15}H_8$	16.337	1.247
189	$C_7H_{13}N_2O_4$	8.692	1.137
	$C_7H_{15}N_3O_3$	9.066	0.969
	$C_7H_{17}N_4O_2$	9.440	0.803
	$C_8HN_2O_4$	9.580	1.213
	$C_8H_3N_3O_3$	9.954	1.048
	$C_8H_5N_4O_2$	10.329	0.885
	$C_8H_{15}NO_4$	9.423	1.198
	$C_8H_{17}N_2O_3$	9.797	1.033
	$C_8H_{19}N_3O_2$	10.171	0.869
	$C_8H_{21}N_4O$	10.546	0.707
	$C_9H_3NO_4$	10.311	1.280
	$C_9H_5N_2O_3$	10.686	1.118
	$C_9H_7N_3O_2$	11.060	0.958
	$C_9H_9N_4O$	11.434	0.799
	$C_9H_{17}O_4$	10.154	1.265
	$C_9H_{19}NO_3$	10.528	1.102
	$C_9H_{21}N_2O_2$	10.903	0.941
	$C_9H_{23}N_3O$	11.277	0.782
	$C_{10}H_5O_4$	11.042	1.353
	$C_{10}H_7NO_3$	11.417	1.194
	$C_{10}H_9N_2O_2$	11.791	1.036
	$C_{10}H_{11}N_3O$	12.165	0.880
	$C_{10}H_{13}N_4$	12.540	0.725
	$C_{10}H_{21}O_3$	11.259	1.177
	$C_{10}H_{23}NO_2$	11.634	1.019
	$C_{11}HN_4$	13.428	0.835
	$C_{11}H_9O_3$	12.148	1.275
	$C_{11}H_{11}NO_2$	12.522	1.120
	$C_{11}H_{13}N_2O$	12.897	0.966
	$C_{11}H_{15}N_3$	13.271	0.814
	$C_{12}HN_2O$	13.785	1.079
	$C_{12}H_3N_3$	14.160	0.930
	$C_{12}H_{13}O_2$	13.253	1.209
	$C_{12}H_{15}NO$	13.628	1.058
	$C_{12}H_{17}N_2$	14.002	0.909
	$C_{13}HO_2$	14.142	1.325
	$C_{13}H_3NO$	14.516	1.178
	$C_{13}H_5N_2$	14.891	1.031
	$C_{13}H_{17}O$	14.359	1.155
	$C_{13}H_{19}N$	14.733	1.009
	$C_{14}H_5O$	15.248	1.281
	$C_{14}H_7N$	15.622	1.133
	$C_{14}H_{21}$	15.464	1.114
	$C_{15}H_9$	16.353	1.250
190	$C_7H_{14}N_2O_4$	8.708	1.139
	$C_7H_{16}N_3O_3$	9.082	0.971
	$C_7H_{18}N_4O_2$	9.456	0.804
	$C_8H_2N_2O_4$	9.596	1.214
	$C_8H_4N_3O_3$	9.970	1.050
	$C_8H_6N_4O_2$	10.345	0.886
	$C_8H_{16}NO_4$	9.439	1.200
	$C_8H_{18}N_2O_3$	9.813	1.035
	$C_8H_{20}N_3O_2$	10.187	0.871
	$C_8H_{22}N_4O$	10.562	0.709
	$C_9H_4NO_4$	10.327	1.282
	$C_9H_6N_2O_3$	10.702	1.120
	$C_9H_8N_3O_2$	1.108	0.960
	$C_9H_{10}N_4O$	11.450	0.801
	$C_9H_{18}O_4$	10.170	1.267
	$C_9H_{20}NO_3$	10.544	1.104
	$C_9H_{22}N_2O_2$	10.919	0.943
	$C_{10}H_6O_4$	11.058	1.355
	$C_{10}H_8NO_3$	11.433	1.196
	$C_{10}H_{10}N_2O_2$	11.807	1.028
	$C_{10}H_{12}N_3O$	12.181	0.882
	$C_{10}H_{14}N_4$	12.556	0.727
	$C_{10}H_{22}O_3$	11.275	1.179

(Contd.)

		M + 1	M + 2
	$C_{11}H_2N_4$	13.444	0.837
	$C_{11}H_{10}O_3$	12.164	1.277
	$C_{11}H_{12}NO_2$	12.538	1.122
	$C_{11}H_{14}N_2O$	12.913	0.969
	$C_{11}H_{16}N_3$	13.287	0.816
	$C_{12}H_2N_2O$	13.801	1.081
	$C_{12}H_4N_3$	14.176	0.933
	$C_{12}H_{14}O_2$	13.269	1.211
	$C_{12}H_{16}NO$	13.644	1.060
	$C_{12}H_{18}N_2$	14.018	0.911
	$C_{13}H_2O_2$	14.158	1.327
	$C_{13}H_4NO$	14.532	1.180
	$C_{13}H_6N_2$	14.907	1.034
	$C_{13}H_{18}O$	14.375	1.158
	$C_{13}H_{20}N$	14.749	1.011
	$C_{14}H_6O$	15.264	1.284
	$C_{14}H_8N$	15.638	1.140
	$C_{14}H_{22}$	15.480	1.117
	$C_{15}H_{10}$	16.369	1.252
191	$C_7H_{15}N_2O_4$	8.724	1.140
	$C_7H_{17}N_3O_3$	9.098	0.972
	$C_7H_{19}N_4O_2$	9.472	0.806
	$C_8H_3N_2O_4$	9.612	1.216
	$C_8H_5N_3O_3$	9.986	1.051
	$C_8H_7N_4O_2$	10.361	0.888
	$C_8H_{17}NO_4$	9.455	1.201
	$C_8H_{19}N_2O_3$	9.829	1.036
	$C_8H_{21}N_3O_2$	10.203	0.873
	$C_9H_5NO_4$	10.343	1.284
	$C_9H_7N_2O_3$	10.718	1.122
	$C_9H_9N_3O_2$	11.092	0.961
	$C_9H_{11}N_4O$	11.466	0.802
	$C_9H_{19}O_4$	10.186	1.268
	$C_9H_{21}NO_3$	10.560	1.106
	$C_{10}H_7O_4$	11.074	1.357
	$C_{10}H_9NO_3$	11.449	1.198
	$C_{10}H_{11}N_2O_2$	11.823	1.040
	$C_{10}H_{13}N_3O$	12.197	0.884
	$C_{10}H_{15}N_4$	12.572	0.729
	$C_{11}HN_3O$	13.086	0.990
	$C_{11}H_3N_4$	13.460	0.839
	$C_{11}H_{11}O_3$	12.180	1.280
	$C_{11}H_{13}NO_2$	12.554	1.124
	$C_{11}H_{15}N_2O$	12.929	0.971
	$C_{11}H_{17}N_3$	13.303	0.818
	$C_{12}HNO_2$	13.443	1.234
	$C_{12}H_3N_2O$	13.817	1.084
	$C_{12}H_5N_3$	14.192	0.935
	$C_{12}H_{15}O_2$	13.285	1.213
	$C_{12}H_{17}NO$	13.660	1.063
	$C_{12}H_{19}N_2$	14.034	0.913
	$C_{13}H_3O_2$	14.174	1.330
	$C_{13}H_5NO$	14.548	1.182
	$C_{13}H_7N_2$	14.923	1.036
	$C_{13}H_{19}O$	14.391	1.160
	$C_{13}H_{21}N$	14.765	1.013
	$C_{14}H_7O$	15.280	1.286
	$C_{14}H_9N$	15.654	1.143
	$C_{14}H_{23}$	15.496	1.119
	$C_{15}H_{11}$	16.385	1.255
192	$C_7H_{16}N_2O_4$	8.470	1.141
	$C_7H_{18}N_3O_3$	9.114	0.974
	$C_7H_{20}N_4O_2$	9.488	0.807
	$C_8H_4N_2O_4$	9.628	1.217
	$C_8H_6N_3O_3$	10.002	1.053
	$C_8H_8N_4O_2$	10.377	0.890
	$C_8H_{18}NO_4$	9.471	1.203
	$C_8H_{20}N_2O_3$	9.845	1.038
	$C_9H_6NO_4$	10.359	1.285
	$C_9H_8N_2O_3$	10.734	1.124
	$C_9H_{10}N_3O_2$	11.108	0.963
	$C_9H_{12}N_4O$	11.482	0.804
	$C_9H_{20}O_4$	10.202	1.270
	$C_{10}H_8O_4$	11.090	1.359
	$C_{10}H_{10}NO_3$	11.465	1.200
	$C_{10}H_{12}N_2O_2$	11.839	1.042
	$C_{10}H_{14}N_3O$	12.213	0.886
	$C_{10}H_{16}N_4$	12.588	0.731
	$C_{11}H_2N_3O$	13.102	0.992
	$C_{11}H_4N_4$	13.476	0.841

(Contd.)

		M + 1	M + 2			M + 1	M + 2
	$C_{11}H_{12}O_3$	12.196	1.281		$C_{11}H_{17}N_2O$	12.961	0.975
	$C_{11}H_{14}NO_2$	12.570	1.126		$C_{11}H_{19}N_3$	13.335	0.823
	$C_{11}H_{16}N_2O$	12.945	0.973		$C_{12}HO_3$	13.100	1.390
	$C_{11}H_{18}N_3$	13.319	0.821		$C_{12}H_3NO_2$	13.475	1.238
	$C_{12}H_2NO_2$	13.459	1.236		$C_{12}H_5N_2O$	13.849	1.088
	$C_{12}H_4N_2O$	13.833	1.086		$C_{12}H_7N_3$	14.224	0.939
	$C_{12}H_6N_3$	14.208	0.937		$C_{12}H_{17}O_2$	13.317	1.218
	$C_{12}H_{16}O_2$	13.301	1.216		$C_{12}H_{19}NO$	13.692	1.067
	$C_{12}H_{18}NO$	13.676	1.065		$C_{12}H_{21}N_2$	14.066	0.918
	$C_{12}H_{20}N_2$	14.050	0.916		$C_{13}H_5O_2$	14.206	1.334
	$C_{13}H_4O_2$	14.190	1.332		$C_{13}H_7NO$	14.580	1.187
	$C_{13}H_6NO$	14.564	1.184		$C_{13}H_9N_2$	14.955	1.041
	$C_{13}H_8N_2$	14.939	1.039		$C_{13}H_{21}O$	14.423	1.165
	$C_{13}H_{20}O$	14.407	1.162		$C_{13}H_{23}N$	14.797	1.018
	$C_{13}H_{22}N$	14.781	1.016		$C_{14}H_9O$	15.312	1.291
	$C_{14}H_8O$	15.296	1.289		$C_{14}H_{11}N$	15.686	1.148
	$C_{14}H_{10}N$	15.670	1.145		$C_{14}H_{25}$	15.528	1.124
	$C_{14}H_{24}$	15.512	1.121		$C_{15}H_{13}$	16.417	1.260
	$C_{15}H_{12}$	16.401	1.257		$C_{16}H$	17.306	1.404
193	$C_7H_{17}N_2O_4$	8.756	1.143	194	$C_7H_{18}N_2O_4$	8.772	1.144
	$C_7H_{19}N_3O_3$	9.130	0.975		$C_8H_6N_2O_4$	9.660	1.220
	$C_8H_5N_2O_4$	9.644	1.219		$C_8H_8N_3O_3$	10.034	1.056
	$C_8H_7N_3O_3$	10.018	1.054		$C_8H_{10}N_4O_2$	10.409	0.893
	$C_8H_9N_4O_2$	10.393	0.891		$C_9H_8NO_4$	10.391	1.289
	$C_8H_{19}NO_4$	9.487	1.204		$C_9H_{10}N_2O_3$	10.766	1.127
	$C_9H_7NO_4$	10.375	1.287		$C_9H_{12}N_3O_2$	11.140	0.967
	$C_9H_9N_2O_3$	10.750	1.125		$C_9H_{14}N_4O$	11.514	0.808
	$C_9H_{11}N_3O_2$	11.124	0.965		$C_{10}H_2N_4O$	12.403	0.908
	$C_9H_{13}N_4O$	11.498	0.806		$C_{10}H_{10}O_4$	11.122	1.362
	$C_{10}HN_4O$	12.387	0.906		$C_{10}H_{12}NO_3$	11.497	1.203
	$C_{10}H_9O_4$	11.106	1.360		$C_{10}H_{14}N_2O_2$	11.871	1.046
	$C_{10}H_{11}NO_3$	11.481	1.201		$C_{10}H_{16}N_3O$	12.245	0.890
	$C_{10}H_{13}N_2O_2$	11.855	1.044		$C_{10}H_{18}N_4$	12.620	0.735
	$C_{10}H_{15}N_3O$	12.229	0.888		$C_{11}H_2N_2O_2$	12.760	1.149
	$C_{10}H_{17}N_4$	12.604	0.733		$C_{11}H_4N_3O$	13.134	0.997
	$C_{11}HN_2O_2$	12.744	1.147		$C_{11}H_6N_4$	13.508	0.845
	$C_{11}H_3N_3O$	13.118	0.995		$C_{11}H_{14}O_3$	12.228	1.285
	$C_{11}H_5N_4$	13.492	0.843		$C_{11}H_{16}NO_2$	12.602	1.130
	$C_{11}H_{13}O_3$	12.212	1.283		$C_{11}H_{18}N_2O$	12.977	0.977
	$C_{11}H_{15}NO_2$	12.586	1.128		$C_{11}H_{20}N_3$	13.351	0.825

(Contd.)

		M + 1	M + 2			M + 1	M + 2
	$C_{12}H_2O_3$	13.116	1.392		$C_{12}H_5NO_2$	13.507	1.242
	$C_{12}H_4NO_2$	13.491	1.240		$C_{12}H_7N_2O$	13.881	1.092
	$C_{12}H_6N_2O$	13.865	1.090		$C_{12}H_9N_3$	14.256	0.944
	$C_{12}H_8N_3$	14.240	0.942		$C_{12}H_{19}O_2$	13.349	1.222
	$C_{12}H_{18}O_2$	13.333	1.220		$C_{12}H_{21}NO$	13.724	1.071
	$C_{12}H_{20}NO$	13.708	1.069		$C_{12}H_{23}N_2$	14.098	0.922
	$C_{12}H_{22}N_2$	14.082	0.920		$C_{13}H_7O_2$	14.238	1.339
	$C_{13}H_6O_2$	14.222	1.336		$C_{13}H_9NO$	14.612	1.191
	$C_{13}H_8NO$	14.596	1.189		$C_{13}H_{11}N_2$	14.987	1.046
	$C_{13}H_{10}N_2$	14.971	1.043		$C_{13}H_{23}O$	14.455	1.169
	$C_{13}H_{22}O$	14.439	1.167		$C_{13}H_{25}N$	14.829	1.023
	$C_{13}H_{24}N$	14.813	1.021		$C_{14}H_{11}O$	15.344	1.296
	$C_{14}H_{10}O$	15.328	1.293		$C_{14}H_{13}N$	15.718	1.153
	$C_{14}H_{12}N$	15.702	1.150		$C_{14}H_{27}$	15.560	1.129
	$C_{14}H_{26}$	15.544	1.126		$C_{15}HN$	16.606	1.291
	$C_{15}H_{14}$	16.433	1.263		$C_{15}H_{15}$	16.449	1.265
	$C_{16}H_2$	17.322	1.407		$C_{16}H_3$	17.338	1.410
195	$C_8H_7N_2O_4$	9.676	1.222	196	$C_8H_8N_2O_4$	9.692	1.223
	$C_8H_9N_3O_3$	10.050	1.058		$C_8H_{10}N_3O_3$	10.066	1.059
	$C_8H_{11}N_4O_2$	10.425	0.895		$C_8H_{12}N_4O_2$	10.441	0.896
	$C_9H_9NO_4$	10.407	1.290		$C_9H_{10}NO_4$	10.423	1.292
	$C_9H_{11}N_2O_3$	10.782	1.129		$C_9H_{12}N_2O_3$	10.798	1.131
	$C_9H_{13}N_3O_2$	11.156	0.969		$C_9H_{14}N_3O_2$	11.172	0.970
	$C_9H_{15}N_4O$	11.530	0.810		$C_9H_{16}N_4O$	11.546	0.812
	$C_{10}HN_3O_2$	12.045	1.066		$C_{10}H_2N_3O_2$	12.061	1.068
	$C_{10}H_3N_4O$	12.419	0.910		$C_{10}H_4N_4O$	12.435	0.912
	$C_{10}H_{11}O_4$	11.138	1.364		$C_{10}H_{12}O_4$	11.154	1.366
	$C_{10}H_{13}NO_3$	11.513	1.205		$C_{10}H_{14}NO_3$	11.529	1.207
	$C_{10}H_{15}N_2O_2$	11.887	1.048		$C_{10}H_{16}N_2O_2$	11.903	1.050
	$C_{10}H_{17}N_3O$	12.261	0.892		$C_{10}H_{18}N_3O$	12.277	0.894
	$C_{10}H_{19}N_4$	12.636	0.737		$C_{10}H_{20}N_4$	12.652	0.739
	$C_{11}HNO_3$	12.401	1.305		$C_{11}H_2NO_3$	12.417	1.307
	$C_{11}H_3N_2O_2$	12.776	1.151		$C_{11}H_4N_2O_2$	12.792	1.153
	$C_{11}H_5N_3O$	13.150	0.999		$C_{11}H_6N_3O$	13.166	1.001
	$C_{11}H_7N_4$	13.524	0.848		$C_{11}H_8N_4$	13.540	0.850
	$C_{11}H_{15}O_3$	12.244	1.287		$C_{11}H_{16}O_3$	12.260	1.289
	$C_{11}H_{17}NO_2$	12.618	1.132		$C_{11}H_{18}NO_2$	12.634	1.134
	$C_{11}H_{19}N_2O$	12.993	0.979		$C_{11}H_{20}N_2O$	13.009	0.981
	$C_{11}H_{21}N_3$	13.367	0.827		$C_{11}H_{22}N_3$	13.383	0.829
	$C_{12}H_3O_3$	13.132	1.394		$C_{12}H_4O_3$	13.148	1.396

(Contd.)

		M + 1	M + 2
	$C_{12}H_6NO_2$	13.523	1.245
	$C_{12}H_8N_2O$	13.897	1.095
	$C_{12}H_{10}N_3$	14.272	0.946
	$C_{12}H_{20}O_2$	13.365	1.224
	$C_{12}H_{22}NO$	13.740	1.074
	$C_{12}H_{24}N_2$	14.114	0.925
	$C_{13}H_8O_2$	14.254	1.341
	$C_{13}H_{10}NO$	14.628	1.194
	$C_{13}H_{12}N_2$	15.003	1.048
	$C_{13}H_{24}O$	14.471	1.172
	$C_{13}H_{26}N$	14.845	1.025
	$C_{14}H_{12}O$	15.360	1.298
	$C_{14}H_{14}N$	15.734	1.155
	$C_{14}H_{28}$	15.576	1.131
	$C_{15}H_2N$	16.622	1.293
	$C_{15}H_{16}$	16.465	1.268
	$C_{16}H_4$	17.354	1.412
197	$C_8H_9N_2O_4$	9.708	1.225
	$C_8H_{11}N_3O_3$	10.082	1.061
	$C_8H_{13}N_4O_2$	10.457	0.898
	$C_9HN_4O_2$	11.345	0.989
	$C_9H_{11}NO_4$	10.439	1.294
	$C_9H_{13}N_2O_3$	10.814	1.132
	$C_9H_{15}N_3O_2$	11.188	0.972
	$C_9H_{17}N_4O$	11.562	0.813
	$C_{10}HN_2O_3$	11.702	1.226
	$C_{10}H_3N_3O_2$	12.077	1.070
	$C_{10}H_5N_4O$	12.451	0.914
	$C_{10}H_{13}O_4$	11.170	1.367
	$C_{10}H_{15}NO_3$	11.545	1.209
	$C_{10}H_{17}N_2O_2$	11.919	1.051
	$C_{10}H_{19}N_3O$	12.294	0.896
	$C_{10}H_{21}N_4$	12.668	0.741
	$C_{11}HO_4$	12.059	1.465
	$C_{11}H_3NO_3$	12.433	1.309
	$C_{11}H_5N_2O_2$	12.808	1.155
	$C_{11}H_7N_3O$	13.182	1.003
	$C_{14}H_9N_4$	13.556	0.852
	$C_{11}H_{17}O_3$	12.276	1.291
	$C_{11}H_{19}NO_2$	12.650	1.136
	$C_{11}H_{21}N_2O$	13.025	0.983
	$C_{11}H_{23}N_3$	13.399	0.831
	$C_{12}H_5O_3$	13.164	1.398
	$C_{12}H_7NO_2$	13.539	1.247
	$C_{12}H_9N_2O$	13.913	1.097
	$C_{12}H_{11}N_3$	14.288	0.948
	$C_{12}H_{21}O_2$	13.381	1.226
	$C_{12}H_{23}NO$	13.756	1.076
	$C_{12}H_{25}N_2$	14.130	0.927
	$C_{13}H_9O_2$	14.270	1.343
	$C_{13}H_{11}NO$	14.644	1.196
	$C_{13}H_{13}N_2$	15.019	1.050
	$C_{13}H_{25}O$	14.487	1.174
	$C_{13}H_{27}N$	14.861	1.028
	$C_{14}HN_2$	15.907	1.182
	$C_{14}H_{13}O$	15.376	1.301
	$C_{14}H_{15}N$	15.750	1.158
	$C_{14}H_{29}$	15.592	1.134
	$C_{15}HO$	16.264	1.436
	$C_{15}H_3N$	16.638	1.296
	$C_{15}H_{17}$	16.481	1.271
	$C_{16}H_5$	17.370	1.415
198	$C_8H_{10}N_2O_4$	9.724	1.227
	$C_8H_{12}N_3O_3$	10.098	1.062
	$C_8H_{14}N_4O_2$	10.473	0.890
	$C_9H_2N_4O_2$	11.361	0.991
	$C_9H_{12}NO_4$	10.455	1.295
	$C_9H_{14}N_2O_3$	10.830	1.134
	$C_9H_{16}N_3O_2$	11.204	0.974
	$C_9H_{18}N_4O$	11.578	0.815
	$C_{10}H_2N_2O_3$	11.718	1.228
	$C_{10}H_4N_3O_2$	12.093	1.072
	$C_{10}H_6N_4O$	12.467	0.916
	$C_{10}H_{14}O_4$	11.186	1.369
	$C_{10}H_{16}NO_3$	11.561	1.211
	$C_{10}H_{18}N_2O_2$	11.935	1.053
	$C_{10}H_{20}N_3O$	122.310	0.898
	$C_{10}H_{22}N_4$	12.684	0.743
	$C_{11}H_2O_4$	12.075	14.667
	$C_{11}H_4NO_3$	12.449	1.311

(Contd.)

		M + 1	M + 2			M + 1	M + 2
	$C_{11}H_6N_2O_2$	12.824	1.158		$C_{10}H_{15}O_4$	11.202	1.371
	$C_{11}H_8N_3O$	13.198	1.005		$C_{10}H_{17}NO_3$	11.577	1.212
	$C_{11}H_{10}N_4$	13.572	0.854		$C_{10}H_{19}N_2O_2$	11.951	1.055
	$C_{11}H_{18}O_3$	12.292	1.293		$C_{10}H_{21}N_3O$	12.326	0.890
	$C_{11}H_{20}NO_2$	12.666	1.138		$C_{10}H_{23}N_4$	12.700	0.745
	$C_{11}H_{22}N_2O$	13.041	0.985		$C_{11}H_2O_4$	12.091	1.469
	$C_{11}H_{24}N_3$	13.415	0.833		$C_{11}H_5NO_3$	12.465	1.313
	$C_{12}H_6O_3$	13.180	1.400		$C_{11}H_7N_2O_2$	12.840	1.160
	$C_{12}H_8NO_2$	13.555	1.249		$C_{11}H_9N_3O$	13.214	1.007
	$C_{12}H_{10}N_2O$	13.929	1.099		$C_{11}H_{11}N_4$	13.588	0.856
	$C_{12}H_{12}N_3$	14.304	0.951		$C_{11}H_{19}O_3$	12.308	1.295
	$C_{12}H_{22}O_2$	13.397	1.228		$C_{11}H_{21}NO_2$	12.682	1.140
	$C_{12}H_{24}NO$	13.772	1.078		$C_{11}H_{23}N_2O$	13.057	0.987
	$C_{12}H_{26}N_2$	14.146	0.929		$C_{11}H_{25}N_3$	13.431	0.836
	$C_{13}H_{10}O_2$	14.286	1.346		$C_{12}H_7O_3$	13.197	1.402
	$C_{13}H_{12}NO$	14.660	1.199		$C_{12}H_9NO_2$	13.571	1.251
	$C_{13}H_{14}N_2$	15.035	1.053		$C_{12}H_{11}N_2O$	13.945	1.101
	$C_{13}H_{26}O$	14.503	1.176		$C_{12}H_{13}N_3$	14.320	0.953
	$C_{13}H_{28}N$	14.877	1.030		$C_{12}H_{23}O_2$	13.413	1.231
	$C_{14}H_2N_2$	15.923	1.485		$C_{12}H_{25}NO$	13.788	1.080
	$C_{14}H_{14}O$	15.392	1.303		$C_{12}H_{27}N_2$	14.162	0.931
	$C_{14}H_{16}N$	15.766	1.160		$C_{13}HN_3$	15.208	1.078
	$C_{14}H_{30}$	15.608	1.136		$C_{13}H_{11}O_2$	14.302	1.348
	$C_{15}H_2O$	16.280	1.438		$C_{13}H_{13}NO$	14.676	1.201
	$C_{15}H_4N$	16.654	1.299		$C_{13}H_{15}N_2$	15.051	1.055
	$C_{15}H_{18}$	16.497	1.273		$C_{13}H_{27}O$	14.519	1.179
	$C_{16}H_6$	17.386	1.418		$C_{13}H_{29}N$	14.893	1.032
199	$C_8H_{11}N_2O_4$	9.740	1.228		$C_{14}HNO$	15.565	1.329
	$C_8H_{13}N_3O_3$	10.114	1.064		$C_{14}H_3N_2$	15.939	1.187
	$C_8H_{15}N_4O_2$	10.489	0.901		$C_{14}H_{15}O$	15.408	1.306
	$C_9HN_3O_3$	11.003	1.152		$C_{14}H_{17}N$	15.782	1.163
	$C_9H_3N_4O_2$	11.377	0.993		$C_{15}H_3O$	16.296	1.441
	$C_9H_{13}NO_4$	10.471	1.297		$C_{15}H_5N$	16.670	1.301
	$C_9H_{15}N_2O_3$	10.846	1.136		$C_{15}H_{19}$	16.513	1.276
	$C_9H_{17}N_3O_2$	11.220	0.976		$C_{16}H_7$	17.402	1.421
	$C_9H_{19}N_4O$	11.594	0.817	200	$C_8H_{12}N_2O_4$	9.756	1.230
	$C_{10}HNO_4$	11.360	1.388		$C_8H_{14}N_3O_3$	10.130	1.066
	$C_{10}H_3N_2O_3$	11.734	1.230		$C_8H_{16}N_4O_2$	10.505	0.903
	$C_{10}H_5N_3O_2$	12.109	1.074		$C_9H_2N_3O_3$	11.019	1.154
	$C_{10}H_7N_4O$	12.483	0.918		$C_9H_4N_4O_2$	11.393	0.995

(Contd.)

		M + 1	M + 2
	$C_9H_{14}NO_4$	10.487	1.299
	$C_9H_{16}N_2O_3$	10.862	1.137
	$C_9H_{18}N_3O_2$	11.236	0.977
	$C_9H_{20}N_4O$	11.610	0.819
	$C_{10}H_2NO_4$	11.376	1.390
	$C_{10}H_4N_2O_3$	11.750	1.232
	$C_{10}H_6N_3O_2$	12.125	1.075
	$C_{10}H_8N_3O$	12.499	0.920
	$C_{10}H_{16}O_4$	11.218	1.373
	$C_{10}H_{18}NO_3$	11.593	1.214
	$C_{10}H_{20}N_2O_2$	11.967	1.057
	$C_{10}H_{22}N_3O$	12.342	0.901
	$C_{10}H_{24}N_4$	12.716	0.747
	$C_{11}H_4O_4$	12.107	1.471
	$C_{11}H_6NO_3$	12.481	1.315
	$C_{11}H_8N_2O_2$	12.856	1.162
	$C_{11}H_{10}N_3O$	13.230	1.009
	$C_{11}H_{12}N_4$	13.604	0.858
	$C_{11}H_{20}O_3$	12.324	1.297
	$C_{11}H_{22}NO_2$	12.698	1.142
	$C_{11}H_{24}N_2O$	13.073	0.989
	$C_{11}H_{26}N_3$	13.447	0.838
	$C_{12}H_8O_3$	13.213	1.404
	$C_{12}H_{10}NO_2$	13.587	1.253
	$C_{12}H_{12}N_2O$	13.961	1.104
	$C_{12}H_{14}N_3$	13.336	0.955
	$C_{12}H_{24}O_2$	13.429	1.233
	$C_{12}H_{26}NO$	13.804	1.082
	$C_{12}H_{28}N_2$	14.178	0.934
	$C_{13}H_2N_3$	15.224	1.081
	$C_{13}H_{12}O_2$	14.318	1.350
	$C_{13}H_{14}NO$	14.692	1.203
	$C_{13}H_{16}N_2$	15.067	1.058
	$C_{13}H_{28}O$	14.535	1.181
	$C_{14}H_2NO$	15.581	1.332
	$C_{14}H_4N_2$	15.955	1.190
	$C_{14}H_{16}O$	15.424	1.308
	$C_{14}H_{18}N$	15.798	1.165
	$C_{15}H_4O$	16.312	1.443
	$C_{15}H_6N$	16.686	1.304
	$C_{15}H_{20}$	16.529	1.279
	$C_{18}H_8$	17.418	1.423
201	$C_8H_{13}N_2O_4$	9.772	1.231
	$C_8H_{15}N_3O_3$	10.146	1.067
	$C_8H_{17}N_4O_2$	10.521	0.905
	$C_9HN_2O_4$	10.661	1.316
	$C_9H_3N_3O_3$	11.035	1.156
	$C_9H_5N_4O_2$	11.409	0.996
	$C_9H_{15}NO_4$	10.503	1.300
	$C_9H_{17}N_2O_3$	10.878	1.139
	$C_9H_{19}N_3O_2$	11.252	0.979
	$C_9H_{21}N_4O$	11.626	0.821
	$C_{10}H_3NO_4$	11.392	1.392
	$C_{10}H_5N_2O_3$	11.766	1.234
	$C_{10}H_7N_3O_2$	12.141	1.077
	$C_{10}H_9N_4O$	12.515	0.922
	$C_{10}H_{17}O_4$	11.234	1.375
	$C_{10}H_{19}NO_3$	11.609	1.216
	$C_{10}H_{21}N_2O_2$	11.983	1.059
	$C_{10}H_{23}N_3O$	12.358	0.903
	$C_{10}H_{25}N_4$	12.732	0.749
	$C_{11}H_5O_4$	12.123	1.473
	$C_{11}H_7NO_3$	12.497	1.317
	$C_{11}H_9N_2O_2$	12.872	1.164
	$C_{11}H_{11}N_3O$	13.246	1.011
	$C_{11}H_{13}N_4$	13.620	0.860
	$C_{11}H_{21}O_3$	12.340	1.299
	$C_{11}H_{23}NO_2$	12.714	1.144
	$C_{11}H_{25}N_2O$	13.089	0.991
	$C_{11}H_{27}N_3$	13.463	0.840
	$C_{12}HN_4$	14.509	0.980
	$C_{12}H_9O_3$	13.229	1.406
	$C_{12}H_{11}NO_2$	13.603	1.255
	$C_{12}H_{13}N_2O$	13.977	1.106
	$C_{12}H_{15}N_3$	14.352	0.958
	$C_{12}H_{25}O_2$	13.445	1.235
	$C_{12}H_{27}NO$	13.820	1.085
	$C_{13}HN_2O$	14.866	1.228
	$C_{13}H_3N_3$	15.240	1.083
	$C_{13}H_{13}O_2$	14.334	1.352

(Contd.)

		M + 1	M + 2			M + 1	M + 2
	$C_{13}H_{15}NO$	14.708	1.206		$C_{12}H_{12}NO_2$	13.619	1.258
	$C_{13}H_{17}N_2$	15.083	1.060		$C_{12}H_{14}N_2O$	13.993	1.108
	$C_{14}HO_2$	15.223	1.478		$C_{12}H_{16}N_3$	14.368	0.960
	$C_{14}H_3NO$	15.597	1.334		$C_{12}H_{26}O_2$	13.461	1.237
	$C_{14}H_5N_2$	15.971	1.192		$C_{13}H_2N_2O$	14.882	1.231
	$C_{14}H_{17}O$	15.440	1.311		$C_{13}H_4N_3$	15.256	1.086
	$C_{14}H_{19}N$	15.814	1.168		$C_{13}H_{14}O_2$	14.350	1.355
	$C_{15}H_5O$	16.328	1.446		$C_{13}H_{16}NO$	14.724	1.208
	$C_{15}H_7N$	16.702	1.307		$C_{13}H_{18}N_2$	15.099	1.063
	$C_{15}H_{21}$	16.545	1.281		$C_{14}H_2O_2$	15.239	1.480
	$C_{16}H_9$	17.434	1.426		$C_{14}H_4NO$	15.613	1.337
202	$C_8H_{14}N_2O_4$	9.788	1.233		$C_{14}H_6N_2$	15.987	1.195
	$C_8H_{16}N_3O_3$	10.162	1.069		$C_{14}H_{18}O$	15.456	1.313
	$C_8H_{18}N_4O_2$	10.537	0.906		$C_{14}H_{20}N$	15.830	1.170
	$C_9H_2N_2O_4$	10.677	1.318		$C_{15}H_6O$	16.344	1.449
	$C_9H_4N_3O_3$	11.051	1.157		$C_{15}H_8N$	16.718	1.309
	$C_9H_6N_4O_2$	11.425	0.998		$C_{15}H_{22}$	16.561	1.284
	$C_9H_{16}NO_4$	10.519	1.302		$C_{16}H_{10}$	17.450	1.429
	$C_9H_{18}N_2O_3$	10.894	1.141	203	$C_8H_{15}N_2O_4$	9.804	1.234
	$C_9H_{20}N_3O_2$	11.268	0.981		$C_8H_{17}N_3O_3$	10.178	1.071
	$C_9H_{22}N_4O$	11.642	0.823		$C_8H_{19}N_4O_2$	10.553	0.908
	$C_{10}H_4NO_4$	11.408	1.394		$C_9H_3N_2O_4$	10.693	1.320
	$C_{10}H_6N_2O_3$	11.782	1.236		$C_9H_5N_3O_3$	11.067	1.159
	$C_{10}H_8N_3O_2$	12.157	1.079		$C_9H_7N_4O_2$	11.441	1.000
	$C_{10}H_{10}N_4O$	12.531	0.924		$C_9H_{17}NO_4$	10.535	1.304
	$C_{10}H_{18}O_4$	11.250	1.376		$C_9H_{19}N_2O_3$	10.910	1.143
	$C_{10}H_{20}NO_3$	11.625	1.218		$C_9H_{21}N_3O_2$	11.284	0.983
	$C_{10}H_{22}N_2O_2$	11.999	1.061		$C_9H_{23}N_4O$	11.658	0.825
	$C_{10}H_{24}N_3O$	12.374	0.905		$C_{10}H_5NO_4$	11.424	1.395
	$C_{10}H_{26}N_4$	12.748	0.751		$C_{10}H_7N_2O_3$	11.798	1.238
	$C_{11}H_6O_4$	12.139	1.474		$C_{10}H_9N_3O_2$	12.173	1.081
	$C_{11}H_8NO_3$	12.513	1.319		$C_{10}H_{11}N_4O$	12.547	0.926
	$C_{11}H_{10}N_2O_2$	12.888	1.166		$C_{10}H_{19}O_4$	11.266	1.378
	$C_{11}H_{12}N_3O$	13.262	1.014		$C_{10}H_{21}NO_3$	11.641	1.220
	$C_{11}H_{14}N_4$	13.636	0.863		$C_{10}H_{23}N_2O_2$	12.015	1.063
	$C_{11}H_{22}O_3$	12.356	1.301		$C_{10}H_{25}N_3O$	12.390	0.907
	$C_{11}H_{21}NO_2$	12.730	1.146		$C_{11}H_7O_4$	12.155	1.476
	$C_{11}H_{26}N_2O$	13.105	0.993		$C_{11}H_9NO_3$	12.529	1.321
	$C_{12}H_2N_4$	14.525	0.982		$C_{11}H_{11}N_2O_2$	12.904	1.168
	$C_{12}H_{10}O_3$	13.245	1.408		$C_{11}H_{13}N_3O$	13.278	1.016

(Contd.)

		M + 1	M + 2
	$C_{11}H_{15}N_4$	13.652	0.865
	$C_{11}H_{23}O_3$	13.372	1.303
	$C_{11}H_{25}NO_2$	12.746	1.148
	$C_{12}HN_3O$	14.167	1.132
	$C_{12}H_3N_4$	14.541	0.984
	$C_{12}H_{11}O_3$	13.261	1.411
	$C_{12}H_{13}NO_2$	13.635	1.260
	$C_{12}H_{15}N_2O$	14.009	1.110
	$C_{12}H_{17}N_3$	14.384	0.962
	$C_{13}HNO_2$	14.523	1.379
	$C_{13}H_3N_2O$	14.898	1.233
	$C_{13}H_5N_3$	15.272	1.088
	$C_{13}H_{15}O_2$	14.366	1.357
	$C_{13}H_{17}NO$	14.740	1.210
	$C_{13}H_{19}N_2$	15.115	1.065
	$C_{14}H_3O_2$	15.255	1.483
	$C_{14}H_5NO$	15.629	1.339
	$C_{14}H_7N_2$	16.003	1.197
	$C_{14}H_{19}O$	15.472	1.316
	$C_{14}H_{21}N$	15.486	1.173
	$C_{15}H_7O$	16.360	1.451
	$C_{15}H_9N$	16.734	1.312
	$C_{15}H_{23}$	16.577	1.286
	$C_{16}H_{11}$	17.466	1.432
204	$C_8H_{16}N_2O_4$	9.820	1.236
	$C_8H_{18}N_3O_3$	10.194	1.072
	$C_8H_{20}N_4O_2$	10.569	0.910
	$C_9H_4N_2O_4$	10.709	1.321
	$C_9H_6N_3O_3$	11.083	1.161
	$C_9H_8N_4O_2$	11.457	1.002
	$C_9H_{18}NO_4$	10.551	1.305
	$C_9H_{20}N_2O_3$	10.926	1.144
	$C_9H_{22}N_3O_2$	11.300	0.985
	$C_9H_{24}N_4O$	11.674	0.826
	$C_{10}H_6NO_4$	11.440	1.397
	$C_{10}H_8N_2O_3$	11.814	1.239
	$C_{10}H_{10}N_3O_2$	12.189	1.083
	$C_{10}H_{12}N_4O$	12.563	0.928
	$C_{10}H_{20}O_4$	11.282	1.380
	$C_{10}H_{22}NO_3$	11.657	1.222
	$C_{10}H_{24}N_2O_2$	12.031	1.065
	$C_{11}H_8O_4$	12.171	1.478
	$C_{11}H_{10}NO_3$	12.545	1.323
	$C_{11}H_{12}N_2O_2$	12.920	1.170
	$C_{11}H_{14}N_3O$	13.294	1.018
	$C_{11}H_{16}N_4$	13.668	0.867
	$C_{11}H_{24}O_3$	12.388	1.305
	$C_{12}H_2N_3O$	14.183	1.134
	$C_{12}H_4N_4$	14.557	0.987
	$C_{12}H_{12}O_3$	13.277	1.413
	$C_{12}H_{14}NO_2$	13.651	1.262
	$C_{12}H_{16}N_2O$	14.025	1.113
	$C_{12}H_{18}N_3$	14.400	0.965
	$C_{13}H_2NO_2$	14.539	1.381
	$C_{13}H_4N_2O$	14.914	1.235
	$C_{13}H_6N_3$	15.288	1.091
	$C_{13}H_{16}O_2$	14.382	1.359
	$C_{13}H_{18}NO$	14.756	1.213
	$C_{13}H_{20}N_2$	15.131	1.067
	$C_{14}H_4O_2$	15.271	1.485
	$C_{14}H_6NO$	15.645	1.642
	$C_{14}H_8N_2$	16.019	1.200
	$C_{14}H_{20}O$	15.488	1.318
	$C_{14}H_{22}N$	15.862	1.176
	$C_{15}H_8O$	16.376	1.454
	$C_{15}H_{10}N$	16.750	1.315
	$C_{15}H_{24}$	16.593	1.289
	$C_{16}H_{12}$	17.482	1.437
205	$C_8H_{17}N_2O_4$	9.836	1.237
	$C_8H_{19}N_3O_3$	10.210	1.074
	$C_8H_{21}N_4O_2$	10.585	0.912
	$C_9H_5N_2O_4$	10.725	1.323
	$C_9H_7N_3O_3$	11.099	1.163
	$C_9H_9N_4O_2$	11.473	1.004
	$C_9H_{19}NO_4$	10.567	1.307
	$C_9H_{21}N_2O_3$	10.942	1.146
	$C_9H_{23}N_3O_2$	11.316	0.987
	$C_{10}H_7NO_4$	11.546	1.399
	$C_{10}H_9N_2O_3$	11.830	1.241
	$C_{10}H_{11}N_3O_2$	12.205	1.085

(Contd.)

		M + 1	M + 2
	$C_{10}H_{13}N_4O$	12.579	0.930
	$C_{10}H_{21}O_4$	11.298	1.382
	$C_{10}H_{23}NO_3$	11.673	1.224
	$C_{11}HN_4O$	13.467	1.040
	$C_{11}H_9O_4$	12.187	1.480
	$C_{11}H_{11}NO_3$	12.561	1.325
	$C_{11}H_{13}N_2O_2$	12.936	1.172
	$C_{11}H_{15}N_3O$	13.310	1.020
	$C_{11}H_{17}N_4$	13.684	0.869
	$C_{12}HN_2O_2$	13.824	1.285
	$C_{12}H_3N_3O$	14.199	1.136
	$C_{12}H_5N_4$	14.573	0.989
	$C_{12}H_{13}O_3$	13.293	1.415
	$C_{12}H_{15}NO_2$	13.667	1.264
	$C_{12}H_{17}N_2O$	14.041	1.148
	$C_{12}H_{19}N_3$	14.416	0.967
	$C_{13}HO_3$	14.181	1.531
	$C_{13}H_3NO_2$	14.555	1.384
	$C_{13}H_5N_2O$	14.930	1.238
	$C_{13}H_7N_3$	15.304	1.093
	$C_{13}H_{17}O_2$	14.398	13.615
	$C_{13}H_{19}NO$	14.772	1.215
	$C_{13}H_{21}N_2$	15.147	1.070
	$C_{14}H_5O_2$	15.287	1.488
	$C_{14}H_7NO$	15.287	1.488
	$C_{14}H_9N_2$	16.035	1.203
	$C_{14}H_{21}O$	15.504	1.321
	$C_{14}H_{23}N$	15.878	1.478
	$C_{15}H_9O$	16.392	1.456
	$C_{15}H_{11}N$	16.766	1.317
	$C_{15}H_{25}$	16.609	1.292
	$C_{16}H_{13}$	17.498	1.437
	$C_{17}H$	18.386	1.591
206	$C_8H_{18}N_2O_4$	9.852	1.239
	$C_8H_{20}N_3O_3$	10.226	1.075
	$C_8H_{22}N_4O_2$	10.601	0.913
	$C_9H_6N_2O_4$	10.741	1.325
	$C_9H_8N_3O_3$	11.115	1.164
	$C_9H_{10}N_4O_2$	11.489	1.006
	$C_9H_{20}NO_4$	10.583	1.309
	$C_9H_{22}N_2O_3$	10.958	1.148
	$C_{10}H_8NO_4$	11.472	1.401
	$C_{10}H_{10}N_2O_3$	11.846	1.243
	$C_{10}H_{12}N_3O_2$	12.221	1.087
	$C_{10}H_{14}N_4O$	12.595	0.932
	$C_{10}H_{22}O_4$	11.314	1.384
	$C_{11}H_2N_4O$	13.483	1.042
	$C_{11}H_{10}O_4$	12.203	1.482
	$C_{11}H_{12}NO_3$	12.577	1.327
	$C_{11}H_{14}N_2O_2$	12.952	1.174
	$C_{11}H_{16}N_3O$	13.326	1.022
	$C_{11}H_{18}N_4$	13.700	0.871
	$C_{12}H_2N_2O_2$	13.840	1.287
	$C_{12}H_4N_3O$	14.215	1.139
	$C_{12}H_6N_4$	14.589	0.991
	$C_{12}H_{14}O_3$	13.309	1.417
	$C_{12}H_{16}NO_2$	13.683	1.266
	$C_{12}H_{18}N_2O$	14.057	1.117
	$C_{12}H_{20}N_3$	14.432	0.969
	$C_{13}H_2O_3$	14.197	1.533
	$C_{13}H_4NO_2$	14.571	1.386
	$C_{13}H_6N_2O$	14.946	1.240
	$C_{13}H_8N_3$	15.320	1.095
	$C_{13}H_{18}O_2$	14.414	1.364
	$C_{13}H_{20}NO$	14.788	1.217
	$C_{13}H_{22}N_2$	15.163	1.072
	$C_{14}H_6O_2$	15.303	1.490
	$C_{14}H_8NO$	15.677	1.347
	$C_{14}H_{10}N_2$	16.051	1.205
	$C_{14}H_{22}O$	15.520	1.323
	$C_{14}H_{24}N$	15.894	1.181
	$C_{15}H_{10}O$	16.408	1.459
	$C_{15}H_{12}N$	16.782	1.320
	$C_{15}H_{26}$	16.625	1.294
	$C_{16}H_{14}$	17.514	1.440
	$C_{17}H_2$	18.402	1.594
207	$C_8H_{19}N_2O_4$	9.868	1.241
	$C_8H_{21}N_3O_3$	10.242	1.077
	$C_9H_7N_2O_4$	10.757	1.326
	$C_9H_9N_3O_3$	11.131	1.166

(Contd.)

		M + 1	M + 2
	$C_9H_{11}N_4O_2$	11.505	1.007
	$C_9H_{21}NO_4$	10.599	1.310
	$C_{10}H_9NO_4$	11.488	1.403
	$C_{10}H_{11}N_2O_3$	11.862	1.245
	$C_{10}H_{13}N_3O_2$	12.237	1.089
	$C_{11}H_{15}N_4O$	12.611	0.934
	$C_{11}HN_3O_2$	13.125	1.196
	$C_{11}H_3N_4O$	13.500	1.045
	$C_{11}H_{11}O_4$	12.219	1.484
	$C_{11}H_{13}NO_3$	12.593	1.329
	$C_{11}H_{15}N_2O_2$	12.968	1.176
	$C_{11}H_{17}N_3O$	13.342	1.024
	$C_{11}H_{19}N_4$	13.716	0.874
	$C_{12}HNO_3$	13.482	1.439
	$C_{12}H_3N_2O_2$	13.856	1.289
	$C_{12}H_5N_3O$	14.231	1.141
	$C_{12}H_7N_4$	14.605	0.994
	$C_{12}H_{15}O_3$	13.325	1.419
	$C_{12}H_{17}NO_2$	13.699	1.268
	$C_{12}H_{19}N_2O$	14.073	1.119
	$C_{12}H_{21}N_3$	14.448	0.971
	$C_{13}H_3O_3$	14.213	1.536
	$C_{13}H_5NO_2$	14.587	1.388
	$C_{13}H_7N_2O$	14.962	1.242
	$C_{13}H_9N_3$	15.336	1.098
	$C_{13}H_{19}O_2$	14.430	1.366
	$C_{13}H_{21}NO$	14.804	1.220
	$C_{13}H_{23}N_2$	15.179	1.075
	$C_{14}H_7O_2$	15.319	1.493
	$C_{14}H_9NO$	15.693	1.349
	$C_{14}H_{11}N_2$	16.067	1.208
	$C_{14}H_{23}O$	15.536	1.326
	$C_{14}H_{25}N$	15.910	1.183
	$C_{15}H_{11}O$	16.424	1.462
	$C_{15}H_{13}N$	16.798	1.323
	$C_{15}H_{27}$	16.641	1.297
	$C_{16}HN$	17.687	1.470
	$C_{16}H_{15}$	17.530	1.443
	$C_{17}H_3$	18.418	1.597
208	$C_8H_{20}N_2O_4$	9.884	1.242
	$C_9H_8N_2O_4$	10.773	1.328
	$C_9H_{10}N_3O_3$	11.147	1.168
	$C_9H_{12}N_4O_2$	11.521	1.009
	$C_{10}H_{10}NO_4$	11.504	1.405
	$C_{10}H_{12}N_2O_3$	11.878	1.247
	$C_{10}H_{14}N_3O_2$	12.253	1.091
	$C_{10}H_{16}N_4O$	12.627	0.936
	$C_{11}H_2N_3O_2$	13.141	1.198
	$C_{11}H_4N_4O$	13.516	1.047
	$C_{11}H_{12}O_4$	12.235	1.486
	$C_{11}H_{14}NO_3$	12.609	1.331
	$C_{11}H_{16}N_2O_2$	12.984	1.178
	$C_{11}H_{18}N_3O$	13.358	1.026
	$C_{11}H_{20}N_4$	13.732	0.876
	$C_{12}H_2NO_3$	13.498	1.442
	$C_{12}H_4N_2O_2$	13.872	1.292
	$C_{12}H_6N_3O$	14.247	1.143
	$C_{12}H_8N_4$	14.621	0.996
	$C_{12}H_{16}O_3$	13.341	1.421
	$C_{12}H_{18}NO_2$	13.715	1.271
	$C_{12}H_{20}N_2O$	14.089	1.122
	$C_{12}H_{22}N_3$	14.464	0.974
	$C_{13}H_4O_3$	14.229	1.538
	$C_{13}H_6NO_2$	14.603	1.391
	$C_{13}H_8N_2O$	14.978	1.245
	$C_{13}H_{10}N_3$	15.352	1.100
	$C_{13}H_{20}O_2$	14.446	1.369
	$C_{13}H_{22}NO$	14.820	1.222
	$C_{13}H_{24}N_2$	15.195	1.077
	$C_{14}H_8O_2$	15.335	1.495
	$C_{14}H_{10}NO$	15.709	1.652
	$C_{14}H_{12}N_2$	16.083	1.210
	$C_{14}H_{24}O$	15.552	1.328
	$C_{14}H_{26}N$	15.926	1.186
	$C_{15}H_{12}O$	16.440	1.464
	$C_{15}H_{14}N$	16.814	1.325
	$C_{15}H_{28}$	16.657	1.300
	$C_{16}H_2N$	17.703	1.473
	$C_{16}H_{16}$	17.456	1.446
	$C_{17}H_4$	18.434	1.599

(Contd.)

		M + 1	M + 2			M + 1	M + 2
209	$C_9H_9N_2O_4$	10.789	1.330		$C_{15}H_{29}$	16.673	1.302
	$C_9H_{11}N_3O_3$	11.163	1.170		$C_{16}HO$	17.345	1.611
	$C_9H_{13}N_4O_2$	11.537	1.011		$C_{16}H_3N$	17.719	1.476
	$C_{10}HN_4O_2$	12.426	1.412		$C_{16}H_{17}$	17.562	1.449
	$C_{10}H_{11}NO_4$	11.520	1.406		$C_{17}H_5$	18.450	1.602
	$C_{10}H_{13}N_2O_3$	11.894	1.249	210	$C_9H_{10}N_2O_4$	10.805	1.332
	$C_{10}H_{15}N_3O_2$	12.269	1.093		$C_9H_{12}N_3O_3$	11.179	1.172
	$C_{10}H_{17}N_4O$	12.643	0.938		$C_9H_{14}N_4O_2$	11.553	1.013
	$C_{11}HN_2O_3$	12.783	1.353		$C_{10}H_2N_4O_2$	12.442	1.114
	$C_{11}H_3N_3O_2$	13.157	1.200		$C_{10}H_{12}NO_4$	11.536	1.408
	$C_{11}H_5N_4O$	13.532	1.049		$C_{10}H_{14}N_2O_3$	11.910	1.251
	$C_{11}H_{13}O_4$	12.251	1.488		$C_{10}H_{16}N_3O_2$	12.285	1.095
	$C_{11}H_{15}NO_3$	12.625	1.333		$C_{10}H_{18}N_4O$	12.659	0.940
	$C_{11}H_{17}N_2O_2$	13.000	1.180		$C_{11}H_2N_2O_3$	12.799	1.355
	$C_{11}H_{19}N_3O$	13.374	1.028		$C_{11}H_4N_3O_2$	13.173	1.202
	$C_{11}H_{21}N_4$	13.748	0.878		$C_{11}H_6N_4O$	13.548	1.051
	$C_{12}HO_4$	13.140	1.595		$C_{11}H_{14}O_4$	12.267	1.190
	$C_{12}H_3NO_3$	13.514	1.444		$C_{11}H_{16}NO_3$	12.641	1.336
	$C_{12}H_5N_2O_2$	13.888	1.294		$C_{11}H_{18}N_2O_2$	13.016	1.182
	$C_{12}H_7N_3O$	14.263	1.145		$C_{11}H_{20}N_3O$	13.390	1.031
	$C_{12}H_9N_4$	14.637	0.998		$C_{11}H_{22}N_4$	13.764	0.880
	$C_{12}H_{17}O_3$	13.357	1.423		$C_{12}H_2O_4$	13.156	1.597
	$C_{12}H_{19}NO_2$	13.731	1.273		$C_{12}H_4NO_3$	13.530	1.446
	$C_{12}H_{21}N_2O$	14.105	1.124		$C_{12}H_6N_2O_2$	13.904	1.296
	$C_{12}H_{23}N_3$	14.480	0.976		$C_{12}H_8N_3O$	14.279	1.148
	$C_{13}H_5O_3$	14.245	1.540		$C_{12}H_{10}N_4$	14.653	1.001
	$C_{13}H_7NO_2$	14.619	1.393		$C_{12}H_{18}O_3$	13.373	1.426
	$C_{13}H_9N_2O$	14.994	1.247		$C_{12}H_{20}NO_2$	13.747	1.275
	$C_{13}H_{11}N_3$	15.368	1.103		$C_{12}H_{22}N_2O$	14.121	1.126
	$C_{13}H_{21}O_2$	14.462	1.371		$C_{12}H_{24}N_3$	14.496	0.978
	$C_{13}H_{23}NO$	14.836	1.224		$C_{13}H_6O_3$	14.261	1.542
	$C_{13}H_{25}N_2$	15.211	1.080		$C_{13}H_8NO_2$	14.635	1.395
	$C_{14}H_9O_2$	15.351	1.497		$C_{13}H_{10}N_2O$	15.010	1.250
	$C_{14}H_{11}NO$	15.725	1.354		$C_{13}H_{12}N_3$	15.384	1.105
	$C_{14}H_{13}N_2$	16.099	1.213		$C_{13}H_{22}O_2$	14.478	1.373
	$C_{14}H_{25}O$	15.568	1.331		$C_{13}H_{24}NO$	14.852	1.227
	$C_{14}H_{27}N$	15.942	1.188		$C_{13}H_{26}N_2$	15.227	1.082
	$C_{15}HN_2$	16.988	1.354		$C_{14}H_{10}O_2$	15.367	1.500
	$C_{15}H_{13}O$	16.456	1.467		$C_{14}H_{12}NO$	15.741	1.357
	$C_{15}H_{15}N$	16.830	1.328		$C_{14}H_{14}N_2$	16.115	1.215

(Contd.)

		M + 1	M + 2
	$C_{14}H_{26}O$	15.584	1.333
	$C_{14}H_{28}N$	15.958	1.191
	$C_{15}H_{2}N_{2}$	17.004	1.357
	$C_{15}H_{14}O$	16.472	1.470
	$C_{15}H_{16}N$	16.846	1.331
	$C_{15}H_{30}$	16.689	1.305
	$C_{16}H_{2}O$	17.361	1.614
	$C_{16}H_{4}N$	17.735	1.479
	$C_{16}H_{18}$	17.578	1.451
	$C_{17}H_{6}$	18.466	1.606
211	$C_{9}H_{11}N_{2}O_{4}$	10.821	1.333
	$C_{9}H_{13}N_{3}O_{3}$	11.195	1.173
	$C_{9}H_{15}N_{4}O_{2}$	11.569	1.015
	$C_{10}HN_{3}O_{3}$	12.084	1.271
	$C_{10}H_{3}N_{4}O_{2}$	12.458	1.116
	$C_{10}H_{13}NO_{4}$	11.552	1.410
	$C_{10}H_{15}N_{2}O_{3}$	11.926	1.253
	$C_{10}H_{17}N_{3}O_{2}$	12.301	1.097
	$C_{10}H_{19}N_{4}O$	12.675	0.942
	$C_{11}HNO_{4}$	12.440	1.511
	$C_{11}H_{3}N_{2}O_{3}$	12.815	1.357
	$C_{11}H_{5}N_{3}O_{2}$	13.189	1.204
	$C_{11}H_{7}N_{4}O$	13.564	1.053
	$C_{11}H_{15}O_{4}$	12.283	1.492
	$C_{11}H_{17}NO_{3}$	12.657	1.338
	$C_{11}H_{19}N_{2}O_{2}$	13.032	1.184
	$C_{11}H_{21}N_{3}O$	13.406	1.033
	$C_{11}H_{23}N_{4}$	13.780	0.882
	$C_{12}H_{3}O_{4}$	13.172	1.599
	$C_{12}H_{5}NO_{3}$	13.546	1.448
	$C_{12}H_{7}N_{2}O_{2}$	13.920	1.298
	$C_{12}H_{9}N_{3}O$	14.295	1.150
	$C_{12}H_{11}N_{4}$	14.669	1.603
	$C_{12}H_{19}O_{3}$	13.389	1.428
	$C_{12}H_{21}NO_{2}$	13.763	1.277
	$C_{12}H_{23}N_{2}O$	14.137	1.128
	$C_{12}H_{25}N_{3}$	14.512	0.981
	$C_{13}H_{7}O_{3}$	14.277	1.545
	$C_{13}H_{9}NO_{2}$	14.651	1.398
	$C_{13}H_{11}N_{2}O$	15.026	1.252
	$C_{13}H_{13}N_{3}$	15.400	1.108
	$C_{13}H_{23}O_{2}$	14.494	1.375
	$C_{13}H_{25}NO$	14.868	1.229
	$C_{13}H_{27}N_{2}$	15.243	1.084
	$C_{14}HN_{3}$	16.289	1.243
	$C_{14}H_{11}O_{2}$	15.383	1.502
	$C_{14}H_{13}NO$	15.757	1.359
	$C_{14}H_{15}N_{2}$	16.131	1.218
	$C_{14}H_{27}O$	15.600	1.335
	$C_{14}H_{29}N$	15.974	1.193
	$C_{15}HNO$	16.646	1.498
	$C_{15}H_{3}N_{2}$	17.020	1.359
	$C_{15}H_{15}O$	16.488	1.472
	$C_{15}H_{17}N$	16.863	1.333
	$C_{15}H_{31}$	16.705	1.308
	$C_{16}H_{3}O$	17.377	1.617
	$C_{16}H_{5}N$	17.751	1.481
	$C_{16}H_{19}$	17.594	1.454
	$C_{17}H_{7}$	18.482	1.609
212	$C_{9}H_{12}N_{2}O_{4}$	10.837	1.335
	$C_{9}H_{14}N_{3}O_{3}$	11.211	1.175
	$C_{9}H_{16}N_{4}O_{2}$	11.585	1.017
	$C_{10}H_{2}N_{3}O_{3}$	12.100	1.273
	$C_{10}H_{4}N_{4}O_{2}$	12.474	1.118
	$C_{10}H_{14}NO_{4}$	11.568	1.412
	$C_{10}H_{16}N_{2}O_{3}$	11.942	1.255
	$C_{10}H_{18}N_{3}O_{2}$	12.317	1.099
	$C_{10}H_{20}N_{4}O$	12.691	0.945
	$C_{11}H_{2}NO_{4}$	12.456	1.513
	$C_{11}H_{4}N_{2}O_{3}$	12.831	1.359
	$C_{11}H_{6}N_{3}O_{2}$	13.205	1.206
	$C_{11}H_{8}N_{4}O$	13.580	1.055
	$C_{11}H_{16}O_{4}$	12.299	1.494
	$C_{14}H_{18}NO_{3}$	12.673	1.340
	$C_{11}H_{20}N_{2}O_{2}$	13.048	1.187
	$C_{11}H_{22}N_{3}O$	13.422	1.035
	$C_{11}H_{24}N_{4}$	13.796	0.885
	$C_{12}H_{4}O_{4}$	13.188	1.601
	$C_{12}H_{6}NO_{3}$	13.562	1.450
	$C_{12}H_{8}N_{2}O_{2}$	13.936	1.301

(Contd.)

		M + 1	M + 2		M + 1	M + 2
	$C_{12}H_{10}N_3O$	14.311	1.152	$C_{11}H_7N_3O_2$	13.221	1.209
	$C_{12}H_{12}N_4$	14.685	1.005	$C_{11}H_9N_4O$	13.596	1.058
	$C_{12}H_{20}O_3$	13.405	1.430	$C_{11}H_{17}O_4$	12.315	1.496
	$C_{12}H_{22}NO_2$	13.779	1.279	$C_{11}H_{19}NO_3$	12.689	1.342
	$C_{12}H_{24}N_2O$	14.153	1.131	$C_{11}H_{21}N_2O_2$	13.064	1.189
	$C_{12}H_{26}N_3$	14.528	0.983	$C_{11}H_{23}N_3O$	13.438	1.037
	$C_{13}H_8O_3$	14.293	1.547	$C_{11}H_{25}N_4$	13.812	0.887
	$C_{13}H_{10}NO_2$	14.667	1.400	$C_{12}H_5O_4$	13.204	1.604
	$C_{13}H_{12}N_2O$	15.042	1.254	$C_{12}H_7NO_3$	13.578	1.452
	$C_{13}H_{14}N_3$	15.416	1.110	$C_{12}H_9N_2O_2$	13.952	1.303
	$C_{13}H_{24}O_2$	14.510	1.378	$C_{12}H_{11}N_3O$	14.327	1.155
	$C_{13}H_{26}NO$	14.884	1.232	$C_{12}H_{13}N_4$	14.701	1.008
	$C_{13}H_{28}N_2$	15.259	1.087	$C_{12}H_{21}O_3$	13.421	1.432
	$C_{14}H_2N_3$	16.305	1.245	$C_{12}H_{23}NO_2$	13.795	1.282
	$C_{14}H_{12}O_2$	15.399	1.505	$C_{12}H_{25}N_2O$	14.169	1.133
	$C_{14}H_{14}NO$	15.773	1.362	$C_{12}H_{27}N_3$	14.544	0.985
	$C_{14}H_{16}N_2$	16.147	1.221	$C_{13}HN_4$	15.590	1.136
	$C_{14}H_{28}O$	15.616	1.338	$C_{13}H_9N_3$	14.309	1.549
	$C_{14}H_{30}N$	15.990	1.196	$C_{13}H_{11}NO_2$	14.683	1.402
	$C_{15}H_2NO$	16.662	1.500	$C_{13}H_{13}N_2O$	15.058	1.257
	$C_{15}H_4N_2$	17.036	1.362	$C_{13}H_{15}N_3$	15.432	1.113
	$C_{15}H_{16}O$	16.504	1.475	$C_{13}H_{25}O_2$	14.526	1.380
	$C_{15}H_{18}N$	16.879	1.336	$C_{13}H_{27}NO$	14.900	1.234
	$C_{15}H_{32}$	16.721	1.310	$C_{13}H_{29}N_2$	15.275	1.089
	$C_{16}H_4O$	17.393	1.620	$C_{14}HN_2O$	15.946	1.389
	$C_{16}H_6N$	17.767	1.484	$C_{14}H_3N_3$	16.321	1.248
	$C_{16}H_{20}$	17.610	1.457	$C_{14}H_{13}O_2$	15.415	1.507
	$C_{17}H_8$	18.498	1.612	$C_{14}H_{15}NO$	15.789	1.565
213	$C_9H_{13}N_2O_4$	10.853	1.337	$C_{14}H_{17}N_2$	16.163	1.223
	$C_9H_{15}N_3O_3$	11.227	1.177	$C_{14}H_{29}O$	15.632	1.340
	$C_9H_{17}N_4O_2$	11.601	1.018	$C_{14}H_{31}N$	16.006	1.198
	$C_{10}HN_2O_4$	11.741	1.431	$C_{15}HO_2$	16.303	1.642
	$C_{10}H_3N_3O_2$	12.116	1.275	$C_{15}H_3NO$	16.678	1.503
	$C_{10}H_5N_4O_2$	12.490	1.120	$C_{15}H_5N_2$	17.052	1.565
	$C_{10}H_{15}NO_4$	11.584	1.414	$C_{15}H_{17}O$	16.520	1.478
	$C_{10}H_{17}N_2O_3$	11.958	1.257	$C_{15}H_{19}N$	16.895	1.339
	$C_{10}H_{19}N_3O_2$	12.333	1.101	$C_{16}H_5O$	17.409	1.622
	$C_{10}H_{21}N_4O$	12.707	0.947	$C_{16}H_7N$	17.783	1.487
	$C_{11}H_3NO_4$	12.472	1.515	$C_{16}H_{21}$	17.626	1.460
	$C_{11}H_5N_2O_3$	12.847	1.361	$C_{17}H_9$	18.514	1.615

(Contd.)

		M + 1	M + 2
214	$C_9H_{14}N_2O_4$	10.869	1.339
	$C_9H_{16}N_3O_3$	11.243	1.179
	$C_9H_{18}N_4O_2$	11.617	1.020
	$C_{10}H_2N_2O_4$	11.757	1.433
	$C_{10}H_4N_3O_3$	12.132	1.277
	$C_{10}H_6N_4O_2$	12.506	1.122
	$C_{10}H_{16}NO_4$	11.600	1.416
	$C_{10}H_{18}N_2O_3$	11.974	1.258
	$C_{10}H_{20}N_3O_2$	12.349	1.103
	$C_{10}H_{22}N_4O$	12.723	0.949
	$C_{11}H_4NO_4$	12.488	1.517
	$C_{11}H_6N_2O_3$	12.863	1.363
	$C_{11}H_8N_3O_2$	13.237	1.211
	$C_{11}H_{10}N_4O$	13.612	1.060
	$C_{11}H_{18}O_4$	12.331	1.498
	$C_{11}H_{20}NO_3$	12.705	1.344
	$C_{11}H_{22}N_2O_2$	13.080	1.191
	$C_{11}H_{24}N_3O$	13.454	1.039
	$C_{11}H_{26}N_4$	13.828	0.889
	$C_{12}H_6O_4$	13.220	1.606
	$C_{12}H_8NO_3$	13.594	1.455
	$C_{12}H_{10}N_2O_2$	13.968	1.305
	$C_{12}H_{12}N_3O$	14.343	1.157
	$C_{12}H_{14}N_4$	14.717	1.010
	$C_{12}H_{22}O_3$	13.437	1.434
	$C_{12}H_{24}NO_2$	13.811	1.284
	$C_{12}H_{26}N_2O$	14.185	1.135
	$C_{12}H_{28}N_3$	14.560	0.988
	$C_{13}H_2N_4$	15.606	1.139
	$C_{13}H_{10}O_3$	14.325	1.552
	$C_{13}H_{12}NO_2$	14.699	1.405
	$C_{13}H_{14}N_2O$	15.074	1.259
	$C_{13}H_{16}N_3$	15.448	1.151
	$C_{13}H_{26}O_2$	14.542	1.382
	$C_{13}H_{28}NO$	14.916	1.236
	$C_{13}H_{30}N_2$	15.291	1.092
	$C_{14}H_2N_2O$	15.962	1.391
	$C_{14}H_4N_3$	16.337	1.251
	$C_{14}H_{14}O_2$	15.431	1.510
	$C_{14}H_{16}NO$	15.805	1.367

		M + 1	M + 2
	$C_{14}H_{18}N_2$	16.179	1.226
	$C_{14}H_{30}O$	15.648	1.343
	$C_{15}H_2O_2$	16.319	1.645
	$C_{15}H_4NO$	16.694	1.506
	$C_{15}H_6N_2$	17.068	1.368
	$C_{15}H_{18}O$	16.536	1.480
	$C_{15}H_{20}N$	16.911	1.342
	$C_{16}H_6O$	17.425	1.625
	$C_{16}H_8N$	17.799	1.490
	$C_{16}H_{22}$	17.642	1.463
	$C_{17}H_{20}$	18.530	1.618
215	$C_9H_{15}N_2O_4$	10.885	1.340
	$C_9H_{17}N_3O_3$	11.259	1.181
	$C_9H_{19}N_4O_2$	11.633	1.022
	$C_{10}H_3N_2O_4$	11.773	1.435
	$C_{10}H_5N_3O_3$	12.148	1.279
	$C_{10}H_7N_4O_2$	12.522	1.124
	$C_{10}H_{17}NO_4$	11.616	1.417
	$C_{10}H_{19}N_2O_3$	11.990	1.260
	$C_{10}H_{21}N_3O_2$	12.365	1.105
	$C_{10}H_{23}N_4O$	12.739	0.951
	$C_{11}H_5NO_4$	12.504	1.519
	$C_{11}H_7N_2O_3$	12.879	1.365
	$C_{11}H_9N_3O_2$	13.253	1.213
	$C_{11}H_{11}N_4O$	13.628	1.062
	$C_{11}H_{19}O_4$	12.347	1.500
	$C_{11}H_{21}NO_3$	12.721	1.346
	$C_{11}H_{23}N_2O_2$	13.096	1.193
	$C_{11}H_{25}N_3O$	13.470	1.041
	$C_{11}H_{27}N_4$	13.844	0.891
	$C_{12}H_7O_4$	13.236	1.608
	$C_{12}H_9NO_3$	13.610	1.457
	$C_{12}H_{11}N_2O_2$	13.984	1.307
	$C_{12}H_{13}N_3O$	14.359	1.159
	$C_{12}H_{15}N$	14.733	1.012
	$C_{12}H_{23}O_3$	13.453	14.362
	$C_{12}H_{25}NO_2$	13.827	1.286
	$C_{12}H_{27}N_2O$	14.201	1.137
	$C_{12}H_{29}N_3$	14.576	0.990
	$C_{13}HN_3O$	15.247	1.285

(Contd.)

		M + 1	M + 2			M + 1	M + 2
	$C_{13}H_3N_4$	15.622	1.141		$C_{11}H_{28}N_4$	13.860	0.893
	$C_{13}H_{11}O_3$	14.341	1.554		$C_{12}H_8O_4$	13.252	1.610
	$C_{13}H_{13}NO_2$	14.715	1.407		$C_{12}H_{10}NO_3$	13.626	1.459
	$C_{13}H_{15}N_2O$	15.090	1.262		$C_{12}H_{12}N_2O_2$	14.000	1.310
	$C_{13}H_{17}N_3$	15.464	1.118		$C_{12}H_{14}N_3O$	14.375	1.161
	$C_{13}H_{27}O_2$	14.558	1.385		$C_{12}H_{16}N_4$	14.749	1.015
	$C_{13}H_{29}NO$	14.932	1.239		$C_{12}H_{24}O_3$	13.469	1.438
	$C_{14}HNO_2$	15.604	1.536		$C_{12}H_{26}NO_2$	13.843	1.288
	$C_{14}H_3N_2O$	15.978	1.394		$C_{12}H_{28}N_2O$	14.217	1.140
	$C_{14}H_5N_3$	16.353	1.253		$C_{13}H_2N_2O$	15.263	1.287
	$C_{14}H_{15}O_2$	15.447	1.512		$C_{13}H_4N_4$	15.638	1.144
	$C_{14}H_{17}NO$	15.821	1.370		$C_{13}H_{12}O_3$	14.357	1.556
	$C_{14}H_{19}N_2$	16.195	1.228		$C_{13}H_{14}NO_2$	14.731	1.409
	$C_{15}H_3O_2$	16.335	1.648		$C_{13}H_{16}N_2O$	15.106	1.264
	$C_{15}H_5NO$	16.710	1.508		$C_{13}H_{18}N_3$	15.480	1.120
	$C_{15}H_7N_2$	17.084	1.370		$C_{13}H_{28}O_2$	14.574	1.387
	$C_{15}H_{19}O$	16.552	1.483		$C_{14}H_2NO_2$	15.620	1.538
	$C_{15}H_{21}N$	16.927	1.344		$C_{14}H_4N_2O$	15.994	1.396
	$C_{17}H_7O$	17.441	1.628		$C_{14}H_6N_3$	16.369	1.256
	$C_{16}H_9N$	17.815	1.493		$C_{14}H_{16}O_2$	15.463	1.515
	$C_{16}H_{23}$	17.658	1.466		$C_{14}H_{18}NO$	15.837	1.372
	$C_{17}H_{11}$	18.546	1.621		$C_{14}H_{20}N_2$	16.211	1.231
216	$C_9H_{16}N_2O_4$	10.901	1.342		$C_{15}H_4O_2$	16.351	1.650
	$C_9H_{18}N_3O_3$	11.275	1.182		$C_{15}H_6NO$	16.726	1.511
	$C_9H_{20}N_4O_2$	11.649	1.024		$C_{15}H_8N_2$	17.100	1.373
	$C_{10}H_4N_2O_4$	11.789	1.437		$C_{15}H_{20}O$	16.568	1.485
	$C_{10}H_6N_3O_3$	12.164	1.281		$C_{15}H_{22}N$	16.943	1.347
	$C_{10}H_8N_4O_2$	12.538	1.126		$C_{16}H_8O$	17.457	1.631
	$C_{10}H_{18}NO_4$	11.632	1.419		$C_{16}H_{10}N$	17.831	1.496
	$C_{10}H_{20}N_2O_3$	12.006	1.262		$C_{16}H_{24}$	17.674	1.468
	$C_{10}H_{22}N_3O_2$	12.381	1.107		$C_{17}H_{12}$	18.562	1.624
	$C_{10}H_{24}N_4O$	12.755	0.953	217	$C_9H_{17}N_2O_4$	10.917	1.344
	$C_{11}H_6NO_4$	12.520	1.521		$C_9H_{19}N_3O_3$	11.291	1.184
	$C_{11}H_8N_2O_3$	12.895	1.367		$C_9H_{21}N_4O_2$	11.665	1.026
	$C_{11}H_{10}N_3O_2$	13.269	1.215		$C_{10}H_5N_2O_4$	11.805	1.439
	$C_{11}H_{12}N_4O$	13.644	1.064		$C_{10}H_7N_3O_3$	12.180	1.283
	$C_{11}H_{20}O_4$	12.363	1.502		$C_{10}H_9N_4O_2$	12.554	1.128
	$C_{11}H_{22}NO_3$	12.737	1.348		$C_{10}H_{19}NO_4$	11.648	1.421
	$C_{11}H_{24}N_2O_2$	13.112	1.195		$C_{10}H_{21}N_2O_3$	12.022	1.264
	$C_{11}H_{26}N_3O$	13.486	1.043		$C_{10}H_{23}N_3O_2$	12.397	1.109

(Contd.)

		M + 1	M + 2
	$C_{10}H_{25}N_4O$	12.771	0.955
	$C_{11}H_7NO_4$	12.536	1.523
	$C_{11}H_9N_2O_3$	12.911	1.369
	$C_{11}H_{11}N_3O_2$	13.285	1.217
	$C_{11}H_{13}N_4O$	13.660	1.066
	$C_{11}H_{21}O_4$	12.379	1.504
	$C_{11}H_{23}NO_3$	12.753	1.350
	$C_{11}H_{25}N_2O_2$	13.128	1.197
	$C_{11}H_{27}N_3O$	13.502	1.046
	$C_{12}HN_4O$	14.548	1.186
	$C_{12}H_9O_4$	13.268	1.612
	$C_{12}H_{11}NO_3$	13.642	1.461
	$C_{12}H_{13}N_2O_2$	14.016	1.312
	$C_{12}H_{15}N_3O$	14.391	1.164
	$C_{12}H_{17}N_4$	14.765	1.017
	$C_{12}H_{25}O_3$	13.485	1.441
	$C_{12}H_{27}NO_2$	13.859	1.291
	$C_{13}HN_2O_2$	14.905	1.435
	$C_{13}H_3N_3O$	15.279	1.290
	$C_{13}H_5N_4$	15.654	1.146
	$C_{13}H_{13}O_3$	14.373	1.558
	$C_{13}H_{15}NO_2$	14.747	1.412
	$C_{13}H_{17}N_2O$	15.122	1.266
	$C_{13}H_{19}N_3$	15.496	1.123
	$C_{14}HO_3$	15.262	1.684
	$C_{14}H_3NO_2$	15.636	1.541
	$C_{14}H_5N_2O$	16.010	1.399
	$C_{14}H_7N_3$	16.385	1.258
	$C_{14}H_{17}O_2$	15.479	1.517
	$C_{14}H_{19}NO$	15.583	1.375
	$C_{14}H_{21}N_2$	16.227	1.233
	$C_{15}H_5O_2$	16.367	1.653
	$C_{15}H_7NO$	16.742	1.514
	$C_{15}H_9N_2$	17.116	1.376
	$C_{15}H_{21}O$	16.584	1.488
	$C_{15}H_{23}N$	16.959	1.350
	$C_{16}H_9O$	17.473	1.634
	$C_{16}H_{11}N$	17.847	1.498
	$C_{16}H_{25}$	17.690	1.471
	$C_{17}H_{13}$	18.578	1.627
	$C_{18}H$	19.467	1.790
218	$C_9H_{18}N_2O_4$	10.933	1.346
	$C_9H_{20}N_3O_3$	11.307	1.186
	$C_9H_{22}N_4O_2$	11.681	1.028
	$C_{10}H_6N_2O_4$	11.821	1.441
	$C_{10}H_8N_3O_3$	12.196	1.285
	$C_{10}H_{10}N_4O_2$	12.570	1.130
	$C_{10}H_{20}NO_4$	11.664	1.423
	$C_{10}H_{22}N_2O_3$	12.038	1.266
	$C_{10}H_{24}N_3O_2$	12.413	1.111
	$C_{10}H_{26}N_4O$	12.787	0.957
	$C_{11}H_8NO_4$	12.552	1.525
	$C_{11}H_{10}N_2O_3$	12.927	1.371
	$C_{11}H_{12}N_3O_2$	13.301	1.219
	$C_{11}H_{14}N_4O$	13.676	1.068
	$C_{11}H_{22}O_4$	12.395	1.506
	$C_{11}H_{24}NO_3$	12.769	1.352
	$C_{11}H_{26}N_2O_2$	13.144	1.199
	$C_{12}H_2N_4O$	14.564	1.188
	$C_{12}H_{10}O_4$	13.284	1.614
	$C_{12}H_{12}NO_3$	13.658	1.463
	$C_{12}H_{14}N_2O_2$	14.032	1.314
	$C_{12}H_{16}N_3O$	14.407	1.166
	$C_{12}H_{18}N_4$	14.781	1.019
	$C_{12}H_{26}O_3$	13.501	1.443
	$C_{13}H_2N_2O_2$	14.921	1.437
	$C_{13}H_4N_3O$	15.295	1.292
	$C_{13}H_6N_4$	15.670	1.149
	$C_{13}H_{14}O_3$	14.389	1.561
	$C_{13}H_{16}NO_2$	14.763	1.414
	$C_{13}H_{18}N_2O$	15.138	1.269
	$C_{13}H_{20}N_3$	15.512	1.125
	$C_{14}H_2O_3$	15.278	1.687
	$C_{14}H_4NO_2$	15.652	1.543
	$C_{14}H_6N_2O$	16.026	1.402
	$C_{14}H_8N_3$	16.401	1.261
	$C_{14}H_{18}O_2$	15.495	1.520
	$C_{14}H_{20}NO$	15.869	1.377
	$C_{14}H_{22}N_2$	16.243	1.236
	$C_{15}H_6O_2$	16.383	1.655

(Contd.)

		M + 1	M + 2
	$C_{15}H_8NO$	16.758	1.516
	$C_{15}H_{10}N_2$	17.132	1.379
	$C_{15}H_{22}O$	16.600	1.491
	$C_{15}H_{24}N$	16.975	1.352
	$C_{16}H_{10}O$	17.489	1.636
	$C_{16}H_{12}N$	17.863	1.501
	$C_{16}H_{26}$	17.706	1.474
	$C_{17}H_{14}$	18.594	1.630
	$C_{18}H_2$	19.483	1.793
219	$C_9H_{19}N_2O_4$	10.949	1.347
	$C_9H_{21}N_3O_3$	11.323	1.188
	$C_9H_{23}N_4O_2$	11.697	1.030
	$C_{10}H_7N_2O_4$	11.837	1.443
	$C_{10}H_9N_3O_3$	12.212	1.287
	$C_{10}H_{11}N_4O_2$	12.586	1.132
	$C_{10}H_{21}NO_4$	11.680	1.425
	$C_{10}H_{23}N_2O_3$	12.054	1.268
	$C_{10}H_{25}N_3O_2$	12.429	1.113
	$C_{11}H_9NO_4$	12.568	1.527
	$C_{11}H_{11}N_2O_3$	12.943	1.373
	$C_{11}H_{13}N_3O_2$	13.317	1.221
	$C_{11}H_{15}N_4O$	13.692	1.071
	$C_{11}H_{23}O_4$	12.411	1.508
	$C_{11}H_{25}NO_3$	12.785	1.354
	$C_{12}HN_3O_2$	14.206	1.338
	$C_{12}H_3N_4O$	14.580	1.190
	$C_{12}H_{11}O_4$	13.300	1.616
	$C_{12}H_{13}NO_3$	13.674	1.466
	$C_{12}H_{15}N_2O_2$	14.048	1.316
	$C_{12}H_{17}N_3O$	14.423	1.168
	$C_{12}H_{19}N_4$	14.797	1.022
	$C_{13}HNO_3$	14.563	1.585
	$C_3H_3N_2O_2$	14.937	1.439
	$C_{13}H_5N_3O$	15.311	1.295
	$C_{13}H_7N_4$	15.686	1.151
	$C_{13}H_{15}O_3$	14.405	1.563
	$C_{13}H_{17}NO_2$	14.779	1.417
	$C_{13}H_{19}N_2O$	15.154	1.271
	$C_{13}H_{21}N_3$	15.528	1.128
	$C_{14}H_3O_3$	15.294	1.689

		M + 1	M + 2
	$C_{14}H_5NO_2$	15.668	1.546
	$C_{14}H_7N_2O$	16.042	1.404
	$C_{14}H_9N_3$	16.417	1.264
	$C_{14}H_{19}O_2$	15.511	1.522
	$C_{14}H_{21}NO$	15.885	1.380
	$C_{14}H_{23}N_2$	16.259	1.239
	$C_{15}H_7O_2$	16.399	1.658
	$C_{15}H_9NO$	16.774	1.519
	$C_{15}H_{11}N_2$	17.148	1.381
	$C_{15}H_{23}O$	16.616	1.493
	$C_{15}H_{25}N$	16.991	1.355
	$C_{16}H_{11}O$	17.505	1.639
	$C_{16}H_{13}N$	17.879	1.504
	$C_{16}H_{27}$	17.722	1.477
	$C_{17}HN$	18.768	1.661
	$C_{17}H_{15}$	18.610	1.632
	$C_{18}H_3$	19.499	1.796
220	$C_9H_{20}N_2O_4$	10.965	1.349
	$C_9H_{22}N_3O_3$	11.339	1.190
	$C_9H_{24}N_4O_2$	11.713	1.032
	$C_{10}H_8N_2O_4$	11.853	1.445
	$C_{10}H_{10}N_3O_3$	12.228	1.288
	$C_{10}H_{12}N_4O_2$	12.602	1.134
	$C_{10}H_{22}NO_4$	11.696	1.427
	$C_{10}H_{24}N_2O_3$	12.070	1.270
	$C_{11}H_{10}NO_4$	12.584	1.529
	$C_{11}H_{12}N_2O_3$	12.959	1.375
	$C_{11}H_{14}N_3O_2$	13.333	1.234
	$C_{11}H_{16}N_4O$	13.708	1.073
	$C_{11}H_{24}O_4$	12.427	1.510
	$C_{12}H_2N_3O_2$	14.222	1.340
	$C_{12}H_4N_4O$	14.596	1.193
	$C_{12}H_{12}O_4$	13.316	1.618
	$C_{12}H_{14}NO_3$	13.690	1.468
	$C_{12}H_{16}N_2O_2$	14.064	1.318
	$C_{12}H_{18}N_3O$	14.439	1.171
	$C_{12}H_{20}N_4$	14.813	1.024
	$C_{13}H_2NO_3$	14.579	1.588
	$C_{13}H_4N_2O_2$	14.953	1.442
	$C_{13}H_6N_3O$	15.327	1.297

(Contd.)

		M + 1	M + 2
	$C_{13}H_8N_4$	15.702	1.154
	$C_{13}H_{16}O_3$	14.421	1.565
	$C_{13}H_{18}NO_2$	14.795	1.419
	$C_{13}H_{20}N_2O$	15.170	1.274
	$C_{13}H_{22}N_3$	15.544	1.130
	$C_{14}H_4O_3$	15.310	1.692
	$C_{14}H_6NO_2$	15.684	1.548
	$C_{14}H_8N_2O$	16.058	1.407
	$C_{14}H_{10}N_3$	16.433	1.267
	$C_{14}H_{20}O_2$	15.527	1.525
	$C_{14}H_{22}NO$	15.901	1.382
	$C_{14}H_{24}N_2$	16.275	1.241
	$C_{15}H_8O_2$	16.415	1.661
	$C_{15}H_{10}NO$	16.790	1.522
	$C_{15}H_{12}N_2$	17.164	1.384
	$C_{15}H_{24}O$	16.632	1.496
	$C_{15}H_{26}N$	17.007	1.358
	C[illegible]$H_{12}O$	17.521	1.642
	C[illegible]N	17.895	1.507
	$C_{16}H_{28}$	17.738	1.480
	$C_{17}H_2N$	18.784	1.664
	$C_{17}H_{16}$	18.626	1.635
	$C_{18}H_4$	19.515	1.799
221	$C_9H_{21}N_2O_4$	10.981	1.351
	$C_9H_{23}N_3O_3$	11.355	1.191
	$C_{10}H_9N_2O_4$	11.869	1.446
	$C_{10}H_{11}N_3O_3$	12.244	1.290
	$C_{10}H_{13}N_4O_2$	12.618	1.136
	$C_{10}H_{23}NO_4$	11.712	1.429
	$C_{11}HN_4O_2$	13.507	1.246
	$C_{11}H_{11}NO_4$	12.600	1.531
	$C_{11}H_{13}N_2O_3$	12.975	1.378
	$C_{11}H_{15}N_3O_2$	13.349	1.226
	$C_{11}H_{17}N_4O$	13.724	1.075
	$C_{12}HN_2O_3$	13.863	1.491
	$C_{12}H_3N_3O_2$	14.238	1.342
	$C_{12}H_5N_4O$	14.612	1.195
	$C_{12}H_{13}O_4$	13.332	1.621
	$C_{12}H_{15}NO_3$	13.706	1.470
	$C_{12}H_{17}N_2O_2$	14.080	1.321
	$C_{12}H_{19}N_3O$	14.455	1.173
	$C_{12}H_{21}N_4$	14.829	1.027
	$C_{13}HO_4$	14.220	1.737
	$C_{13}H_3NO_3$	14.595	1.590
	$C_{13}H_5N_2O_2$	14.969	1.444
	$C_{13}H_7N_3O$	15.343	1.300
	$C_{13}H_9N_4$	15.718	1.156
	$C_{13}H_{17}O_3$	14.437	1.568
	$C_{13}H_{19}NO_2$	14.811	1.421
	$C_{13}H_{21}N_2O$	15.186	1.276
	$C_{13}H_{23}N_3$	15.560	1.133
	$C_{14}H_5O_3$	15.326	1.694
	$C_{14}H_7NO_2$	15.700	1.551
	$C_{14}H_9N_2O$	16.074	1.409
	$C_{14}H_{11}N_3$	16.449	1.269
	$C_{14}H_{21}O_2$	15.543	1.527
	$C_{14}H_{23}NO$	15.917	1.385
	$C_{14}H_{25}N_2$	16.291	1.244
	$C_{15}H_9O_2$	16.431	1.663
	$C_{15}H_{11}NO$	16.806	1.524
	$C_{15}H_{13}N_2$	17.180	1.387
	$C_{15}H_{25}O$	16.648	1.499
	$C_{15}H_{27}N$	17.023	1.361
	$C_{16}HN_2$	18.069	1.538
	$C_{16}H_{13}O$	17.537	1.645
	$C_{16}H_{15}N$	17.911	1.510
	$C_{16}H_{29}$	17.754	1.483
	$C_{18}HO$	18.425	1.799
	$C_{18}H_3N$	18.800	1.667
	$C_{18}H_5$	19.531	1.802
222	$C_9H_{22}N_2O_4$	10.997	1.353
	$C_{10}H_{10}N_2O_4$	11.885	1.448
	$C_{10}H_{12}N_3O_3$	12.260	1.292
	$C_{10}H_{14}N_4O_2$	12.634	1.138
	$C_{11}H_2N_4O_2$	13.523	1.248
	$C_{11}H_{12}NO_4$	12.616	1.533
	$C_{11}H_{14}N_2O_3$	12.991	1.380
	$C_{11}H_{16}N_3O_2$	13.365	1.228
	$C_{11}H_{18}N_4O$	13.740	1.077
	$C_{12}H_2N_2O_3$	13.879	1.493

(Contd.)

		M + 1	M + 2			M + 1	M + 2
	$C_{12}H_4N_3O_2$	14.254	1.345		$C_{11}H_3N_4O_2$	13.539	1.250
	$C_{12}H_6N_4O$	14.628	1.197		$C_{11}H_{13}NO_4$	12.632	1.535
	$C_{12}H_{14}O_4$	13.348	1.623		$C_{11}H_{15}N_2O_3$	13.007	1.382
	$C_{12}H_{16}NO_3$	13.722	1.472		$C_{11}H_{17}N_3O_2$	13.381	1.230
	$C_{12}H_{18}N_2O_2$	14.096	1.323		$C_{11}H_{19}N_4O$	13.756	1.079
	$C_{12}H_{20}N_3O$	14.471	1.175		$C_{12}HNO_4$	13.521	1.645
	$C_{12}H_{22}N_4$	14.845	1.029		$C_{12}H_3N_2O_3$	13.895	1.495
	$C_{13}H_2O_4$	14.236	1.739		$C_{12}H_5N_3O_2$	14.270	1.347
	$C_{13}H_4NO_3$	14.611	1.592		$C_{12}H_7N_4O$	14.644	1.200
	$C_{13}H_6N_2O_2$	14.985	1.446		$C_{12}H_{15}O_4$	13.364	1.625
	$C_{13}H_8N_3O$	15.359	1.302		$C_{12}H_{17}NO_3$	13.738	1.474
	$C_{13}H_{10}N_4$	15.734	1.159		$C_{12}H_{19}N_2O_2$	14.112	1.325
	$C_{13}H_{18}O_3$	14.453	1.570		$C_{12}H_{21}N_3O$	14.487	1.178
	$C_{13}H_{20}NO_2$	14.827	1.424		$C_{12}H_{23}N_4$	14.861	1.031
	$C_{13}H_{22}N_2O$	15.202	1.279		$C_{13}H_3O_4$	14.252	1.742
	$C_{13}H_{24}N_3$	15.576	1.135		$C_{13}H_5NO_3$	14.627	1.595
	$C_{14}H_6O_3$	15.342	1.697		$C_{13}H_7N_2O_2$	15.001	1.449
	$C_{14}H_8NO_2$	15.716	1.553		$C_{13}H_9N_3O$	15.375	1.304
	$C_{14}H_{10}N_2O$	16.090	1.412		$C_{13}H_{11}N_4$	15.750	1.161
	$C_{14}H_{12}N_3$	16.465	1.272		$C_{13}H_{19}O_3$	14.469	1.572
	$C_{14}H_{22}O_2$	15.559	1.530		$C_{13}H_{21}NO_2$	14.843	1.426
	$C_{14}H_{24}NO$	15.933	1.387		$C_{13}H_{23}N_2O$	15.218	1.281
	$C_{14}H_{26}N_2$	16.307	1.246		$C_{13}H_{25}N_3$	15.592	1.138
	$C_{15}H_{10}O_2$	16.447	1.666		$C_{14}H_7O_4$	15.358	1.699
	$C_{15}H_{12}NO$	16.822	1.527		$C_{14}H_9NO_2$	15.732	1.556
	$C_{15}H_{14}N_2$	17.196	1.390		$C_{14}H_{11}N_2O$	16.106	1.414
	$C_{15}H_{26}O$	16.664	1.501		$C_{14}H_{13}N_3$	16.481	1.274
	$C_{15}H_{28}N$	17.039	1.363		$C_{14}H_{23}O_2$	15.575	1.532
	$C_{16}H_2N_2$	18.085	1.540		$C_{14}H_{25}NO$	15.949	1.390
	$C_{16}H_{14}O$	17.553	1.648		$C_{14}H_{27}N_2$	16.323	1.249
	$C_{16}H_{16}N$	17.927	1.513		$C_{15}HN_3$	17.369	1.419
	$C_{16}H_{30}$	17.770	1.485		$C_{15}H_{11}O_2$	16.463	1.669
	$C_{17}H_2O$	18.441	1.802		$C_{15}H_{13}NO$	16.838	1.530
	$C_{17}H_4N$	18.816	1.670		$C_{15}H_{15}N_2$	17.212	1.392
	$C_{17}H_{18}$	18.658	1.641		$C_{15}H_{27}O$	16.680	1.504
	$C_{18}H_6$	19.547	1.805		$C_{15}H_{29}N$	17.055	1.366
223	$C_{10}H_{11}N_2O_4$	11.901	1.450		$C_{16}HNO$	17.726	1.677
	$C_{10}H_{13}N_3O_3$	12.276	1.294		$C_{16}H_3N_2$	18.101	1.543
	$C_{10}H_{15}N_4O_2$	12.650	1.140		$C_{16}H_{15}O$	17.569	1.650
	$C_{11}HN_3O_3$	13.164	1.401		$C_{16}H_{17}N$	17.943	1.516

(Contd.)

		M + 1	M + 2			M + 1	M + 2
	$C_{16}H_{31}$	17.786	1.488		$C_{15}H_{12}O_2$	16.479	1.671
	$C_{17}H_3O$	18.457	1.805		$C_{15}H_{14}NO$	16.854	1.532
	$C_{17}H_5N.$	18.832	1.673		$C_{15}H_{16}N_2$	17.228	1.395
	$C_{17}H_{19}$	18.674	1.644		$C_{15}H_{28}O$	16.696	1.507
	$C_{18}H_7$	19.563	1.808		$C_{15}H_{30}N$	17.071	1.369
224	$C_{10}H_{12}N_2O_4$	11.917	1.452		$C_{16}H_2NO$	17.742	1.680
	$C_{10}H_{14}N_3O_3$	12.292	1.296		$C_{16}H_4N_2$	18.117	1.546
	$C_{10}H_{16}N_4O_2$	12.666	1.142		$C_{16}H_{16}O$	17.585	1.653
	$C_{11}H_2N_3O_3$	13.180	1.404		$C_{16}H_{18}N$	17.959	1.519
	$C_{11}H_4N_4O_2$	13.555	1.252		$C_{16}H_{32}$	17.802	1.491
	$C_{11}H_{14}NO_4$	12.648	1.537		$C_{17}H_4O$	18.473	1.808
	$C_{11}H_{16}N_2O_3$	13.023	1.384		$C_{17}H_6N$	18.848	1.676
	$C_{11}H_{18}N_3O_2$	13.397	1.232		$C_{17}H_{20}$	18.690	1.647
	$C_{11}H_{20}N_4O$	13.772	1.082		$C_{18}H_8$	19.579	1.182
	$C_{12}H_2NO_4$	13.537	1.647	225	$C_{10}H_{13}N_2O_4$	11.933	1.454
	$C_{12}H_4N_2O_3$	13.911	1.498		$C_{10}H_{15}N_3O_3$	12.308	1.298
	$C_{12}H_6N_3O_2$	14.286	1.349		$C_{10}H_{17}N_4O_2$	12.682	1.144
	$C_{12}H_8N_4O$	14.660	1.202		$C_{11}HN_2O_4$	12.822	1.558
	$C_{12}H_{16}O_4$	13.380	1.627		$C_{11}H_3N_3O_3$	13.196	1.406
	$C_{12}H_{18}NO_3$	13.754	1.477		$C_{11}H_5N_4O_2$	13.571	1.255
	$C_{12}H_{20}N_2O_2$	14.128	1.328		$C_{11}H_{15}NO_4$	12.664	1.539
	$C_{12}H_{22}N_3O$	14.503	1.180		$C_{11}H_{17}N_2O_3$	13.039	1.386
	$C_{12}H_{24}N_4$	14.877	1.034		$C_{11}H_{19}N_3O_2$	13.413	1.234
	$C_{13}H_4O_4$	14.268	1.744		$C_{11}H_{21}N_4O$	13.788	1.084
	$C_{13}H_6NO_3$	14.643	1.597		$C_{12}H_3NO_4$	13.553	1.650
	$C_{13}H_8N_2O_2$	15.017	1.451		$C_{12}H_5N_2O_3$	13.927	1.500
	$C_{13}H_{10}N_3O$	15.391	1.307		$C_{12}H_7N_3O_2$	14.302	1.351
	$C_{13}H_{12}N_4$	15.766	1.164		$C_{12}H_9N_4O$	14.676	1.204
	$C_{13}H_{20}O_3$	14.485	1.575		$C_{12}H_{17}O_4$	13.396	1.629
	$C_{13}H_{22}NO_2$	14.860	1.428		$C_{12}H_{19}NO_3$	13.770	1.479
	$C_{13}H_{24}N_2O$	15.234	1.283		$C_{12}H_{21}N_2O_2$	14.144	1.330
	$C_{13}H_{26}N_3$	15.608	1.140		$C_{12}H_{23}N_3O$	14.519	1.182
	$C_{14}H_8O_3$	15.374	1.701		$C_{12}H_{25}N_4$	14.893	1.036
	$C_{14}H_{10}NO_2$	15.748	1.559		$C_{13}H_5O_4$	14.284	1.746
	$C_{14}H_{12}N_2O$	16.122	1.417		$C_{13}H_7NO_2$	14.659	1.599
	$C_{14}H_{14}N_3$	16.497	1.277		$C_{13}H_9N_2O_2$	15.033	1.454
	$C_{14}H_{24}O_2$	15.591	1.535		$C_{13}H_{11}N_3O$	15.407	1.309
	$C_{14}H_{26}NO$	15.965	1.392		$C_{13}H_{13}N_4$	15.782	1.167
	$C_{14}H_{28}N_2$	16.339	1.252		$C_{13}H_{21}O_3$	14.501	1.577
	$C_{15}H_2N_3$	17.385	1.422		$C_{13}H_{23}NO_2$	14.876	1.431

(Contd.)

		M + 1	M + 2
	$C_{13}H_{25}N_2O$	15.250	1.286
	$C_{13}H_{27}N_3$	15.624	1.143
	$C_{14}HN_4$	16.670	1.305
	$C_{14}H_9O_3$	15.390	1.704
	$C_{11}H_{11}NO_2$	15.764	1.561
	$C_{14}H_{13}N_2O$	16.138	1.420
	$C_{14}H_{15}N_3$	16.513	1.279
	$C_{14}H_{25}O_2$	15.607	1.537
	$C_{14}H_{27}NO$	15.981	1.395
	$C_{14}H_{29}N_2$	16.355	1.254
	$C_{15}HN_2O$	17.027	1.561
	$C_{15}H_3N_3$	17.401	1.424
	$C_{15}H_{13}O_2$	16.495	1.674
	$C_{15}H_{15}NO$	16.870	1.535
	$C_{15}H_{17}N_2$	17.244	1.398
	$C_{15}H_{29}O$	16.712	1.509
	$C_{15}H_{31}N$	17.087	1.371
	$C_{16}HO_2$	17.384	1.819
	$C_{16}H_3NO$	17.758	1.683
	$C_{16}H_5N_2$	18.133	1.549
	$C_{16}H_{17}O$	17.601	1.656
	$C_{16}H_{19}N$	17.975	1.521
	$C_{16}H_{33}$	17.818	1.494
	$C_{17}H_5O$	18.489	1.811
	$C_{17}H_7N$	18.864	1.679
	$C_{17}H_{21}$	18.706	1.650
	$C_{18}H_9$	19.595	1.815
226	$C_{10}H_{14}N_2O_4$	11.949	1.456
	$C_{10}H_{16}N_3O_3$	12.324	1.300
	$C_{10}H_{18}N_4O_2$	12.698	1.146
	$C_{11}H_2N_2O_4$	12.838	1.560
	$C_{11}H_4N_3O_3$	13.212	1.408
	$C_{11}H_6N_4O_2$	13.587	1.257
	$C_{11}H_{16}NO_4$	12.680	1.541
	$C_{11}H_{18}N_2O_3$	13.055	1.388
	$C_{11}H_{20}N_3O_2$	13.429	1.236
	$C_{11}H_{22}N_4O$	13.804	1.086
	$C_{12}H_4NO_4$	13.569	1.652
	$C_{12}H_6N_2O_3$	13.943	1.502
	$C_{12}H_8N_3O_2$	14.318	1.354
	$C_{12}H_{10}N_4O$	14.692	1.207
	$C_{12}H_{18}O_4$	13.412	1.631
	$C_{12}H_{20}NO_3$	13.786	1.481
	$C_{12}H_{22}N_2O_2$	14.160	1.332
	$C_{12}H_{24}N_3O$	14.535	1.185
	$C_{12}H_{26}N_4$	14.909	1.038
	$C_{13}H_6O_4$	14.300	1.749
	$C_{13}H_8NO_3$	14.675	1.602
	$C_3H_{10}N_2O_2$	15.049	1.456
	$C_{13}H_{12}N_3O$	15.423	1.312
	$C_{13}H_{14}N_4$	15.798	1.169
	$C_{13}H_{22}O_3$	14.517	1.579
	$C_{13}H_{24}NO_2$	14.892	1.433
	$C_{13}H_{26}N_2O$	15.266	1.288
	$C_{13}H_{28}N_3$	15.640	1.145
	$C_{14}H_2N_4$	16.686	1.308
	$C_{14}H_{10}O_3$	15.406	1.706
	$C_{14}H_{12}NO_2$	15.780	1.564
	$C_{14}H_{14}N_2O$	16.154	1.422
	$C_{14}H_{16}N_3$	16.529	1.282
	$C_{14}H_{26}O_2$	15.623	1.540
	$C_{14}H_{28}NO$	15.997	1.398
	$C_{14}H_{30}N_2$	16.371	1.257
	$C_{15}H_2N_2O$	17.043	1.564
	$C_{15}H_4N_3$	17.417	1.427
	$C_{15}H_{14}O_2$	16.511	1.677
	$C_{15}H_{16}NO$	16.886	1.538
	$C_{15}H_{18}N_2$	17.260	1.401
	$C_{15}H_{30}O$	16.728	1.512
	$C_{15}H_{32}N$	17.103	1.374
	$C_{16}H_2O_2$	17.400	1.821
	$C_{16}H_4NO$	17.774	1.686
	$C_{16}H_6N_2$	18.149	1.552
	$C_{16}H_{18}O$	17.617	1.659
	$C_{16}H_{20}N$	17.991	1.524
	$C_{16}H_{34}$	17.834	1.497
	$C_{17}H_6O$	18.505	1.813
	$C_{17}H_8N$	18.880	1.682
	$C_{17}H_{22}$	18.722	1.653
	$C_{18}H_{10}$	19.611	1.818

(Contd.)

		M + 1	M + 2			M + 1	M + 2
227	$C_{10}H_{15}N_2O_4$	11.965	1.458		$C_{15}H_{15}O_2$	16.527	1.679
	$C_{10}H_{17}N_3O_3$	12.340	1.302		$C_{15}H_{17}NO$	16.902	1.541
	$C_{10}H_{19}N_4O_2$	12.714	1.148		$C_{15}H_{19}N_2$	17.276	1.403
	$C_{11}H_3N_2O_4$	12.854	1.562		$C_{15}H_{31}O$	16.744	1.515
	$C_{11}H_5N_3O_3$	13.228	1.410		$C_{15}H_{33}N$	17.119	1.377
	$C_{11}H_7N_4O_2$	13.603	1.259		$C_{16}H_3O_2$	17.416	1.824
	$C_{11}H_{17}NO_4$	12.696	1.543		$C_{16}H_5NO$	17.790	1.689
	$C_{11}H_{19}N_2O_3$	13.071	1.390		$C_{16}H_7N_2$	18.165	1.555
	$C_{11}H_{21}N_3O_2$	13.445	1.238		$C_{16}H_{19}O$	17.633	1.662
	$C_{11}H_{23}N_4O$	13.820	1.088		$C_{16}H_{21}N$	18.007	1.527
	$C_{12}H_5NO_4$	13.585	1.654		$C_{17}H_7O$	18.521	1.816
	$C_{12}H_7N_2O_3$	13.959	1.504		$C_{17}H_9N$	18.896	1.685
	$C_{12}H_9N_3O_2$	14.334	1.356		$C_{17}H_{23}$	18.738	1.656
	$C_{12}H_{11}N_4O$	14.708	1.209		$C_{18}H_{11}$	19.627	1.821
	$C_{12}H_{19}O_4$	13.428	1.633	228	$C_{10}H_{16}N_2O_4$	11.981	1.460
	$C_{12}H_{21}NO_3$	13.802	1.483		$C_{10}H_{18}N_3O_3$	12.356	1.304
	$C_{12}H_{23}N_2O_2$	14.176	1.334		$C_{10}H_{20}N_4O_2$	12.730	1.150
	$C_{12}H_{25}N_3O$	14.551	1.187		$C_{11}H_4N_2O_4$	12.870	1.564
	$C_{12}H_{27}N_4$	14.925	1.041		$C_{11}H_6N_3O_3$	13.244	1.412
	$C_{13}H_7O_4$	14.316	1.751		$C_{11}H_8N_4O_2$	13.619	1.261
	$C_{13}H_9NO_3$	14.691	1.604		$C_{11}H_{18}NO_4$	12.712	1.545
	$C_{13}H_{11}N_2O_2$	15.065	1.458		$C_{11}H_{20}N_2O_3$	13.087	1.392
	$C_{13}H_{13}N_3O$	15.439	1.314		$C_{11}H_{22}N_3O_2$	13.461	1.241
	$C_{13}H_{15}N_4$	15.814	1.172		$C_{11}H_{24}N_4O$	13.836	1.090
	$C_{13}H_{23}O_3$	14.533	1.582		$C_{12}H_6NO_4$	13.601	1.656
	$C_{13}H_{25}NO_2$	14.908	1.436		$C_{12}H_8N_2O_3$	13.975	1.507
	$C_{13}H_{27}N_2O$	15.282	1.291		$C_{12}H_{10}N_3O_2$	14.350	1.358
	$C_{13}H_{29}N_3$	15.656	1.148		$C_{12}H_{12}N_4O$	14.724	1.212
	$C_{14}HN_3O$	16.328	1.450		$C_{12}H_{20}O_4$	13.444	1.636
	$C_{14}H_3N_4$	16.702	1.310		$C_{12}H_{22}NO_3$	13.818	1.485
	$C_{14}H_{11}O_3$	15.422	1.709		$C_{12}H_{24}N_2O_2$	14.192	1.337
	$C_{14}H_{13}NO_2$	15.796	1.566		$C_{12}H_{26}N_3O$	14.567	1.189
	$C_{14}H_{15}N_2O$	16.170	1.425		$C_{12}H_{28}N_4$	14.941	1.043
	$C_{14}H_{17}N_3$	16.545	1.285		$C_{13}H_8O_4$	14.332	1.753
	$C_{14}H_{27}O_2$	15.639	1.542		$C_{13}H_{10}NO_3$	14.707	1.606
	$C_{14}H_{29}NO$	16.013	1.400		$C_{13}H_{12}N_2O_2$	15.081	1.461
	$C_{14}H_{31}N_2$	16.387	1.260		$C_{13}H_{14}N_3O$	15.455	1.317
	$C_{15}HNO_2$	16.685	1.705		$C_{13}H_{16}N_4$	15.830	1.174
	$C_{15}H_3N_2O$	17.059	1.567		$C_{13}H_{24}O_3$	14.549	1.584
	$C_{15}H_5N_3$	17.433	1.430		$C_{13}H_{26}NO_2$	14.924	1.438

(Contd.)

		M + 1	M + 2			M + 1	M + 2
	$C_{13}H_{28}N_2O$	15.298	1.293		$C_{12}H_{13}N_4O$	14.740	1.214
	$C_{13}H_{30}N_3$	15.672	1.150		$C_{12}H_{21}O_4$	13.460	1.638
	$C_{14}H_2N_3O$	16.344	1.452		$C_{12}H_{23}NO_3$	13.834	1.488
	$C_{14}H_4N_4$	16.718	1.313		$C_{12}H_{25}N_2O_2$	14.208	1.339
	$C_{14}H_{12}O_3$	15.438	1.711		$C_{12}H_{27}N_3O$	14.583	1.192
	$C_{14}H_{14}NO_2$	15.812	1.569		$C_{12}H_{29}N_4$	14.957	1.046
	$C_{14}H_{16}N_2O$	16.186	1.427		$C_{13}HN_4O$	15.629	1.343
	$C_{14}H_{18}N_3$	16.561	1.287		$C_{13}H_9O_4$	14.348	1.755
	$C_{14}H_{28}O_2$	15.655	1.545		$C_{13}H_{11}NO_3$	14.723	1.609
	$C_{14}H_{30}NO$	16.029	1.403		$C_{13}H_{13}N_2O_2$	15.097	1.463
	$C_{14}H_{32}N_2$	16.403	1.262		$C_{13}H_{15}N_3O$	15.471	1.319
	$C_{15}H_2NO_2$	16.701	1.707		$C_{13}H_{17}N_4$	15.846	1.177
	$C_{15}H_4N_2O$	17.075	1.569		$C_{13}H_{25}O_3$	14.565	1.586
	$C_{15}H_6N_3$	17.449	1.433		$C_{13}H_{27}NO_2$	14.940	1.440
	$C_{15}H_{16}O_2$	16.543	1.682		$C_{13}H_{29}N_2O$	15.314	1.296
	$C_{15}H_{18}NO$	16.918	1.543		$C_{13}H_{31}N_3$	15.688	1.153
	$C_{15}H_{20}N_2$	17.292	1.406		$C_{14}HN_2O_2$	15.985	1.595
	$C_{15}H_{32}O$	16.760	1.517		$C_{14}H_3N_3O$	16.360	1.455
	$C_{16}H_4O_2$	17.432	1.827		$C_{14}H_5N_4$	16.734	1.316
	$C_{16}H_6NO$	17.806	1.692		$C_{14}H_{13}O_3$	15.454	1.714
	$C_{16}H_8N_2$	18.181	1.558		$C_{14}H_{15}NO_2$	15.828	1.571
	$C_{16}H_{20}O$	17.649	1.665		$C_{14}H_{17}N_2O$	16.202	1.430
	$C_{16}H_{22}N$	18.023	1.530		$C_{14}H_{19}N_3$	16.577	1.290
	$C_{17}H_8O$	18.537	1.819		$C_{14}H_{29}O_2$	15.671	1.547
	$C_{17}H_{10}N$	18.912	1.688		$C_{14}H_{31}NO$	16.045	1.405
	$C_{17}H_{24}$	18.754	1.659		$C_{15}HO_3$	16.342	1.849
	$C_{18}H_{12}$	19.643	1.824		$C_{15}H_3NO_2$	16.717	1.710
229	$C_{10}H_{17}N_2O_4$	11.997	1.462		$C_{15}H_5N_2O$	17.091	1.572
	$C_{10}H_{19}N_3O_3$	12.372	1.306		$C_{15}H_7N_3$	17.465	1.435
	$C_{10}H_{21}N_4O_2$	12.746	1.152		$C_{15}H_{17}O_2$	16.559	1.684
	$C_{11}H_5N_2O_4$	12.886	1.566		$C_{15}H_{19}NO$	16.934	1.546
	$C_{11}H_7N_3O_3$	13.260	1.414		$C_{15}H_{21}N_2$	17.308	1.409
	$C_{11}H_9N_4O_2$	13.635	1.263		$C_{16}H_5O_2$	17.448	1.830
	$C_{11}H_{19}NO_4$	12.728	1.547		$C_{16}H_7NO$	17.822	1.695
	$C_{11}H_{21}N_2O_3$	13.103	1.394		$C_{16}H_9N_2$	18.197	1.561
	$C_{11}H_{23}N_3O_2$	13.477	1.243		$C_{16}H_{21}O$	17.665	1.667
	$C_{11}H_{25}N_4O$	13.852	1.093		$C_{16}H_{23}N$	18.039	1.533
	$C_{12}H_7NO_4$	13.617	1.658		$C_{17}H_9O$	18.553	1.822
	$C_{12}H_9N_2O_3$	13.991	1.509		$C_{17}H_{11}N$	18.928	1.691
	$C_{12}H_{11}N_3O_2$	14.366	1.361		$C_{17}H_{25}$	18.770	1.662

(Contd.)

		M + 1	M + 2			M + 1	M + 2
	$C_{18}H_{13}$	19.659	1.827		$C_{15}H_6N_2O$	17.107	1.575
	$C_{19}H$	20.547	2.000		$C_{15}H_8N_3$	17.481	1.438
230	$C_{10}H_{18}N_2O_4$	12.013	1.464		$C_{15}H_{18}O_2$	16.575	1.687
	$C_{10}H_{20}N_3O_3$	12.388	1.308		$C_{15}H_{20}NO$	16.950	1.549
	$C_{10}H_{22}N_4O_2$	12.762	1.154		$C_{15}H_{22}N_2$	17.324	1.412
	$C_{11}H_6N_2O_4$	12.902	1.569		$C_{16}H_6O_2$	17.464	1.832
	$C_{11}H_8N_3O_3$	13.276	1.116		$C_{16}H_8NO$	17.838	1.697
	$C_{11}H_{10}N_4O_2$	13.651	1.266		$C_{16}H_{10}N_2$	18.213	1.564
	$C_{11}H_{20}NO_4$	12.744	1.549		$C_{16}H_{22}O$	17.681	1.670
	$C_{11}H_{22}N_2O_3$	13.119	1.396		$C_{16}H_{24}N$	18.055	1.536
	$C_{11}H_{24}N_3O_2$	13.493	1.245		$C_{17}H_{10}O$	18.569	1.825
	$C_{11}H_{26}N_4O$	13.868	1.095		$C_{17}H_{12}N$	18.944	1.694
	$C_{12}H_8NO_4$	13.633	1.660		$C_{17}H_{26}$	18.786	1.665
	$C_{12}H_{10}N_2O_3$	14.007	1.511		$C_{18}H_{14}$	19.675	1.830
	$C_{12}H_{12}N_3O_2$	14.382	1.363		$C_{19}H_2$	20.563	2.003
	$C_{12}H_{14}N_4O$	14.756	1.216	231	$C_{10}H_{19}N_2O_4$	12.029	1.466
	$C_{12}H_{22}O_4$	13.476	1.640		$C_{10}H_{21}N_3O_3$	12.404	1.310
	$C_{12}H_{24}NO_3$	13.850	1.490		$C_{10}H_{23}N_4O_2$	12.778	1.456
	$C_{12}H_{26}N_2O_2$	14.224	1.341		$C_{11}H_7N_2O_4$	12.918	1.571
	$C_{12}H_{28}N_3O$	14.599	1.194		$C_{11}H_9N_3O_3$	13.292	1.418
	$C_{12}H_{30}N_4$	14.973	1.048		$C_{11}H_{11}N_4O_2$	13.667	1.268
	$C_{13}H_2N_4O$	15.645	1.345		$C_{11}H_{21}NO_4$	12.760	1.551
	$C_{13}H_{10}O_4$	14.364	1.758		$C_{11}H_{23}N_2O_3$	13.135	1.398
	$C_{13}H_{12}NO_3$	14.739	1.611		$C_{11}H_{25}N_3O_2$	13.509	1.247
	$C_{13}H_{14}N_2O_2$	15.113	1.466		$C_{11}H_{27}N_4O$	13.884	1.097
	$C_{13}H_{16}N_3O$	15.487	1.322		$C_{12}H_9NO_4$	13.649	1.663
	$C_{13}H_{18}N_4$	15.862	1.179		$C_{12}H_{11}N_2O_3$	14.023	1.513
	$C_{13}H_{26}O_3$	14.581	1.589		$C_{12}H_{13}N_3O_2$	14.398	1.365
	$C_{13}H_{28}NO_2$	14.956	1.443		$C_{12}H_{15}N_4O$	14.772	1.219
	$C_{13}H_{30}N_2O$	15.330	1.298		$C_{12}H_{23}O_4$	13.492	1.642
	$C_{14}H_2N_2O_2$	16.001	1.598		$C_{12}H_{25}NO_3$	13.866	1.492
	$C_{14}H_4N_3O$	16.376	1.457		$C_{12}H_{27}N_2O_2$	14.240	1.343
	$C_{14}H_6N_4$	16.750	1.318		$C_{12}H_{29}N_3O$	14.615	1.196
	$C_{14}H_{14}O_3$	15.470	1.716		$C_{13}HN_3O_2$	15.286	1.491
	$C_{14}H_{16}NO_2$	15.844	1.574		$C_{13}H_3N_4O$	15.661	1.348
	$C_{14}H_{18}N_2O$	16.218	1.132		$C_{13}H_{11}O_4$	14.380	1.760
	$C_{14}H_{20}N_3$	16.593	1.293		$C_{13}H_{13}NO_3$	14.755	1.613
	$C_{14}H_{30}O_2$	15.687	1.550		$C_{13}H_{15}N_2O_2$	15.129	1.468
	$C_{15}H_2O_3$	16.358	1.852		$C_{13}H_{17}N_3O$	15.503	1.324
	$C_{15}H_4NO_2$	16.733	1.713		$C_{13}H_{19}N_4$	15.878	1.182

(Contd.)

		M + 1	M + 2			M + 1	M + 2
	$C_{13}H_{27}O_3$	14.597	1.591		$C_{12}H_{14}N_3O_2$	14.414	1.368
	$C_{13}H_{29}NO_2$	14.972	1.445		$C_{12}H_{16}N_4O$	14.788	1.221
	$C_{14}HNO_3$	15.643	1.743		$C_{12}H_{24}O_4$	13.508	1.644
	$C_{14}H_3N_2O_2$	16.017	1.501		$C_{12}H_{26}NO_3$	13.882	1.494
	$C_{14}H_5N_3O$	16.392	1.460		$C_{12}H_{28}N_2O_2$	14.256	1.346
	$C_{14}H_7N_4$	16.766	1.321		$C_{13}H_2N_3O_2$	15.302	1.494
	$C_{14}H_{15}O_3$	15.486	1.719		$C_{13}H_4N_4O$	15.677	1.351
	$C_{14}H_{17}NO_2$	15.860	1.576		$C_{12}H_{12}O_4$	14.396	1.762
	$C_{14}H_{19}N_2O$	16.234	1.435		$C_{13}H_{14}NO_3$	14.771	1.616
	$C_{14}H_{21}N_3$	16.609	1.295		$C_{13}H_{16}N_2O_2$	15.145	1.470
	$C_{15}H_3O_3$	16.374	1.854		$C_{13}H_{18}N_3O$	15.519	1.327
	$C_{15}H_5NO_2$	16.749	1.715		$C_{13}H_{20}N_4$	15.894	1.484
	$C_{15}H_7N_2O$	17.123	1.577		$C_{13}H_{28}O_3$	14.613	1.593
	$C_{15}H_9N_3$	17.497	1.441		$C_{14}H_2NO_3$	15.659	1.745
	$C_{15}H_{19}O_2$	16.591	1.690		$C_{14}H_4N_2O_2$	16.033	1.603
	$C_{15}H_{21}NO$	16.966	1.515		$C_{14}H_6N_2O$	16.408	1.463
	$C_{15}H_{23}N_2$	17.340	1.414		$C_{14}H_8N_4$	16.782	1.324
	$C_{16}H_7O_2$	17.480	1.835		$C_{14}H_{16}O_3$	15.502	1.721
	$C_{16}H_9NO$	17.854	1.700		$C_{14}H_{18}NO_2$	15.876	1.579
	$C_{16}H_{11}N_2$	18.229	1.567		$C_{14}H_{20}N_2O$	16.250	1.438
	$C_{16}H_{23}O$	17.697	1.673		$C_{14}H_{22}N_3$	16.625	1.298
	$C_{16}H_{25}N$	18.071	1.539		$C_{15}H_4O_3$	16.390	1.857
	$C_{17}H_{11}O$	18.585	1.828		$C_{15}H_6NO_2$	16.765	1.718
	$C_{17}H_{13}N$	18.960	1.697		$C_{15}H_8N_2O$	17.139	1.580
	$C_{17}H_{27}$	18.802	1.668		$C_{15}H_{10}N_3$	17.513	1.444
	$C_{18}HN$	19.848	1.864		$C_{15}H_{20}O_2$	16.607	1.692
	$C_{18}H_{15}$	19.691	1.834		$C_{15}H_{22}NO$	16.982	1.554
	$C_{19}H_3$	20.579	2.001		$C_{15}H_{24}N_2$	17.356	1.417
232	$C_{10}H_{20}N_2O_4$	12.045	1.468		$C_{16}H_8O_2$	17.496	1.838
	$C_{10}H_{22}N_3O_3$	12.420	1.312		$C_{16}H_{10}NO$	17.870	1.703
	$C_{10}H_{24}N_4O_2$	12.974	1.458		$C_{16}H_{12}N_2$	18.245	1.569
	$C_{11}H_8N_2O_4$	12.934	1.573		$C_{16}H_{24}O$	17.713	1.676
	$C_{11}H_{10}N_3O_3$	13.308	1.421		$C_{16}H_{26}N$	18.087	1.542
	$C_{11}H_{12}N_4O_2$	13.683	1.270		$C_{17}H_{12}O$	18.601	1.831
	$C_{11}H_{22}NO_4$	12.776	1.553		$C_{17}H_{14}N$	18.976	1.700
	$C_{11}H_{24}N_2O_3$	13.151	1.400		$C_{17}H_{28}$	18.818	1.671
	$C_{11}H_{26}N_3O_2$	13.525	1.249		$C_{18}H_2N$	19.864	1.867
	$C_{11}H_{28}N_4O$	13.900	1.099		$C_{18}H_{16}$	19.707	1.837
	$C_{12}H_{10}NO_4$	13.665	1.665		$C_{19}H_4$	20.595	2.001
	$C_{12}H_{12}N_2O$	14.039	1.515	233	$C_{10}H_{21}N_2O_4$	12.061	1.469

(Contd.)

		M + 1	M + 2
	$C_{10}H_{23}N_3O_3$	12.436	1.314
	$C_{10}H_{25}N_4O_2$	12.810	1.160
	$C_{11}H_9N_2O_4$	12.950	1.575
	$C_{11}H_{11}N_3O_3$	13.324	1.423
	$C_{11}H_{13}N_4O_2$	13.699	1.272
	$C_{11}H_{23}NO_4$	12.792	1.555
	$C_{11}H_{25}N_2O_3$	13.167	1.403
	$C_{11}H_{27}N_3O_2$	13.541	1.251
	$C_{12}HN_4O_2$	14.587	1.392
	$C_{12}H_{11}NO_4$	13.681	1.667
	$C_{12}H_{13}N_2O_3$	14.055	1.518
	$C_{12}H_{15}N_3O_2$	14.430	1.370
	$C_{12}H_{17}N_4O$	14.804	1.223
	$C_{12}H_{25}O_4$	13.524	1.646
	$C_{12}H_{27}NO_3$	13.898	1.496
	$C_{13}HN_2O_3$	14.944	1.641
	$C_{13}H_3N_3O_2$	15.318	1.496
	$C_{13}H_5N_4O$	15.693	1.353
	$C_{13}H_{13}O_4$	14.412	1.765
	$C_{13}H_{15}NO_3$	14.787	1.618
	$C_{13}H_{17}N_2O_2$	15.161	1.473
	$C_{13}H_{19}N_3O$	15.535	1.329
	$C_{13}H_{21}N_4$	15.910	1.187
	$C_{14}HO_4$	15.301	1.891
	$C_{14}H_3NO_3$	15.675	1.748
	$C_{14}H_5N_2O_2$	16.050	1.606
	$C_{14}H_7N_3O$	16.424	1.465
	$C_{14}H_9N_4$	15.798	1.326
	$C_{14}H_{17}O_3$	15.518	1.724
	$C_{14}H_{19}NO_2$	15.892	1.581
	$C_{14}H_{21}N_2O$	16.266	1.440
	$C_{14}H_{23}N_3$	16.641	1.301
	$C_{15}H_5O_3$	16.406	1.860
	$C_{15}H_7NO_2$	16.781	1.721
	$C_{15}H_9N_2O$	17.155	1.583
	$C_{15}H_{11}N_3$	17.529	1.447
	$C_{15}H_{21}O_2$	16.623	1.695
	$C_{15}H_{23}NO$	16.998	1.557
	$C_{15}H_{25}N_2$	17.372	1.420
	$C_{16}H_9O_2$	17.512	1.841
	$C_{16}H_{11}NO$	17.886	1.706
	$C_{16}H_{13}N_2$	18.261	1.572
	$C_{16}H_{25}O$	17.729	1.679
	$C_{16}H_{27}N$	18.103	1.544
	$C_{17}HN_2$	19.149	1.733
	$C_{17}H_{13}O$	18.617	1.834
	$C_{17}H_{15}N$	18.992	1.703
	$C_{17}H_{29}$	18.834	1.674
	$C_{18}HO$	19.506	1.998
	$C_{18}H_3N$	19.880	1.870
	$C_{18}H_{17}$	19.723	1.840
	$C_{19}H_5$	20.611	2.013
234	$C_{10}H_{22}N_2O_4$	12.077	1.471
	$C_{10}H_{24}N_3O_3$	12.452	1.316
	$C_{10}H_{26}N_4O_2$	12.826	1.162
	$C_{11}H_{10}N_2O_4$	12.966	1.577
	$C_{11}H_{12}N_3O_3$	13.340	1.425
	$C_{11}H_{14}N_4O_2$	13.715	1.274
	$C_{11}H_{24}NO_4$	12.808	1.557
	$C_{11}H_{26}N_2O_3$	13.183	1.405
	$C_{12}H_2N_4O_2$	14.603	1.394
	$C_{12}H_{12}NO_4$	13.697	1.669
	$C_{12}H_{14}N_2O_3$	14.071	1.520
	$C_{12}H_{16}N_3O_2$	14.446	1.372
	$C_{12}H_{18}N_4O$	14.820	1.226
	$C_{12}H_{26}O_4$	13.540	1.648
	$C_{13}H_2N_2O_3$	14.960	1.643
	$C_{13}H_4N_3O_2$	15.334	1.499
	$C_{13}H_6N_4O$	15.709	1.356
	$C_{13}H_{14}O_4$	14.428	1.767
	$C_{13}H_{16}NO_3$	14.803	1.620
	$C_{13}H_{18}N_2O_2$	15.177	1.475
	$C_{13}H_{20}N_3O$	15.551	1.332
	$C_{13}H_{22}N_4$	15.926	1.189
	$C_{14}H_2O_4$	15.317	1.893
	$C_{14}H_4NO_3$	15.691	1.750
	$C_{14}H_6N_2O_2$	16.066	1.608
	$C_{14}H_8N_3O$	16.440	1.468
	$C_{14}H_{10}N_4$	16.814	1.329
	$C_{14}H_{18}O_3$	15.534	1.726

(Contd.)

		M + 1	M + 2
	$C_{14}H_{20}NO_2$	15.908	1.584
	$C_{14}H_{22}N_2O$	16.282	1.443
	$C_{14}H_{24}N_3$	16.657	1.303
	$C_{15}H_6O_3$	16.422	1.862
	$C_{15}H_8NO_2$	16.797	1.723
	$C_{15}H_{10}N_2O$	17.171	1.586
	$C_{15}H_{12}N_3$	17.545	1.449
	$C_{15}H_{22}O_2$	16.639	1.698
	$C_{15}H_{24}NO$	17.014	1.560
	$C_{15}H_{26}N_2$	17.388	1.423
	$C_{16}H_{10}O_2$	17.528	1.844
	$C_{16}H_{12}NO$	17.902	1.709
	$C_{16}H_{14}N_2$	18.277	1.575
	$C_{16}H_{26}O$	17.745	1.681
	$C_{16}H_{28}N$	18.119	1.547
	$C_{17}H_2N_2$	19.165	1.736
	$C_{17}H_{14}O$	18.633	1.837
	$C_{17}H_{16}N$	19.008	1.707
	$C_{17}H_{30}$	18.850	1.677
	$C_{18}H_2O$	19.522	2.001
	$C_{18}H_4N$	19.896	1.874
	$C_{18}H_{18}$	19.739	1.843
	$C_{19}H_6$	20.627	2.017
235	$C_{10}H_{23}N_2O_4$	12.093	1.473
	$C_{10}H_{25}N_3O_3$	12.468	1.318
	$C_{11}H_{11}N_2O_4$	12.982	1.579
	$C_{11}H_{13}N_3O_3$	13.356	1.427
	$C_{11}H_{15}N_4O_2$	13.731	1.277
	$C_{11}H_{25}NO_4$	12.824	1.559
	$C_{12}HN_3O_3$	14.245	1.544
	$C_{12}H_3N_4O_2$	14.619	1.397
	$C_{12}H_{13}NO_4$	13.713	1.671
	$C_{12}H_{15}N_2O_3$	14.087	1.522
	$C_{12}H_{17}N_3O_2$	14.462	1.374
	$C_{12}H_{19}N_4O$	14.836	1.228
	$C_{13}HNO_4$	14.602	1.791
	$C_{13}H_3N_2O_3$	14.976	1.646
	$C_{13}H_5N_3O_2$	15.350	1.501
	$C_{13}H_7N_4O$	15.725	1.358
	$C_{13}H_{15}O_4$	14.444	1.769
	$C_{13}H_{17}NO_3$	14.819	1.623
	$C_{13}H_{19}N_2O_2$	15.193	1.478
	$C_{13}H_{21}N_3O$	15.567	1.334
	$C_{13}H_{23}N_4$	15.942	1.192
	$C_{14}H_3O_4$	15.333	1.896
	$C_{14}H_5NO_3$	15.707	1.753
	$C_{14}H_7N_2O_2$	16.082	1.611
	$C_{14}H_9N_3O$	16.456	1.471
	$C_{14}H_{11}N_4$	16.830	1.332
	$C_{14}H_{19}O_3$	15.550	1.729
	$C_{14}H_{21}NO_2$	15.924	1.586
	$C_{14}H_{23}N_2O$	16.298	1.446
	$C_{14}H_{25}N_3$	16.673	1.306
	$C_{15}H_7O_3$	16.438	1.865
	$C_{15}H_9NO_2$	16.813	1.726
	$C_{15}H_{11}N_2O$	17.187	1.588
	$C_{15}H_{13}N_3$	17.561	1.442
	$C_{15}H_{23}O_2$	16.655	1.700
	$C_{15}H_{25}NO$	17.030	1.562
	$C_{15}H_{27}N_2$	17.404	1.425
	$C_{16}HN_3$	18.450	1.606
	$C_{16}H_{11}O_2$	17.544	1.846
	$C_{16}H_{13}NO$	17.918	1.712
	$C_{16}H_{15}N_2$	18.293	1.578
	$C_{16}H_{27}O$	17.761	1.684
	$C_{16}H_{29}N$	18.135	1.550
	$C_{17}HNO$	18.807	1.869
	$C_{17}H_3N_2$	19.181	1.739
	$C_{17}H_{15}O$	18.649	1.840
	$C_{17}H_{17}N$	19.024	1.710
	$C_{17}H_{31}$	18.866	1.680
	$C_{18}H_3O$	19.538	2.004
	$C_{18}H_3N$	19.912	1.877
	$C_{18}H_{19}$	19.755	1.846
	$C_{19}H_7$	20.643	2.120
236	$C_{10}H_{24}N_2O_4$	12.109	1.475
	$C_{11}H_{12}N_2O_4$	12.998	1.581
	$C_{11}H_{14}N_3O_3$	13.372	1.429
	$C_{11}H_{16}N_4O_2$	13.747	1.279
	$C_{12}H_{12}N_3O_3$	14.261	1.546

(Contd.)

		M + 1	M + 2
	$C_{12}H_4N_4O_2$	14.635	1.399
	$C_{12}H_{14}NO_4$	13.729	1.674
	$C_{12}H_{16}N_2O_3$	14.103	1.524
	$C_{12}H_{18}N_3O_2$	14.478	1.377
	$C_{12}H_{20}N_4O$	14.852	1.230
	$C_{13}H_2NO_4$	14.618	1.794
	$C_{13}H_4N_2O_3$	14.992	1.648
	$C_{13}H_6N_3O_2$	15.366	1.504
	$C_{13}H_8N_4O$	15.741	1.361
	$C_{13}H_{16}O_4$	14.460	1.772
	$C_{13}H_{18}NO_3$	14.835	1.625
	$C_{13}H_{20}N_2O_2$	15.209	1.480
	$C_{13}H_{22}N_3O$	15.583	1.337
	$C_{13}H_{24}N_4$	15.958	1.494
	$C_{14}H_4O_4$	15.349	1.898
	$C_{14}H_6NO_3$	15.723	1.755
	$C_{14}H_8N_2O_2$	16.098	1.613
	$C_{14}H_{10}N_3O$	16.472	1.473
	$C_{14}H_{12}N_4$	16.846	1.334
	$C_{14}H_{20}O_3$	15.566	1.731
	$C_{14}H_{22}NO_2$	15.940	1.589
	$C_{14}H_{24}N_2O$	16.314	1.448
	$C_{14}H_{26}N_3$	16.689	1.309
	$C_{15}H_8O_3$	16.454	1.868
	$C_{15}H_{10}NO_2$	16.829	1.729
	$C_{15}H_{12}N_2O$	17.203	1.591
	$C_{15}H_{14}N_3$	17.577	1.455
	$C_{15}H_{24}O_2$	16.671	1.703
	$C_{15}H_{26}NO$	17.046	1.565
	$C_{15}H_{28}N_2$	17.420	1.428
	$C_{16}H_2N_3$	18.466	1.609
	$C_{16}H_{12}O_2$	17.560	1.849
	$C_{16}H_{14}NO$	17.934	1.715
	$C_{16}H_{16}N_2$	18.309	1.581
	$C_{16}H_{28}O$	17.777	1.687
	$C_{16}H_{30}N$	18.151	1.553
	$C_{17}H_2NO$	18.823	1.872
	$C_{17}H_4N_2$	19.197	1.742
	$C_{17}H_{16}O$	18.665	1.843
	$C_{17}H_{18}N$	19.040	1.713
	$C_{17}H_{32}$	18.882	1.683
	$C_{18}H_4O$	19.554	2.007
	$C_{18}H_6N$	19.928	1.880
	$C_{18}H_{20}$	19.771	1.849
	$C_{19}H_8$	20.659	2.023
237	$C_{11}H_{13}N_2O_4$	13.014	1.583
	$C_{11}H_{15}N_3O_3$	13.388	1.431
	$C_{11}H_{17}N_4O_2$	13.763	1.281
	$C_{12}HN_2O_4$	13.902	1.697
	$C_{12}H_3N_3O_3$	19.277	1.548
	$C_{12}H_5N_4O_2$	14.651	1.401
	$C_{12}H_{15}NO_4$	13.745	1.676
	$C_{12}H_{17}N_2O_3$	14.119	1.527
	$C_{12}H_{19}N_3O_2$	14.494	1.379
	$C_{12}H_{21}N_4O$	14.868	1.233
	$C_{13}H_3NO_4$	14.634	1.796
	$C_{13}H_5N_2O_3$	15.008	1.650
	$C_{13}H_7N_3O_2$	15.382	1.506
	$C_{13}H_9N_4O$	15.757	1.363
	$C_{13}H_{17}O_4$	14.476	1.774
	$C_{13}H_{19}NO_3$	14.851	1.628
	$C_{13}H_{21}N_2O_2$	15.225	1.483
	$C_{13}H_{23}N_3O$	15.599	1.339
	$C_{13}H_{25}N_4$	15.974	1.197
	$C_{14}H_5O_4$	15.365	1.901
	$C_{14}H_7NO_3$	15.739	1.758
	$C_{14}H_9N_2O_2$	16.114	1.616
	$C_{14}H_{11}N_3O$	16.488	1.476
	$C_{14}H_{13}N_4$	16.862	1.337
	$C_{14}H_{21}O_3$	15.582	1.734
	$C_{14}H_{23}NO_2$	15.956	1.591
	$C_{14}H_{25}N_2O$	16.330	1.451
	$C_{14}H_{27}N_3$	16.705	1.311
	$C_{15}HN_4$	17.751	1.485
	$C_{15}H_9O_3$	16.470	1.870
	$C_{15}H_{11}NO_2$	16.845	1.731
	$C_{15}H_{13}N_2O$	17.219	1.594
	$C_{15}H_{15}N_3$	17.593	1.458
	$C_{15}H_{25}O_2$	16.687	1.706
	$C_{15}H_{27}NO$	17.062	1.568

(Contd.)

		M + 1	M + 2
	$C_{15}H_{29}N_2$	17.436	1.431
	$C_{16}HN_2O$	18.108	1.745
	$C_{16}H_3N_3$	18.482	1.612
	$C_{16}H_{13}O_2$	17.576	1.852
	$C_{16}H_{15}NO$	17.950	1.717
	$C_{16}H_{17}N_2$	18.325	1.584
	$C_{16}H_{29}O$	17.793	1.690
	$C_{16}H_{31}N$	18.167	1.556
	$C_{17}HO_2$	18.464	2.006
	$C_{17}H_3NO$	18.839	1.875
	$C_{17}H_5N_2$	19.213	1.745
	$C_{17}H_{17}O$	18.681	1.846
	$C_{17}H_{19}N$	19.056	1.716
	$C_{17}H_{33}$	18.898	1.686
	$C_{18}H_5O$	19.570	2.010
	$C_{18}H_7N$	19.944	1.883
	$C_{18}H_{21}$	19.787	1.853
	$C_{19}H_9$	20.675	2.026
238	$C_{11}H_{14}N_2O_4$	13.030	15.851
	$C_{11}H_{16}N_3O_3$	13.404	1.433
	$C_{11}H_{18}N_4O_2$	13.779	1.283
	$C_{12}H_2N_2O_4$	13.918	1.699
	$C_{12}H_4N_3O_3$	14.293	1.551
	$C_{12}H_6N_4O_2$	14.667	1.404
	$C_{12}H_{16}NO_4$	13.761	1.678
	$C_{12}H_{18}N_2O_3$	14.135	1.530
	$C_{12}H_{20}N_3O_2$	14.510	1.381
	$C_{12}H_{22}N_4O$	14.884	1.235
	$C_{13}H_4NO_4$	14.650	1.798
	$C_{13}H_6N_2O_3$	15.024	1.653
	$C_{13}H_8N_3O_2$	15.398	1.508
	$C_{13}H_{10}N_4O$	15.773	1.366
	$C_{13}H_{18}O_4$	14.492	1.776
	$C_{13}H_{20}NO_3$	14.867	1.630
	$C_{13}H_{22}N_2O_2$	15.241	1.485
	$C_{13}H_{24}N_3O$	15.615	1.342
	$C_{13}H_{26}N_4$	15.990	1.200
	$C_{14}H_6O_4$	15.381	1.903
	$C_{14}H_8NO_3$	15.755	1.760
	$C_{14}H_{10}N_2O_2$	16.130	1.619
	$C_{14}H_{12}N_3O$	16.504	1.478
	$C_{14}H_{14}N_4$	16.878	1.340
	$C_{14}H_{22}O_3$	15.598	1.736
	$C_{14}H_{24}NO_2$	15.972	1.594
	$C_{14}H_{26}N_2O$	16.346	1.453
	$C_{14}H_{28}N_3$	16.721	1.314
	$C_{15}H_2N_4$	17.767	1.488
	$C_{15}H_{10}O_3$	16.486	1.873
	$C_{15}H_{12}NO_2$	16.861	1.734
	$C_{15}H_{14}N_2O$	17.235	1.597
	$C_{15}H_{16}N_3$	17.609	1.461
	$C_{15}H_{26}O_2$	16.703	1.708
	$C_{15}H_{28}NO$	17.078	1.570
	$C_{15}H_{30}N_2$	17.452	1.434
	$C_{16}H_2N_2O$	18.124	1.748
	$C_{16}H_4N_3$	18.498	1.615
	$C_{16}H_{14}O_2$	17.592	1.855
	$C_{16}H_{16}NO$	17.966	1.720
	$C_{16}H_{18}N_2$	18.341	1.587
	$C_{16}H_{30}O$	17.809	1.693
	$C_{16}H_{32}N$	18.183	1.559
	$C_{17}H_2O_2$	18.480	2.009
	$C_{17}H_4NO$	18.855	1.878
	$C_{17}H_6N_2$	19.229	1.748
	$C_{17}H_{18}O$	18.697	1.849
	$C_{17}H_{20}N$	19.072	1.719
	$C_{17}H_{34}$	18.914	1.690
	$C_{18}H_6O$	19.586	2.013
	$C_{18}H_8N$	19.960	1.886
	$C_{18}H_{22}$	19.803	1.856
	$C_{10}H_{10}$	20.691	2.030
239	$C_{11}H_{15}N_2O_4$	13.046	1.587
	$C_{11}H_{17}N_3O_3$	13.420	1.436
	$C_{11}H_{19}N_4O_2$	13.795	1.285
	$C_{12}H_3N_2O_4$	13.934	1.701
	$C_{12}H_5N_3O_3$	14.309	1.553
	$C_{12}H_7N_4O_2$	14.683	1.406
	$C_{12}H_{17}NO_4$	13.777	1.680
	$C_{12}H_{19}N_2O_3$	14.151	1.531
	$C_{12}H_{21}N_3O_2$	14.526	1.384

(Contd.)

		M + 1	M + 2			M + 1	M + 2
	$C_{12}H_{23}N_4O$	14.900	1.238		$C_{17}H_{21}N$	19.088	1.722
	$C_{13}H_5NO_4$	14.666	1.801		$C_{17}H_{35}$	18.930	1.693
	$C_{13}H_7N_2O_3$	15.040	1.655		$C_{18}H_7O$	19.602	2.017
	$C_{13}H_9N_3O_2$	15.414	1.511		$C_{18}H_9N$	19.976	1.889
	$C_{13}H_{11}N_4O$	15.789	1.368		$C_{18}H_{23}$	19.819	1.859
	$C_{13}H_{19}O_4$	14.508	1.778		$C_{19}H_{11}$	20.707	2.033
	$C_{13}H_{21}NO_3$	14.883	1.632	240	$C_{11}H_{16}N_2O_4$	13.062	1.589
	$C_{13}H_{23}N_2O_2$	15.257	1.487		$C_{11}H_{18}N_3O_3$	13.436	1.438
	$C_{13}H_{25}N_3O$	15.631	1.344		$C_{11}H_{20}N_4O_2$	13.811	1.288
	$C_{13}H_{27}N_4$	16.006	1.202		$C_{12}H_4N_2O_4$	13.950	1.703
	$C_{14}H_7O_4$	15.397	1.906		$C_{12}H_6N_3O_3$	14.325	1.555
	$C_{14}H_9NO_3$	15.771	1.763		$C_{12}H_8N_4O_2$	14.699	1.408
	$C_{14}H_{11}N_2O_2$	16.146	1.621		$C_{12}H_{18}NO_4$	13.793	1.682
	$C_{14}H_{13}N_3O$	16.520	1.481		$C_{12}H_{20}N_2O_3$	14.167	1.534
	$C_{14}H_{15}N_4$	16.894	1.342		$C_{12}H_{22}N_3O_2$	14.542	1.386
	$C_{14}H_{23}O_3$	15.614	1.739		$C_{12}H_{24}N_4O$	14.916	1.240
	$C_{14}H_{25}NO_2$	15.988	1.597		$C_{13}H_6NO_4$	14.682	1.803
	$C_{14}H_{27}N_2O$	16.362	1.456		$C_{13}H_8N_2O_3$	15.056	1.658
	$C_{14}H_{29}N_3$	16.737	1.317		$C_{13}H_{10}N_3O_2$	15.430	1.513
	$C_{15}HN_3O$	17.408	1.626		$C_{13}H_{12}N_4O$	15.805	1.371
	$C_{15}H_3N_4$	17.783	1.491		$C_{13}H_{20}O_4$	14.524	1.781
	$C_{15}H_{11}O_3$	16.502	1.876		$C_{13}H_{22}NO_3$	14.899	1.635
	$C_{15}H_{13}NO_2$	16.877	1.737		$C_{13}H_{24}N_2O_2$	15.273	1.490
	$C_{15}H_{15}N_2O$	17.251	1.599		$C_{13}H_{26}N_3O$	15.647	1.347
	$C_{15}H_{17}N_3$	17.625	1.464		$C_{13}H_{28}N_4$	16.022	1.205
	$C_{15}H_{27}O_2$	16.719	1.711		$C_{14}H_8O_4$	15.413	1.908
	$C_{15}H_{29}NO$	17.094	1.573		$C_{14}H_{10}NO_3$	15.787	1.765
	$C_{15}H_{31}N_2$	17.468	1.437		$C_{14}H_{12}N_2O_2$	16.162	1.624
	$C_{16}HNO_2$	17.765	1.885		$C_{14}H_{14}N_3O$	16.536	1.484
	$C_{16}H_3N_2O$	18.140	1.751		$C_{14}H_{16}N_4$	16.910	1.345
	$C_{16}H_5N_3$	18.514	1.618		$C_{14}H_{24}O_3$	15.630	1.741
	$C_{16}H_{15}O_2$	17.608	1.858		$C_{14}H_{26}NO_2$	16.004	1.599
	$C_{16}H_{17}NO$	17.982	1.723		$C_{14}H_{28}N_2O$	16.378	1.459
	$C_{16}H_{19}N_2$	18.357	1.590		$C_{14}H_{20}N_3$	16.753	1.319
	$C_{16}H_{31}O$	17.825	1.696		$C_{15}H_2N_3O$	17.424	1.629
	$C_{16}H_{33}N$	18.199	1.562		$C_{15}H_4N_4$	17.799	1.494
	$C_{17}H_3O_2$	18.496	2.012		$C_{15}H_{12}O_3$	16.518	1.678
	$C_{17}H_5NO$	18.871	1.881		$C_{15}H_{14}NO_2$	16.893	1.739
	$C_{17}H_7N_2$	19.245	1.751		$C_{15}H_{16}N_2O$	17.267	1.602
	$C_{17}H_{19}O$	18.713	1.852		$C_{15}H_{18}N_3$	17.641	1.466

(Contd.)

		M + 1	M + 2			M + 1	M + 2
	$C_{15}H_{28}O_2$	16.735	1.714		$C_{14}HN_4O$	16.709	1.512
	$C_{15}H_{30}NO$	17.110	1.576		$C_{14}H_9O_4$	15.429	1.910
	$C_{15}H_{32}N_2$	17.484	1.439		$C_{14}H_{11}NO_3$	15.803	1.768
	$C_{16}H_2NO_2$	17.781	1.688		$C_{14}H_{13}N_2O_2$	16.178	1.626
	$C_{16}H_4N_2O$	18.156	1.754		$C_{14}H_{15}N_3O$	16.552	1.486
	$C_{16}H_6N_3$	18.530	1.621		$C_{14}H_{17}N_4$	16.926	1.348
	$C_{16}H_{16}O_2$	17.624	1.861		$C_{14}H_{25}O_3$	15.646	1.744
	$C_{16}H_{18}NO$	17.998	1.726		$C_{14}H_{27}NO_2$	16.020	1.602
	$C_{16}H_{20}N_2$	18.373	1.593		$C_{14}H_{29}N_2O$	16.394	1.461
	$C_{16}H_{32}O$	17.841	1.698		$C_{14}H_{31}N_3$	16.769	1.322
	$C_{16}H_{34}N$	18.215	1.565		$C_{15}HN_2O_2$	17.066	1.768
	$C_{17}H_4O_2$	18.512	2.015		$C_{15}H_3N_3O$	17.440	1.632
	$C_{17}H_6NO$	18.887	1.884		$C_{15}H_5N_4$	17.815	1.496
	$C_{17}H_8N_2$	19.261	1.754		$C_{15}H_{13}O_3$	16.534	1.881
	$C_{17}H_{20}O$	18.729	1.855		$C_{15}H_{15}NO_2$	16.909	1.742
	$C_{17}H_{22}N$	19.104	1.725		$C_{15}H_{17}N_2O$	17.283	1.605
	$C_{17}H_{36}$	18.946	1.696		$C_{15}H_{19}N_3$	17.657	1.469
	$C_{18}H_8O$	19.618	2.020		$C_{15}H_{29}O_2$	16.751	1.716
	$C_{18}H_{10}N$	19.992	1.693		$C_{15}H_{31}NO$	17.126	1.579
	$C_{18}H_{24}$	19.835	1.862		$C_{15}H_{33}N_2$	17.500	1.442
	$C_{19}H_{12}$	20.723	2.036		$C_{16}HO_3$	17.423	2.026
241	$C_{11}H_{17}N_2O_4$	13.078	1.591		$C_{16}H_3NO_2$	17.797	1.891
	$C_{11}H_{19}N_3O_3$	13.452	1.140		$C_{16}H_5N_2O$	18.172	1.757
	$C_{11}H_{21}N_4O_2$	13.827	1.290		$C_{16}H_7N_3$	18.546	1.624
	$C_{12}H_5N_2O_4$	13.966	1.706		$C_{16}H_{17}O_2$	17.640	1.863
	$C_{12}H_7N_3O_3$	14.341	1.558		$C_{16}H_{19}NO$	18.014	1.729
	$C_{12}H_9N_4O_2$	14.715	1.411		$C_{16}H_{21}N_2$	18.389	1.596
	$C_{12}H_{19}NO_4$	13.809	1.685		$C_{16}H_{33}O$	17.857	1.701
	$C_{12}H_{21}N_2O_3$	14.183	1.536		$C_{16}H_{35}N$	18.231	1.568
	$C_{12}H_{23}N_3O_2$	14.558	1.388		$C_{17}H_5O_2$	18.528	2.018
	$C_{12}H_{25}N_4O$	14.932	1.242		$C_{17}H_7NO$	18.903	1.887
	$C_{13}H_7NO_4$	14.698	1.805		$C_{17}H_9N_2$	19.277	1.757
	$C_{13}H_9N_2O_3$	15.072	1.660		$C_{17}H_{21}O$	18.745	1.858
	$C_{13}H_{11}N_3O_2$	15.446	1.516		$C_{17}H_{23}N$	19.120	1.728
	$C_{13}H_{13}N_4O$	15.821	1.373		$C_{18}H_9O$	19.634	2.023
	$C_{13}H_{21}O_4$	14.540	1.783		$C_8H_{11}N$	20.008	1.896
	$C_{13}H_{23}NO_3$	14.915	1.637		$C_{18}H_{25}$	19.851	1.865
	$C_{13}H_{25}N_2O_2$	15.289	1.492		$C_{19}H_{13}$	20.739	2.040
	$C_{13}H_{27}N_3O$	15.663	1.349		$C_{20}H$	21.628	2.222
	$C_{13}H_{29}N_4$	16.038	1.207	242	$C_{11}H_{18}N_2O_4$	13.094	1.593

(Contd.)

		M + 1	M + 2
	$C_{11}H_{20}N_3O_3$	13.468	1.442
	$C_{11}H_{22}N_4O_2$	13.843	1.292
	$C_{12}H_6N_2O_4$	13.982	1.708
	$C_{12}H_8N_3O_3$	14.357	1.560
	$C_{12}H_{10}N_2O_2$	14.731	1.413
	$C_{12}H_{20}NO_4$	13.825	1.687
	$C_{12}H_{22}N_2O_3$	14.199	1.538
	$C_{12}H_{24}N_3O_2$	14.574	1.391
	$C_{12}H_{26}N_4O$	14.948	1.245
	$C_{13}H_8NO_4$	14.714	1.808
	$C_{13}H_{10}N_2O_3$	15.088	1.662
	$C_{13}H_{12}N_3O_2$	15.462	1.518
	$C_{13}N_{14}N_4O$	15.837	1.676
	$C_{13}H_{22}O_4$	14.556	1.785
	$C_{13}H_{24}NO_3$	14.931	1.639
	$C_{13}H_{26}N_2O_2$	15.305	1.495
	$C_{13}H_{28}N_3O$	15.679	1.652
	$C_{13}H_{30}N_4$	16.054	1.210
	$C_{14}H_2N_4O$	16.725	1.515
	$C_{14}H_{10}O_4$	15.445	1.913
	$C_{14}H_{12}NO_3$	15.819	1.770
	$C_{14}H_{14}N_2O_2$	16.194	1.629
	$C_{14}H_{16}N_3O$	16.568	1.489
	$C_{14}H_{18}N_4$	16.942	1.351
	$C_{14}H_{26}O_3$	15.662	1.746
	$C_{14}H_{28}NO_2$	16.036	1.604
	$C_{14}H_{30}N_2O$	16.410	1.464
	$C_{14}H_{32}N_3$	16.785	1.325
	$C_{15}H_2N_2O_2$	17.082	1.771
	$C_{15}H_4N_3O$	17.456	1.634
	$C_{15}H_6N_4$	17.831	1.499
	$C_{15}H_{14}O_3$	16.550	1.883
	$C_{15}H_{16}NO_2$	16.925	1.745
	$C_{15}H_{18}N_2O$	17.299	1.608
	$C_{15}H_{20}N_3$	17.673	1.472
	$C_{15}H_{30}O_2$	16.767	1.719
	$C_{15}H_{32}NO$	17.142	1.581
	$C_{15}H_{34}N_2$	17.516	1.445
	$C_{16}H_2O_3$	17.439	2.029
	$C_{16}H_4NO_2$	17.813	1.893
	$C_{16}H_6N_2O$	18.188	1.760
	$C_{16}H_8N_3$	18.562	1.627
	$C_{16}H_{18}O_2$	17.656	1.866
	$C_{16}H_{20}NO$	18.030	1.732
	$C_{16}H_{22}N_2$	18.405	1.599
	$C_{16}H_{34}O$	17.873	1.704
	$C_{17}H_6O_2$	18.544	2.021
	$C_{17}H_8NO$	18.919	1.890
	$C_{17}H_{10}N_2$	19.293	1.760
	$C_{17}H_{22}O$	18.761	1.861
	$C_{17}H_{24}N$	19.136	1.731
	$C_{18}H_{10}O$	19.650	2.026
	$C_{18}H_{12}N$	20.024	1.699
	$C_{18}H_{26}$	19.867	1.868
	$C_{19}H_{14}$	20.755	2.043
	$C_{20}H_2$	21.644	2.226
243	$C_{11}H_{19}N_2O_4$	13.110	1.596
	$C_{11}H_{21}N_3O_3$	13.484	1.444
	$C_{11}H_{23}N_4O_2$	13.859	1.294
	$C_{12}H_7N_2O_4$	13.998	1.710
	$C_{12}H_9N_3O_3$	14.373	1.562
	$C_{12}H_{11}N_4O_2$	14.747	1.415
	$C_{12}H_{21}NO_4$	13.841	1.689
	$C_{12}H_{23}N_2O_3$	14.215	1.540
	$C_{12}H_{25}N_3O_2$	14.590	1.393
	$C_{12}H_{27}N_4O$	14.964	1.247
	$C_{13}H_9NO_4$	14.730	1.810
	$C_{13}H_{11}N_2O_3$	15.104	1.665
	$C_{13}H_{13}N_3O_2$	15.478	1.521
	$C_{13}H_{15}N_4O$	15.853	1.378
	$C_{13}H_{23}O_4$	14.572	1.788
	$C_{13}H_{25}NO_3$	14.947	1.642
	$C_{13}H_{27}N_2O_2$	15.321	1.497
	$C_{13}H_{29}N_3O$	15.695	1.354
	$C_{13}H_{31}N_4$	16.070	1.212
	$C_{14}HN_3O_2$	16.367	1.656
	$C_{14}H_3N_4O$	16.741	1.517
	$C_{14}H_{11}O_4$	15.461	1.915
	$C_{14}H_{13}NO_3$	15.835	1.773
	$C_{14}H_{15}N_2O_2$	16.210	1.632

(Contd.)

		M + 1	M + 2
	$C_{14}H_{17}N_3O$	16.584	1.492
	$C_{14}H_{19}N_4$	16.958	1.353
	$C_{14}H_{27}O_3$	15.678	1.749
	$C_{14}H_{29}NO_2$	16.052	1.607
	$C_{14}H_{31}N_2O$	16.426	1.466
	$C_{14}H_{33}N_3$	16.801	1.327
	$C_{15}HNO_3$	16.724	1.912
	$C_{15}H_3N_2O_2$	17.098	1.774
	$C_{15}H_5N_3O$	17.472	1.637
	$C_{15}H_7N_4$	17.847	1.502
	$C_{15}H_{15}O_3$	16.566	1.886
	$C_{15}H_{17}NO_2$	16.941	1.748
	$C_{15}H_{19}N_2O$	17.315	1.611
	$C_{15}H_{21}N_3$	17.689	1.475
	$C_{15}H_{31}O_2$	16.783	1.722
	$C_{15}H_{33}NO$	17.158	1.584
	$C_{16}H_3O_3$	17.455	2.031
	$C_{16}H_5NO_2$	17.829	1.896
	$C_{16}H_7N_2O$	18.204	1.763
	$C_{16}H_9N_3$	18.578	1.630
	$C_{16}H_{19}O_2$	17.672	1.869
	$C_{16}H_{21}NO$	18.046	1.735
	$C_{16}H_{23}N_2$	18.421	1.602
	$C_{17}H_7O_2$	18.560	2.024
	$C_{17}H_9NO$	18.935	1.893
	$C_{17}H_{11}N_2$	19.309	1.764
	$C_{17}H_{23}O$	18.777	1.864
	$C_{17}H_{25}N$	19.152	1.734
	$C_{18}H_{11}O$	19.666	2.029
	$C_{18}H_{13}N$	20.040	1.902
	$C_{18}H_{27}$	19.883	1.872
	$C_{19}HN$	20.929	2.078
	$C_{19}H_{15}$	20.771	2.046
	$C_{20}H_3$	21.660	2.229
244	$C_{11}H_{20}N_2O_4$	13.126	1.598
	$C_{11}H_{22}N_3O_3$	13.500	1.446
	$C_{11}H_{24}N_4O_2$	13.875	1.296
	$C_{12}H_8N_2O_4$	14.014	1.712
	$C_{12}H_{10}N_3O_3$	14.389	1.564
	$C_{12}H_{12}N_4O_2$	14.763	1.418
	$C_{12}H_{22}NO_4$	13.857	1.691
	$C_{12}H_{24}N_2O_3$	14.231	1.543
	$C_{12}H_{26}N_3O_2$	14.606	1.395
	$C_{12}H_{28}N_4O$	14.980	1.250
	$C_{13}H_{10}NO_4$	14.746	1.812
	$C_{13}H_{12}N_2O_3$	15.120	1.667
	$C_{13}H_{14}N_3O_2$	15.494	1.523
	$C_{13}H_{16}N_4O$	15.869	1.381
	$C_{13}H_{24}O_4$	14.588	1.790
	$C_{13}H_{26}NO_3$	14.963	1.644
	$C_{13}H_{28}N_2O_2$	15.337	1.500
	$C_{13}H_{30}N_3O$	15.711	1.357
	$C_{13}H_{32}N_4$	16.086	1.215
	$C_{14}H_2N_3O_2$	16.383	1.659
	$C_{14}H_4N_4O$	16.757	1.520
	$C_{14}H_{12}O_4$	15.477	1.918
	$C_{14}H_{14}NO_3$	15.851	1.775
	$C_{14}H_{16}N_2O_2$	16.226	1.634
	$C_{14}H_{18}N_3O$	16.600	1.494
	$C_{14}H_{20}N_4$	16.974	1.356
	$C_{14}H_{28}O_3$	15.694	1.751
	$C_{14}H_{30}NO_2$	16.068	1.609
	$C_{14}H_{32}N_2O$	16.442	1.469
	$C_{15}H_2NO_3$	16.740	1.914
	$C_{15}H_4N_2O_2$	17.114	1.776
	$C_{15}H_6N_3O$	17.488	1.640
	$C_{15}H_8N_4$	17.863	1.505
	$C_{15}H_{16}O_3$	16.582	1.889
	$C_{15}H_{18}NO_2$	16.957	1.750
	$C_{15}H_{20}N_2O$	17.331	1.613
	$C_{15}H_{22}N_3$	17.705	1.478
	$C_{15}H_{32}O_2$	16.799	1.724
	$C_{16}H_4O_3$	17.471	2.034
	$C_{16}H_6NO_2$	17.845	1.899
	$C_{16}H_8N_2O$	18.220	1.765
	$C_{16}H_{10}N_3$	18.594	1.633
	$C_{16}H_{20}O_2$	17.688	1.872
	$C_{16}H_{22}NO$	18.062	1.738
	$C_{16}H_{24}N_2$	18.437	1.605
	$C_{17}H_8O_2$	18.576	2.027

(Contd.)

		M + 1	M + 2			M + 1	M + 2
	$C_{17}H_{10}NO$	18.951	1.896		$C_{15}H_3NO_3$	16.756	1.917
	$C_{17}H_{12}N_2$	19.325	1.767		$C_{15}H_5N_2O_2$	17.130	1.779
	$C_{17}H_{24}O$	18.793	1.867		$C_{15}H_7N_3O$	17.504	1.643
	$C_{17}H_{26}N$	19.168	1.737		$C_{15}H_9N_4$	17.879	1.508
	$C_{18}H_{12}O$	19.682	2.032		$C_{15}H_{17}O_3$	16.598	1.891
	$C_{18}H_{14}N$	20.056	1.905		$C_{15}H_{19}NO_2$	16.973	1.753
	$C_{18}H_{28}$	19.899	1.875		$C_{15}H_{21}N_2O$	17.347	1.616
	$C_{19}H_2N$	20.945	2.082		$C_{15}H_{23}N_3$	17.721	1.481
	$C_{19}H_{16}$	20.787	2.050		$C_{16}H_5O_3$	17.487	2.037
	$C_{20}H_4$	21.676	2.233		$C_{16}H_7NO_2$	17.861	1.902
245	$C_{11}H_{21}N_2O_4$	13.142	1.600		$C_{16}H_9N_2O$	18.236	1.768
	$C_{11}H_{23}N_3O_3$	13.516	1.448		$C_{16}H_{11}N_3$	18.610	1.636
	$C_{11}H_{25}N_4O_2$	13.891	1.299		$C_{16}H_{21}O_2$	17.704	1.875
	$C_{12}H_9N_2O_4$	14.030	1.715		$C_{16}H_{23}NO$	18.078	1.740
	$C_{12}H_{11}N_3O_3$	14.405	1.567		$C_{16}H_{25}N_2$	18.453	1.608
	$C_{12}H_{13}N_4O_2$	14.779	1.420		$C_{17}H_9O_2$	18.592	2.030
	$C_{12}H_{23}NO_4$	13.873	1.693		$C_{17}H_{11}NO$	18.967	1.899
	$C_{12}H_{25}N_2O_3$	14.247	1.545		$C_{17}H_{13}N_2$	19.341	1.770
	$C_{12}H_{27}N_3O_2$	14.622	1.398		$C_{17}H_{25}O$	18.809	1.870
	$C_{12}H_{29}N_4O$	14.996	1.252		$C_{17}H_{27}N$	19.184	1.740
	$C_{13}HN_4O_2$	15.668	1.550		$C_{18}HN_2$	20.230	1.940
	$C_{13}H_{11}NO_4$	14.762	1.815		$C_{18}H_{13}O$	19.698	2.035
	$C_{13}H_{13}N_2O_3$	15.136	1.670		$C_{18}H_{15}N$	20.072	1.909
	$C_{13}H_{15}N_3O_2$	15.510	1.526		$C_{18}H_{29}$	19.915	1.878
	$C_{13}H_{17}N_4O$	15.885	1.383		$C_{19}H_{17}$	20.803	2.053
	$C_{13}H_{25}O_4$	14.604	1.792		$C_{19}HO$	20.586	2.209
	$C_{13}H_{27}NO_3$	14.979	1.647		$C_{19}H_3N$	20.961	2.085
	$C_{13}H_{29}N_2O_2$	15.353	1.502		$C_{20}H_5$	21.692	2.236
	$C_{13}H_{31}N_3O$	15.727	1.359	246	$C_{11}H_{22}N_2O_4$	13.158	1.602
	$C_{14}HN_2O_3$	16.025	1.802		$C_{11}H_{24}N_3O_3$	13.532	1.451
	$C_{14}H_3N_3O_2$	16.399	1.662		$C_{11}H_{26}N_4O_2$	13.907	1.301
	$C_{14}H_5N_4O$	16.773	1.523		$C_{12}H_{10}N_2O_4$	14.047	1.717
	$C_{14}H_{13}O_4$	15.493	1.920		$C_{12}H_{12}N_3O_3$	14.421	1.569
	$C_{14}H_{15}NO_3$	15.867	1.778		$C_{12}H_{14}N_2O_2$	14.795	1.422
	$C_{14}H_{17}N_2O_2$	16.242	1.637		$C_{12}H_{24}NO_4$	13.889	1.696
	$C_{14}H_{19}N_3O$	16.616	1.497		$C_{12}H_{26}N_2O_3$	14.263	1.547
	$C_{14}H_{21}N_4$	16.990	1.359		$C_{12}H_{28}N_3O_2$	14.638	1.400
	$C_{14}H_{29}O_3$	15.710	1.754		$C_{12}H_{30}N_4O$	15.012	1.254
	$C_{14}H_{31}NO_2$	16.084	1.612		$C_{13}H_2N_4O_2$	15.684	1.552
	$C_{15}HO_4$	16.381	2.056		$C_{13}H_{12}NO_4$	14.778	1.817

(Contd.)

		M + 1	M + 2
	$C_{13}H_{14}N_2O_3$	15.152	1.672
	$C_{13}H_{16}N_3O_2$	15.526	1.528
	$C_{13}H_{18}N_4O$	15.901	1.386
	$C_{13}H_{26}O_4$	14.620	1.795
	$C_{13}H_{28}NO_3$	14.995	1.649
	$C_{13}H_{30}N_2O_2$	15.369	1.505
	$C_{14}H_2N_2O_3$	16.041	1.805
	$C_{14}H_4N_3O_2$	16.415	1.664
	$C_{14}H_6N_4O$	16.789	1.525
	$C_{14}H_{14}O_4$	15.509	1.923
	$C_{14}H_{16}NO_3$	15.883	1.780
	$C_{14}H_{18}N_2O_2$	16.258	1.639
	$C_{14}H_{20}N_3O$	16.632	1.500
	$C_{14}H_{22}N_4$	17.006	1.361
	$C_{14}H_{30}O_3$	15.726	1.756
	$C_{15}H_2O_4$	16.397	2.059
	$C_{15}H_4NO_3$	16.772	1.920
	$C_{15}H_6N_2O_2$	17.146	1.782
	$C_{15}H_8N_3O$	17.520	1.646
	$C_{15}H_{10}N_4$	17.895	1.511
	$C_{15}H_{18}O_3$	16.614	1.894
	$C_{15}H_{20}NO_2$	16.989	1.756
	$C_{15}H_{22}N_2O$	17.363	1.619
	$C_{15}H_{24}N_3$	17.737	1.483
	$C_{16}H_6O_3$	17.503	2.040
	$C_{16}H_8NO_2$	17.877	1.905
	$C_{16}H_{10}N_2O$	18.252	1.771
	$C_{16}H_{12}N_3$	18.626	1.639
	$C_{16}H_{22}O_2$	17.720	1.878
	$C_{16}H_{24}NO$	18.094	1.743
	$C_{16}H_{26}N_2$	18.469	1.611
	$C_{17}H_{10}O_2$	18.608	2.033
	$C_{17}H_{12}NO$	18.983	1.902
	$C_{17}H_{14}N_2$	19.357	1.773
	$C_{17}H_{26}O$	18.825	1.873
	$C_{17}H_{28}N$	19.200	1.743
	$C_{18}H_2N_2$	20.246	1.943
	$C_{18}H_{14}O$	19.714	2.039
	$C_{18}H_{16}N$	20.088	1.912
	$C_{18}H_{30}$	19.931	1.881

		M + 1	M + 2
	$C_{19}H_2O$	20.602	2.212
	$C_{19}H_4N$	20.977	2.089
	$C_{19}H_{18}$	20.819	2.056
	$C_{20}H_6$	21.708	2.239
247	$C_{11}H_{23}N_2O_4$	13.174	1.604
	$C_{11}H_{25}N_3O_3$	13.548	1.453
	$C_{11}H_{27}N_4O_2$	13.923	1.303
	$C_{12}H_{11}N_2O_4$	14.063	1.719
	$C_{12}H_{13}N_3O_3$	14.437	1.571
	$C_{12}H_{15}N_4O_2$	14.811	1.425
	$C_{12}H_{25}NO_4$	13.905	1.698
	$C_{12}H_{27}N_2O_3$	14.279	1.549
	$C_{12}H_{29}N_3O_2$	14.654	1.402
	$C_{13}HN_3O_3$	15.325	1.698
	$C_{13}H_3N_4O_2$	15.700	1.555
	$C_{13}H_{13}NO_4$	14.794	1.820
	$C_{13}H_{15}N_2O_3$	15.168	1.674
	$C_{13}H_{17}N_3O_2$	15.542	1.531
	$C_{13}H_{19}N_4O$	15.917	1.388
	$C_{13}H_{27}O_4$	14.636	1.797
	$C_{13}H_{29}NO_3$	15.011	1.651
	$C_{14}HNO_4$	15.682	1.949
	$C_{14}H_3N_2O_3$	16.057	1.807
	$C_{14}H_5N_3O_2$	16.431	1.667
	$C_{14}H_7N_4O$	16.805	1.528
	$C_{14}H_{15}O_4$	15.525	1.925
	$C_{14}H_{17}NO_3$	15.899	1.783
	$C_{14}H_{19}N_2O_2$	16.274	1.642
	$C_{14}H_{21}N_3O$	16.648	1.502
	$C_{14}H_{23}N_4$	17.022	1.364
	$C_{15}H_3O_4$	16.413	2.061
	$C_{15}H_5NO_3$	16.788	1.922
	$C_{15}H_7N_2O_2$	17.162	1.785
	$C_{15}H_9N_3O$	17.536	1.648
	$C_{15}H_{11}N_4$	17.911	1.514
	$C_{15}H_{19}O_3$	16.630	1.897
	$C_{15}H_{21}NO_2$	17.005	1.758
	$C_{15}H_{23}N_2O$	17.379	1.622
	$C_{15}H_{25}N_3$	17.753	1.486
	$C_{16}H_7O_3$	17.519	2.043

(Contd.)

		M + 1	M + 2			M + 1	M + 2
	$C_{16}H_9NO_2$	17.893	1.908		$C_{14}H_{16}O_4$	15.541	1.928
	$C_{16}H_{11}N_2O$	18.268	1.774		$C_{14}H_{18}NO_3$	15.915	1.785
	$C_{16}H_{13}N_3$	18.642	1.642		$C_{14}H_{20}N_2O_2$	16.29	1.645
	$C_{16}H_{23}O_2$	17.736	1.880		$C_{14}H_{22}N_3O$	16.664	1.505
	$C_{16}H_{25}NO$	18.110	1.746		$C_{14}H_{24}N_4$	17.038	1.367
	$C_{16}H_{27}N_2$	18.485	1.614		$C_{15}H_4O_4$	16.429	2.064
	$C_{17}HN_3$	19.531	1.806		$C_{15}H_6NO_3$	16.804	1.925
	$C_{17}H_{11}O_2$	18.624	2.036		$C_{15}H_8N_2O_2$	17.178	1.787
	$C_{17}H_{13}NO$	18.999	1.905		$C_{15}H_{10}N_3O$	17.552	1.651
	$C_{17}H_{15}N_2$	19.373	1.776		$C_{15}H_{12}N_4$	17.927	1.516
	$C_{17}H_{27}O$	18.841	1.876		$C_{15}H_{20}O_3$	16.646	1.899
	$C_{17}H_{29}N$	19.216	1.746		$C_{15}H_{22}NO_2$	17.021	1.761
	$C_{18}HNO$	19.887	2.072		$C_{15}H_{22}N_2O$	17.395	1.624
	$C_{18}H_3N_2$	20.262	1.946		$C_{15}H_{26}N_3$	17.769	1.489
	$C_{18}H_{15}O$	19.730	2.042		$C_{16}H_8O_3$	17.535	2.045
	$C_{18}H_{17}N$	20.104	1.915		$C_{16}H_{10}NO_2$	17.909	1.911
	$C_{18}H_{31}$	19.947	1.884		$C_{16}H_{12}N_2O$	18.284	1.777
	$C_{19}H_3O$	20.619	2.215		$C_{16}H_{14}N_3$	18.658	1.645
	$C_{19}H_5N$	20.993	2.092		$C_{16}H_{24}O_2$	17.752	1.883
	$C_{19}H_{19}$	20.835	2.060		$C_{16}H_{26}NO$	1.813	1.749
	$C_{20}H_7$	21.724	2.243		$C_{16}H_{28}N_2$	18.501	1.617
248	$C_{11}H_{24}N_2O_4$	13.190	1.606		$C_{17}H_2N_3$	19.547	1.609
	$C_{11}H_{26}N_3O_3$	13.564	1.455		$C_{17}H_{12}O_2$	18.640	2.039
	$C_{11}H_{28}N_4O_2$	13.939	1.305		$C_{17}H_{14}NO$	19.015	1.908
	$C_{12}H_{12}N_2O_4$	14.079	1.721		$C_{17}H_{16}N_2$	19.389	1.779
	$C_{12}H_{14}N_3O_3$	14.453	1.574		$C_{17}H_{28}O$	18.857	1.879
	$C_{12}H_{16}N_4O_2$	14.827	1.427		$C_{17}H_{30}N$	19.232	1.749
	$C_{12}H_{26}NO_4$	13.921	1.700		$C_{18}H_2NO$	19.903	2.075
	$C_{12}H_{28}N_2O_3$	14.295	1.552		$C_{18}H_4N_2$	20.278	1.949
	$C_{13}H_2N_3O_3$	15.341	1.700		$C_{18}H_{16}O$	19.746	2.045
	$C_{13}H_4N_4O_2$	15.716	1.557		$C_{18}H_{18}N$	20.120	1.918
	$C_{13}H_{14}NO_4$	14.810	1.822		$C_{18}H_{32}$	19.963	1.888
	$C_{13}H_{16}N_2O_3$	15.184	1.677		$C_{19}H_4O$	20.635	2.219
	$C_{13}H_{18}N_3O_2$	15.558	1.533		$C_{19}H_6N$	21.009	2.095
	$C_{13}H_{20}N_4O$	15.933	1.391		$C_{19}H_{20}$	20.851	2.063
	$C_{13}H_{28}O_4$	14.652	1.799		$C_{20}H_8$	21.740	2.246
	$C_{14}H_2NO_4$	15.698	1.952	249	$C_{11}H_{25}N_2O_4$	13.206	1.608
	$C_{14}H_4N_2O_3$	16.073	1.810		$C_{11}H_{27}N_3O_3$	13.580	1.457
	$C_{14}H_6N_3O_2$	16.447	1.670		$C_{12}H_{13}N_2O_4$	14.095	1.724
	$C_{14}H_8N_4O$	16.821	1.531		$C_{12}H_{15}N_3O_3$	14.469	1.576

(Contd.)

	M + 1	M + 2
$C_{12}H_{17}N_4O_2$	14.843	1.430
$C_{12}H_{27}NO_4$	13.937	1.702
$C_{13}HN_2O_4$	14.983	1.847
$C_{13}H_3N_3O_3$	15.357	1.703
$C_{13}H_5N_4O_2$	15.732	1.560
$C_{13}H_{15}NO_4$	14.826	1.824
$C_{13}H_{17}N_2O_3$	15.200	1.679
$C_{13}H_{19}N_3O_2$	15.574	1.536
$C_{13}H_{21}N_4O$	15.949	1.393
$C_{14}H_3NO_4$	15.714	1.954
$C_{14}H_5N_2O_3$	16.089	1.812
$C_{14}H_7N_3O_2$	16.463	1.672
$C_{14}H_9N_4O$	16.837	1.533
$C_{14}H_{17}O_4$	15.557	1.930
$C_{14}H_{19}NO_3$	15.931	1.788
$C_{14}H_{21}N_2O_2$	16.306	1.647
$C_{14}H_{23}N_3O$	16.680	1.508
$C_{14}H_{25}N_4$	17.054	1.370
$C_{15}H_5O_4$	16.445	2.067
$C_{15}H_7NO_3$	16.820	1.928
$C_{15}H_9N_2O_2$	17.194	1.790
$C_{15}H_{11}N_3O$	17.568	1.654
$C_{15}H_{13}N_4$	17.943	1.519
$C_{15}H_{21}O_3$	16.662	1.902
$C_{15}H_{23}NO_2$	17.037	1.764
$C_{15}H_{25}N_2O$	17.411	1.627
$C_{15}H_{27}N_3$	17.785	1.492
$C_{16}HN_4$	18.831	1.677
$C_{16}H_9O_3$	17.551	2.048
$C_{16}H_{11}NO_2$	17.925	1.913
$C_{16}H_{13}N_2O$	18.300	1.780
$C_{16}H_{15}N_3$	18.674	1.648
$C_{16}H_{25}O_2$	17.768	1.887
$C_{16}H_{27}NO$	18.142	1.752
$C_{16}H_{29}N_2$	18.517	1.619
$C_{17}HN_2O$	19.188	1.941
$C_{17}H_3N_3$	19.563	1.812
$C_{17}H_{13}O_2$	18.656	2.042
$C_{17}H_{15}NO$	19.031	1.911
$C_{17}H_{17}N_2$	19.405	1.782

		M + 1	M + 2
	$C_{17}H_{29}O$	18.873	1.882
	$C_{17}H_{31}N$	19.248	1.752
	$C_{18}HO_2$	19.545	2.206
	$C_{128}H_3NO$	19.919	2.079
	$C_{18}H_5N_2$	20.294	1.953
	$C_{18}H_{17}O$	19.762	2.048
	$C_{18}H_{19}N$	2.014	1.922
	$C_{18}H_{33}$	19.979	1.891
	$C_{19}H_5O$	20.651	2.222
	$C_{19}H_7N$	21.025	2.099
	$C_{19}H_{21}$	20.867	2.066
	$C_{20}H_9$	21.756	2.250
250	$C_{11}H_{26}N_2O_4$	13.222	1.610
	$C_{12}H_{14}N_2O_4$	14.111	1.726
	$C_{12}H_{16}N_3O_3$	14.485	1.578
	$C_{12}H_{18}N_4O_2$	14.859	1.432
	$C_{13}H_2N_2O_4$	14.999	1.849
	$C_{13}H_4N_3O_3$	15.373	1.705
	$C_{13}H_6N_4O_2$	15.748	1.562
	$C_{13}H_{16}NO_4$	14.842	1.827
	$C_{13}H_{18}N_2O_3$	15.216	1.682
	$C_{13}H_{20}N_3O_2$	15.590	1.538
	$C_{13}H_{22}N_4O$	15.965	1.396
	$C_{14}H_4NO_4$	15.730	1.957
	$C_{14}H_6N_2O_3$	16.105	1.815
	$C_{13}H_8N_3O_2$	16.479	1.675
	$C_{14}H_{10}N_4O$	16.853	1.536
	$C_{14}H_{18}N_4$	15.573	1.933
	$C_{14}H_{20}NO_3$	15.947	1.791
	$C_{14}H_{22}N_2O_2$	16.322	1.650
	$C_{14}H_{24}N_3O$	16.696	1.510
	$C_{14}H_{26}N_4$	17.070	1.372
	$C_{15}H_6O_4$	16.461	2.069
	$C_{15}H_8NO_3$	16.836	1.930
	$C_{15}H_{10}N_2O_2$	17.210	1.793
	$C_{15}H_{12}N_3O$	17.584	1.657
	$C_{15}H_{14}N_4$	17.959	1.522
	$C_{15}H_{22}O_3$	16.678	1.905
	$C_{15}H_{24}NO_2$	17.053	1.767
	$C_{15}H_{26}N_2O$	17.427	1.630

(Contd.)

	M + 1	M + 2		M + 1	M + 2
$C_{15}H_{28}N_3$	17.801	1.495	$C_{17}H_{18}N_2$	19.421	1.785
$C_{16}H_2N_4$	18.847	1.680	$C_{17}H_{30}O$	18.889	1.885
$C_{16}H_{10}O_3$	17.567	2.051	$C_{17}H_{32}N$	19.264	1.755
$C_{16}H_{12}NO_2$	17.941	1.916	$C_{18}H_2O_2$	19.561	2.209
$C_{16}H_{14}N_2O$	18.31	1.783	$C_{18}H_4NO$	19.935	2.082
$C_{16}H_{16}N_3$	18.690	1.651	$C_{18}H_6N_2$	20.310	1.956
$C_{16}H_{26}O_2$	17.784	1.889	$C_{18}H_{18}O$	19.778	2.051
$C_{16}H_{28}NO$	18.158	1.755	$C_{18}H_{20}N$	20.152	1.925
$C_{16}H_{30}N_2$	18.533	1.622	$C_{18}H_{34}$	19.995	1.894
$C_{17}H_2N_2O$	19.204	1.944	$C_{19}H_6O$	20.667	2.225
$C_{17}H_4N_3$	19.579	1.815	$C_{19}H_8N$	21.041	2.102
$C_{17}H_{14}O_2$	18.672	2.045	$C_{19}H_{22}$	20.883	2.070
$C_{17}H_{16}NO$	19.047	1.914	$C_{20}H_{10}$	21.772	2.253

Index

Alkaloids, fragmentation pattern, 140
Alternate CI-EI, 15
Amino acids, fragmentation pattern, 121
Analytical mass spectrometry, 143
Applications of GC-MS, 165
Applications of LC/MS, 171
Applications of MS in biological research, 174
Applications of tandem mass spectrometry, 150
Applications, 5
Array detector, 37
Atmosphere pressure chemical ionization (APCI), 24, 171
Atmosphere pressure ionization, 22

Batch inlet system, 38
Benzene, fragmentation, 80
Beynon table, molecular formula, 53
Biological mass spectrometry, 174
Bupivacaine, analysis, 148
Buspione, analysis, 155

Camphor, mass spectrum, 131
Carvacrol, mass spectrum, 133
Catechin, fragmentation pattern, 139
Chemical ionization, 11
Chromatographic inlet system, 38
Citronellal, mass spectrum, 128
Citronellol, mass spectrum, 132
Continuous flow FAB coupling, 168
Cotinine, analysis, 148
Cyclic alcohol fragmentation pattern, 84
Cyclohexane, fragmentation, 74
Cyclohexanol, fragmentation pattern, 85
Cyclohexanone, fragmentation pattern, 92
Cyclohexene, fragmentation, 77

Daly detector, 37
Data system, 39
Desorption chemical ionization, 16
Detectors, 35
Determination of molecular formula, 49
Dioxins, 6
Direct liquid introduction interface, 168
Direct probe inlet, 38
Double focusing mass analyzers, 31

Electron ionization, 9
Electron multiplier, 36
Electrospray interface, 171
Electrospray ionization (ESI),
Eriodictyol, fragmentation pattern, 139
Factors influencing the fragmentation, 59
Faraday cup, 35
Fast atom bombardment, 20
Field desorption ionization, 18
Field desorption, 18
Field ionization, 19
Flavonoids, fragmentation pattern, 139
Fluorouracil, analysis, 147
Fragment ions, 44
Fragmentation of organic compounds, 57
Fragmentation pattern for organic functional groups, 71
Fused silica capillary GC columns, 163

Gas chromatography, 161
Gas phase ionization, 8
GC-MS, 160
General structure of mass spectrometer, 8
Geranial, mass spectrum, 128
Geraniol, mass spectrum, 133

Handy rules of fragmentation, 68
Hard source ionization, 9
Heterocyclic compounds, fragmentation pattern, 118
Historical development in mass spectrometry, 4
History of mass spectrometry, 2

Hybrid mass spectrometer, 153
Hydrocarbon, fragmentation, 71
Hydrogen migration, 67

Imipramine, analysis, 147
Index of hydrogen deficiency (IHD), 54
Inductive effect, 60
Interface used in GC-MS, 162
Interface using aerosols and additional ion generation, 164
Interface using desorption techniques, 167
Introduction to mass spectrometer, 7
Introduction to mass spectrometry, 1
Ion cyclotron resonance, 34
Ion source, 8
Ions formed by ion molecule interaction, 48
Ions with odd or even numbers of electrons, 58
Isobutane, fragmentation, 73
Isotope ratio MS, 174
Isotopic abundances, 207
Isotopic ions, 41

J.J. Thomson, 4
Jet orifice separator, 162

Ketones, aliphatic, 90
Ketones, aromatic, 92
Ketones, cyclic, 90
Ketones, fragmentation pattern, 90, 129

Lactones, fragmentation pattern, 102
Laser desorption, 25
LC/MS, 166
Limitations of GC-MS, 164
Linalol, mass spectrum, 133
Luteolin, fragmentation pattern, 139

MALDI, 26
Mass analyzers, 28
McLafferty rearrangements, 45, 65
Membrane separator, 164
Menthone, mass spectrum, 130
Metastable ions, 46
Methyl t-butyl ketone, mass spectrum, 2
Molecular ions, 40
Morphine, fragmentation pattern, 141
Moving belt interface, 167
MS-MS instrumentation, 151
Multicenter fragmentation, 63
Multiple charged ions, 45
Multiple ion detection, 144

Naphthalene, mass spectrum, 82
Natural products, fragmentation pattern, 121
Nebornene, fragmentation, 79
Negative ion chemical ionization, 16
Negative ions, 47
Neighbouring electron participation, 61
Neutral loss scanning, 157
Nicotine, fragmentation pattern, 140
Nitrogen rule, 50

Ortho effect, 65

Particle bombardment, 19
Particle interface coupling, 169
Phenol, fragmentation pattern, 87
Photoionization, 28
Piperitone, mass spectrum, 129
Precursor ion scanning, 155
Product ion scanning, 155
Protein characterization, 176
Protein quantification, 178
QIT, 33
Quadrupole mass analyzers, 32
Quantatative analysis, 143
Quantitative analysis, 146
Quercetin, fragmentation pattern, 139
Questions, 145
Quinine, fragmentation pattern, 140

Rearrangement ions, 45
Relative strength of the bonds, 60
Resonance effect, 62
Retro Diels-Alder reaction, 67, 136
Scintillator, 37
Secondary ion mass spectrometry, 21
Selected reaction monitoring (SRM), 157
Single focusing mass analyzer, 31
Single ion detection,
Source ionization, 9
Stability of the fragments, 60
Steroids, fragmentation pattern, 124
Stevenson's rule, 58

Tandem mass spectrometry, 149
Terpenes, fragmentation pattern, 126
Terpineol, mass spectrum, 135
Thermal ionization (TIMS), 28
Thermospray interface ion source, 170
Thioanisole, mass spectrum, 105
Thiophenol, mass spectrum, 88
Thymol, mass spectrum, 134
Time of flight mass analyzers, 32
Toluene, fragmentation, 81
Toxifolin, fragmentation pattern, 139
Triple quadrupole mass analyzer, 153
Triterpenoids, fragmentation pattern, 136
Tropylium cation, 80
Types of ions, 40

^{235}U, 161

Vacuum system, 39
Valine, 165
Vinylic cleavage, 76

Websites on mass spectrometry, 196
Whole number rule, 3

Xe, 160

Yb, 161

Zn, 160
Zr, 160